Representing Epilepsy

REPRESENTATIONS: HEALTH, DISABILITY, CULTURE

Series Editor
Stuart Murray, University of Leeds

This series provides a ground-breaking and innovative selection of titles that showcase the newest interdisciplinary research on the cultural representations of health and disability in the contemporary social world. Bringing together both subjects and working methods from literary studies, film and cultural studies, medicine and sociology, 'Representations' is scholarly and accessible, addressed to researchers across a number of academic disciplines, and practitioners and members of the public with interests in issues of public health.

The key term in the series will be representations. Public interest in questions of health and disability has never been stronger, and as a consequence cultural forms across a range of media currently produce a never-ending stream of narratives and images that both reflect this interest and generate its forms. The crucial value of the series is that it brings the skilled study of cultural narratives and images to bear on such contemporary medical concerns. It offers and responds to new research paradigms that advance understanding at a scholarly level of the interaction between medicine, culture and society; it also has a strong commitment to public concerns surrounding such issues, and maintains a tone and point of address that seek to engage a general audience.

Other books in the series

Representing Autism: Culture, Narrative, Fascination
Stuart Murray

Idiocy: A Cultural History
Patrick McDonagh

Representing Epilepsy

Myth and Matter

Jeannette Stirling

LIVERPOOL UNIVERSITY PRESS

First published 2010 by
Liverpool University Press
4 Cambridge Street
Liverpool L69 7ZU

British Library Cataloguing-in-Publication data
A British Library CIP record is available

ISBN 978-1-84631-237-3

Typseset in Iowan Old Style by R. J. Footring Ltd, Derby
Printed in Great Britain by the MPG Books Group, Bodmin and King's Lynn

Contents

Acknowledgements

This book has a long and complicated genesis. Parts of it began life as research for my doctoral dissertation, completed at the University of Sydney in 2001. Since then, ongoing research and conversations with colleagues both in Australia and from the US persuaded me that there was more to be said on the subject of epilepsy. My thanks for eventually embarking on this project must go firstly to Lisa Cartwright, University of California, San Diego, who on a long walk around London in 2005 tried her best to convince me that the time was right. You convinced me. And I meant to get started that year Lisa, I really did, but things are not always as straightforward as we would perhaps like. The project might have continued to languish if it had not been for Kate Bowles, friend, colleague and fellow traveller to the south coast and southern highlands campuses of the University of Wollongong: so many kilometres, so many opportunities to talk about our research and why it matters to us. Thank you Kate; you provided the impetus for me to act on all that talk.

Thanks must also go to Pete Randles for reading early sections of the book – again and again – and providing such excellent feedback: friendship and collegiality of the highest order. Thank you to Celeste Rossetto for taking the time, when time was tricky, to read, talk and listen as the project took shape. I always had hope that a chapter might just work when you told me that you laughed or for a moment forgot 'the other stuff'.

As I have said, this book has had a long and complicated genesis. It began back in 1971 when I entered into a circuit of culture that figured me 'epileptic'. As complex as this journey has been for me, it has also and necessarily involved my children. Damion, Ben and Jem, what can

I say? I know it has not always been easy. Thank you for the joy, your unrestrained appreciation for the absurd and for the excellent music when the urge to dance overtakes us all. Where would we be without the dancing? And, of course, the laughter. John never lost sight of me when the journey was at its most complicated and on more than one occasion put his professional identity on the line. I noticed. My siblings, Terry, Bonnie and Chris, have known me the longest and it is one of my life's great pleasures that through this part of the journey we are yet again part of each other's lives.

Jeannette Stirling
Kangaroo Valley

Introduction

> Since at that second, that is at the very last conscious moment before the fit, he had time to say to himself clearly and consciously: 'Yes, for this moment one might give one's whole life!' Then without doubt that moment was really worth the whole of life.
> (Fyodor Dostoevsky, *The Idiot*, 1868, p. 220)

> Write your story as it needs to be written. Write it honestly and tell it as best you can. I'm not sure that there are any other rules. Not ones that matter.
> (Neil Gaiman, *Neil Gaiman's Journal*, 15 June 2004)

I

This is a book about representations of epilepsy. To a point, it is also about those who experience the condition; or, more accurately, any one of the multiple forms the condition may take. Specifically, though, it is about trade routes between culture and medicine and an unacknowledged traffic between systems of representation that accrete to produce the complex and layered meanings adhering to epilepsy and 'the epileptic'. Throughout the following pages, I explore the notion that medical stories of epilepsy from the late nineteenth century through to the present are as much forged by the cultural conditions and representational politics of the times as they are by the science of western medicine. It is, perhaps, a bold claim and testing its limits will require multiple border crossings. These border crossings will be made through time, and across discursive boundaries, and will engage with various genres of epilepsy narrative. Crossing borders can be a risky business; transgressing long-accepted boundaries, perilous. Nevertheless, it is only through a close examination of the territories revealed by these crossings that a rethinking of the cultural and, indeed, medical signification of epilepsy becomes possible. I am interested in the kinds of narratives we develop about the condition – the kinds of narratives we *can* develop, given epilepsy's long service and celebrity as a figurative device that has come to signify some sort of catastrophic upheaval in codes of propriety and the symbolic order.

But to begin somewhere near the beginning. Some years ago, when watching the BBC television series *Brain Story*,[1] three segments of the first episode caught my attention. They were stories about temporal lobe epilepsy which, although presented in sequence, by no means provided a seamless or cohesive account of the condition. Nor did they need to, I suppose; however, the promotional material for the series advertised a 'fascinating new insight' into the mind, and the episode in question as exploring the possibility that all human experience 'will eventually be explained in terms of the physical processes of the brain'. Despite the promise of the advertising, for me the temporal lobe stories presented ended up generating more questions than they answered.

The first story was told by a Harvard medical researcher, Dr Shahram Khoshbin, about his thirty-year project to understand links between temporal lobe epilepsy and creativity. Using the artist Vincent van Gogh as his starting point, Khoshbin also explored possible connections between temporal lobe epilepsy and spiritual experience. His story was framed by the series presenter's claim that even the most profound spiritual experience may somehow be attributed to neuronal malfunction. Khoshbin argued that van Gogh's paintings certainly indicate that he 'saw the world differently' and that this different perspective was likely due to his epilepsy. The temporal lobe, he told viewers, is that part of the brain located just behind the temples and it is where we sort out and comprehend sensory information. Any sort of anomalous activity in this part of the brain will necessarily have an impact on thought processes, emotions and perception. It is these anomalous perceptual changes, Khoshbin suggested, that endowed van Gogh's artistic vision with its particular quality. He argued that the artist's intense religiosity in later life was also 'probably' due to his temporal lobe condition.

Much has been written about van Gogh's seizure episodes since his suicide in 1890, most notably by the French neurologist Henri Gastaut.[2] While the fact of van Gogh's seizures is not at issue, the causes of these episodes are. Despite Gastaut's conclusion that the artist's recorded behavioural disturbances and psychiatric disorders were manifestations of a temporal lobe epilepsy condition, other physicians have remained unconvinced. The neurologist Dietrich Blumer, for instance, while not discounting Gastaut's hypothesis, points out that the 'nearly 30 different diagnoses' made retrospectively include numerous psychiatric disorders, lead poisoning and Ménière's disease.[3] He argues that neurosyphilis may have also played a part in van Gogh's suite of symptoms. Both Blumer and John Hughes note that van Gogh experienced seizures only after drinking absinthe – an identified epileptogenic – which, for van Gogh, was often accompanied by cognac. Gastaut also acknowledged absinthe as a contributory factor to the artist's seizures. Hughes argues that this factor must preclude a diagnosis of epilepsy because van Gogh's seizure episodes were not spontaneous but rather the consequence of alcohol withdrawal.[4] Given the ongoing debate about whether or not van Gogh had epilepsy or a seizure disorder associated with other complex factors in his life and physiology, his value to Khoshbin's project is doubtful, to say the least.

Nevertheless, in order to develop his theories about the impact of epilepsy on van Gogh's life and creativity, Khoshbin observes his patients with temporal lobe epilepsy to better understand 'exactly' how the condition 'distorts their perception'. He said that his patients all told similar stories of enhanced awareness and appreciation of colours and, sometimes, of intense spiritual experience. The biomedical importance of Khoshbin's observations was reinforced twice during this segment by voice-over comments from the series presenter advising viewers that, if left untreated, in some instances temporal lobe epilepsy can 'permanently change the way a person perceives the world'. As an editorial strategy the comments served to provide the story with tension and elucidate the risks at play in Khoshbin's narrative.

The second story in this sequence was told by Reen Carter, Dr Khoshbin's patient and someone who had had temporal lobe epilepsy for most of her life. She spoke about her vivid appreciation of colours and love of rain because 'it brings out the colours in the buildings' near her home and this allowed her to enjoy this sensory experience even more. At one point in her story she told of how the red and green arrows in her college library elevator so entranced her that she once spent three hours riding between floors just to prolong that intense pleasure. Spending three hours in an elevator notwithstanding, her story conveyed the feeling that these sensorially enriched pleasures were important to her sense of self and place in the world.

Reen Carter also told of her lifelong spirituality and said that from a very early age she felt as though she 'had a destiny to do something'.

She shared with the interviewer one of her more profound religious visions and her belief that God was somehow reassuring her of her faith via this vision. To ensure that we were in no doubt about the essential pathology underlying her sensory life, the series presenter informed viewers at this point that 'Like van Gogh, Reen Carter has had temporal lobe epilepsy all her life'. It is an oddly unambiguous statement, given that a little earlier in the sequence we were told that van Gogh's temporal lobe epilepsy was only 'probable' and, as the medical literature suggests, his symptoms did not manifest until adulthood. Pathologisation was further reinforced when various aspects of Reen Carter's story were preceded by camera close-ups of an electroencephalographic (EEG) readout of her brain's electrical activity. One of these close-ups was immediately followed by a widening shot of her reclining, eyes closed, leads from the EEG machine attached to her head. The image suggested complete acceptance and compliance with the medical story of her sensory life. Her work with the neurologist researching her condition – and presumably her medication regime – had led her to understand the spiritual aspect of her inner experience as largely due to temporal lobe activity. She said with some determination: 'When I look back at the vision of Jesus on the cross I believe that I had a seizure'. A little later, she added somewhat wistfully (and subversively): 'My religion is more now in the practical sense [pause] but I keep hoping that something will come back to me'.

The third story in the sequence was about the research of Dr Michael Persinger, who, through his ongoing project in the Behavioural Neuroscience Program at Laurentian University in Canada, had been stimulating the temporal lobes of healthy volunteers to better understand connections between brain function and spiritual experience. In short, he was trying to manufacture, under controlled laboratory conditions, the sort of sensory phenomena experienced by Reen Carter. Persinger argued that this capacity to clinically reproduce at least some aspects of those sensory experiences neuroscientists associate with intense spiritual events means that:

> They are no longer just the privileged experiences of the few or individuals who have been anointed to interpret these experiences. All people have them – it's part of our brain – and like any talent, some people will have more of these experiences than others. The critical thing is that now science has the technology to find out how these experiences actually work.

Although at the time of writing this book Persinger and his team were yet to produce a clearly definable spiritual episode in his research subjects, they had nonetheless been able to recreate under laboratory conditions a number of the sensations thought to accompany spiritual phenomena.

In 2003 British author Richard Dawkins became a participant in Persinger's project in order to test the researcher's claims for the BBC programme *Horizon*. He spent forty minutes in the testing laboratory and reported sensations of 'slight dizzyness', slight changes to respiration and some twitches in his lower limbs. After exiting the testing laboratory, he said of the experience:

> Unfortunately I didn't get the sensation of a presence. It pretty much felt as though I was in total darkness with a helmet on my head and pleasantly relaxed, and occasionally feeling the sensations which I described as they occurred into the microphone. But I would be hard put to it to swear that those were not things that could happen to me any time on a dark night. I'm very disappointed. It would have been deeply interesting to me to have experienced something of what religious people do experience in the way of a mystical experience, a communion with the universe. I would have liked to have experienced that.[5]

Persinger attributed Dawkins' lack of spiritual experience under test conditions to a lack of temporal lobe sensitivity:

> We developed a questionnaire a few years ago called temporal lobe sensitivity and what we found is a continuum of sensitivities from people who are not temporal lobe sensitive to those who are very sensitive, and the experience end being the temporal lobe epileptic. In the case of Dr Dawkins his temporal lobe sensitivity is much, much lower than most people we run than the average person, much, much lower.[6]

If nothing else, Persinger's comments suggest some of the fundamental problems in projects to map and standardise human brain function.

There were several features of these three stories that snagged my attention – not least the apparent contradiction generated by Khoshbin's project to identify temporal lobe phenomena in order to treat them (it was, after all, a premise of the series that in some instances untreated temporal lobe conditions can 'permanently change the way a person perceives the world') and Persinger's project to democratise the phenomena by making what Khoshbin referred to as 'distorted perceptions' available to the many rather than their being just the 'privileged experiences of the few'. Although both projects exhibited a central impulse to identify and therefore control the phenomena under discussion, there appeared to be instability in ascribed meaning. On the one hand, they were states that demanded medical intervention; on the other, they were desirable 'talents' available only to the privileged and those 'anointed to interpret' them.

I was curious. The stories that both researchers told about temporal lobe epilepsy sounded familiar. My first thought was that this was because they were both telling stories about hypothetical links between temporal lobe epilepsy, creativity and spirituality of the kind that had been circulating in western culture for some time. I had been a patient recruited to a neurological research project conducted at a medical facility in Toronto, Canada, in 1972, which covered much the same ground as these projects, albeit with more rudimentary technology than that deployed by Persinger. I was surprised that the medical temporal lobe story I was hearing in a new century had changed so little over those intervening decades and was keen to find out why this should be the case. I then thought that perhaps this is the only kind of temporal lobe epilepsy story western medicine *can* tell.

It would appear that these researchers were locked into what Stuart Hall and other cultural theorists have called the 'circuit of culture':[7] in this case, a medical culture that over the past century and a half (a timeframe that marks the development of neurology – the study of the physical brain – as a discrete discourse within western medicine) has assembled and come to rely on a specific and entrenched system of representation to create epilepsy narratives. The idea of culture that sparked my imagination here grew out of a cultural studies model that focuses on the production, circulation and consumption of meaning. These meanings, so the argument goes, have material consequences in that they generate, organise and regulate our social practices.

This concept is no less relevant to the culture of western medicine than it is to wider culture. Language, Hall tells us, is of primary importance in producing and circulating ideas and ideologies, power, values and feelings within culture. Medical culture is constituted by a language rich in metaphor, metonymy and symbolism. It is a language that constructs a particular order and way of thinking about the body. It is a language that determines the manner in which normality and abnormality are attributed to the body. It is *not* a language that develops in a vacuum – somehow hived off from and untrammelled by the metaphors, images and symbolism circulating through wider cultural frameworks. Medicine's symbolic language is invariably drawn from its wider cultural context. And, as Hall points out, culture is what 'distinguishes the "human" element in social life from what is simply biologically driven'.[8] By drawing on this idea of the cultural circuit, it becomes possible to move beyond the medical/cultural language dichotomy, to an engagement with the multiple sites where meanings of epilepsy are produced, disseminated and understood.

II

Peter Wolf argues that an examination of the cultural history of epilepsy is crucial to understanding its social and historical significance.[9] To this end, a growing body of scholarly work over the past fifteen years or so has examined representations of the condition in literature and film. Jennie Kerson *et al.* observe that, generally, film portrayals of characters with epilepsy conform to entrenched models of cultural superstition or veer towards the sensational.[10] In her comprehensive review of epilepsy in film, Dr Sallie Baxendale from the Institute of Neurology in London suggests that, despite a general view that cultural representations of epilepsy have become more enlightened in recent times, this, in fact, is not the case. She argues: 'Although it is not for the medical profession to dictate or censor cinematic content, a keen eye on these depictions will help us to understand and perhaps combat some of the stereotypes and myths that continue to surround epilepsy in the 21st century'.[11] I wonder, though, whether a cultural system of representation that pays close attention to the medical model would necessarily combat the stereotypes that Baxendale identifies in her research. This is a question that will be explored at length in the following chapters.

In setting up this question for more extensive examination, it is worth taking a moment to consider an overview of the cultural history that endows epilepsy with its complex value as a unit of signification. At various times in this history it has been deployed as a curse. As well as the plague, scurvy, leprosy and carbuncles, the Protestant reformer Martin Luther is said to have called epilepsy down from the heavens to express his views about the Catholic Church more fulsomely.[12] The condition has been posited as an indicator of moral character and intellectual capability, as well as the hidden cause of explosive and unpredictable disruption. Indeed, its signifying potential has made epilepsy and the figure of the epileptic something of a stock device in literature and film. The dramatic possibilities of the seized body in the extremes of a *grand mal* seizure or visionary transcendence have proved valuable to plot progression in some instances, or in others to enrich some aspect of characterisation. More often than not, though, cultural representations of epilepsy locate the affected character in the borderlands between normality and abnormality; as a figurative device, 'the epileptic' is inevitably poised on an unstable threshold between order and an ever-threatening chaos.

William Shakespeare recognised the dramatic possibilities of the condition. In *King Lear*, Kent vents his rage at Oswald's part in the unfolding tragedy with an inventively diverse range of insults. Among other things, Oswald is a 'knave, beggar, coward, pandar, and the son and heir of a mongrel bitch' (2.2.20).[13] Still with spleen to vent, Kent finally curses Oswald with 'a plague upon [his] epileptic visage' (2.2.77). In this text, as with others, epilepsy becomes a metonym for inner corruption. For Sigmund Freud the epileptic body was the living exemplar of the *unheimlich* or uncanny: a body both recognisably human and alive but at the same time possessed of unpredictable and unknowable capabilities. Yet regardless of how characters with epilepsy have been historically deployed in western cultural texts, they are invariably represented as being somehow 'other'.

Male characters are often imbued with violent and dangerous impulses: for example, Shakespeare's Othello; Monks in Charles Dickens' *Oliver Twist*; Smerdyakov in Dostoevsky's *The Brothers Karamazov*; and, more recently, James Walter Wayland, the homicidal protagonist in the 1997 film *Deceiver*. Female characters with the condition tend to be marginalised, infantilised or eroticised. Guster, Mr and Mrs Snagsby's maid in Dickens' *Bleak House*, is thought to be a bit of a bargain in the employment market: because of her 'fits', she 'goes cheap'. The transgressive sexuality of Lucette Le Sueur (Lucetta Templeman) in Thomas Hardy's *The Mayor of Casterbridge* is quite another matter. She is glamorous, passionate and a woman desired by both Michael Henchard and her eventual husband, Donald Farfrae. Carmen Sternwood, the sexually provocative character in Raymond Chandler's *The Big Sleep*, sets the tone for the characterisation of Gabe in the 1992 Australian film *Romper Stomper*.

At various times western medicine has taken up and reinforced these types of cultural formations. Ideas of epileptic violence and deviant eroticism provided a strong current for many of the debates about the 'dangers' posed by those with epilepsy for 'normal' society in the pages of late nineteenth-century medical journals. Belief that folk with epilepsy could suddenly run amok, leaving death and chaos in their wake, regularly featured in the editorial pages of the *Lancet*. Under the heading 'Homicidal epilepsy', a medical writer for the journal issued a 'loud warning' to those 'superintendents of promiscuous hospitals, in which epilepsy is largely represented, never to admit or retain such cases when illusions of the aggressive kind are manifested'.[14] An 1892 article in the *British Medical Journal* presented as evidence of the potential violence in all epileptics prone to 'irritability' the 'case of a young man who some years ago shot a girl without any reason. He said afterwards that he was quite unaware of what he had done, and, as corroborating his statement, he had a fit in the course of his trial.'[15] In 1900, an Australian physician, F. Norton Manning, took a publishing opportunity in the *Australasian Medical Gazette* to inform his medical colleagues that 'the religious and the malicious are curiously intermingled in the epileptic'.[16]

Within the pages of these late nineteenth- and early twentieth-century medical journals, women with epilepsy were frequently represented as manifesting inappropriate sexuality. Tellingly, what constituted inappropriate female sexuality here was often demarcated along cultural boundaries. In a robust engagement with the work of his French colleague Jean-Martin Charcot on the subject, the British neurologist William Gowers argued that, unlike their French counterparts, the seizure episodes suffered by the good British stock of hystero-epileptics at the National Hospital for the Paralysed and Epileptic, Queen Square, London, had never been accompanied 'so far as I have seen ... by any erotic manifestations'. It seemed that the rather more prosaic English woman experienced nothing more florid than some feelings of illness and choking sensations when subjected to pressure on her ovaries from a researching physician's hand.[17] I engage these debates in detail in Chapter 2. It is enough to say for the moment that traffic back and forth between medical and cultural sites of representation at the end of the nineteenth century and well into the twentieth century remained lively.

In the twenty-first century, this trafficking in representation is noticeable in the medical narratives about temporal lobe epilepsy presented by *Brain Story*. The importation of cultural meaning into these stories is evident in Persinger's use of words like 'privileged' and 'anointed'. He is implicitly referencing – maybe ironically, maybe not – a cultural tradition of the ecstatic and visionary epileptic. Historically, religious figures such as the Prophet Mohammed, Saint Francis of Assisi and Jeanne d'Arc have been associated with epilepsy because of their visionary experiences. Accounts of their lives indicate that all heard 'divine' voices while experiencing these visions. The biblical account of Saint Paul's conversion to Christianity on the road to Damascus describes his prostration after seeing a flash of light from the sky. As he lies on the ground blinded by the light, he hears the voice of Jesus asking 'Saul, Saul why are you persecuting me?' (Acts 9:1–20). When he finally reaches Damascus, Paul's sight is restored by the disciple Ananias and he is subsequently baptised into the Christian faith.[18] In fiction, the figure of the ecstatic epileptic is exemplified by Dostoevsky's Prince Myshkin. The temporal lobe stories presented by *Brain Story* fold back into culture via the medium of television and would appear to reinforce and perpetuate cultural stereotypes already in circulation.

III

Despite a climate of free trade in representation, from a medical perspective the relationship between the discipline and its cultural framework is an uneasy one in the twenty-first century. Historically, this uneasiness can be understood, at least in part, by the privileged status medical discourse occupies in western systems of knowledge production about the body. Medical authority in this area began to formalise around the mid nineteenth century, when the body became subject to the subtle but relentless impulses of normalisation. To progress the project of making the body intelligible to medical interpretation, analysis and control, the medical sciences developed what Michel Foucault calls an anatomico-metaphysical register. He argues that the scrutiny and medical definition of bodies through the middle decades of the nineteenth century eventually stabilised classificatory principles and by the closing decades of the century had established a 'natural order of disorder'.[19] The biomedical register was instrumental in developing this taxonomy of disorder. Crucial to its ongoing maintenance is medicine's authority to produce verifiable 'truths' deemed innocent of all cultural bias about the body and embodied experience.

It is possible to see how the anatomico-metaphysical register operates in *Brain Story* by examining its deployment in the medical stories of temporal lobe experience. It is also possible to discern some of the pressure points marking the boundaries of its field of signification. Khoshbin and Persinger project a model of medical research that is culturally neutral. They also present as scientific observers unsullied by cultural values and suppositions. Khoshbin's undertaking to unravel 'exactly' how his patients' temporal lobe conditions 'distort' their perceptions and belief systems assumes a standardised brain, a brain that perceives free from cultural influences. In this schema, only the researcher has the objective (non-acculturated) wherewithal to arbitrate on what constitutes appropriate (non-distorted, according to the observer's referential framework) sensory perceptions. The power to define the line that demarcates distorted from non-distorted perceptions clearly rests with the researcher in this story. For Khoshbin, the medical observer is as culturally neutral as the brain being observed. In his story, the language of spirituality and creativity is re-registered as the language of diagnosis and treatment.

In ranging through some of the benefits he hopes his research will ultimately yield, Persinger argues that experiencing temporal lobe phenomena under laboratory conditions is optimal because it is safe: 'You know it's a laboratory.... You know the experimenter's doing it or something that's involved with the experimenter.' These conditions, he suggests, allow the experimentally affected subjects access to an 'easy, pat explanation' for their altered states. On the other hand, he argues, experiencing these phenomena in culture, one can look only *to* culture for explanations and therefore usually attribute these experiences to 'the gods'. It is difficult to argue with the logical progression of Persinger's argument, but the question arises: so what?

It is not at all clear that the temporal lobe events of the kind that Persinger produced in the laboratory can be meaningfully equated with so-called 'in culture' occurrences in a way that provides useful insight into the subjective experiences of temporal lobe phenomena, a point that would appear to be confirmed by Dawkins' experience. As Khoshbin points out, the temporal lobe has an associative function. It is the part of the brain where we integrate and meaningfully decode sensory information. If we know that perceptual changes are being stimulated by medical technology in a research laboratory, then of course we will understand sensory experience as a generative part of that process. If we experience the same sort of altered state 'out there', in the world, we may indeed attribute it to 'the gods'. However, just as in the laboratory situation, what these 'gods' are will depend on our cultural references and empirical framework.

Spiritual belief systems aside, we may also attribute sensory anomalies to the over-rich food we enjoyed so much a few hours before, or a one-too-many glass of wine, or any number of other recreational substances that we may partake of from time to time. As the medical literature suggests, some of van Gogh's creative perceptions were as likely fuelled by his love of absinthe as they were by temporal lobe activity. And it is of course entirely possible that at least a modicum of his creativity had absolutely nothing to do with pathology, temporarily induced or otherwise. My point here is that the living brain is not firing off neurones, stimulating sensation, processing sensory data in some sort of hermetically neutral environment, experimental or cultural. The temporal lobe integrates sensory information and makes sense of it according to our cultural frameworks, just as western medical researchers make sense of the data they collect and interpret.

Deciphering meaning from an EEG spike/wave pattern of the brain's neuronal activity is a complex process and Khoshbin makes it clear in his temporal lobe story that he can know what his EEG readings of temporal lobe activity mean in terms of subjective experience only because his patients tell him how they feel. Persinger makes the same point. The medical literature indicates that it is exceptionally rare to capture EEG readings of the brain simultaneous with the kind of complex events that comprise Reen Carter's story about her own sensory experiences, and it is unclear from the story that Khoshbin tells whether or not any of his patients' EEG readings are coincidental with religious visions or heightened sensory states. While the EEG research being conducted by Khoshbin and Persinger may go some way in charting the neuronal activity underlying certain sensory changes, both the subjective experience of these sensory events and the medical explanations of their meaning to neuroscience will always and necessarily be articulated through a complex weave of medical language shot through with layers of metaphor and metonym drawn from culture.

One of the more interesting and explicit examples of the representational trade between culture and medicine in the latter part of the twentieth century, and one relevant to the epilepsy narratives presented in *Brain Story*, is provided by the work of Gastaut. The French neurologist first began publishing his research on epilepsy conditions in 1953. A decade after his 1956 paper on van Gogh's symptoms, he published an article exploring the links between epilepsy and creativity in relation to the work of Gustave Flaubert. Of the three artists he wrote about in his research, he argued that Dostoevsky was the most accessible to contemporary medical interest because there was so much detailed knowledge of his epilepsy and some of these accounts had been recorded by physicians treating the author. By 1978, however, Gastaut was to recant his earlier endorsements of Dostoevsky's ecstatic aura.

For many years he had accepted and 'even help[ed] to create'[20] a generalisable medical model of temporal lobe phenomena based on the Russian author's accounts of the moment that precedes and signals the onset of some seizure forms. Despite his earlier wholehearted endorsement of Dostoevsky's description of intense pleasure and bliss as features of some of the author's pre-seizure experiences, Gastaut had come to question the validity of his acceptance. He argued that Dostoevsky's philosophical leanings influenced the way that he wrote about epilepsy in his literary works and experienced it in his own life. Moreover, his literary genius had persuaded neurologists to believe in an ecstatic or euphoric aura despite an absence to date of its appearance in clinical practice. Gastaut concluded that medical authors (himself included) who had allowed themselves to be influenced by Dostoevsky and to be 'abused by the demon of analogy and the desire for symmetry'[21] now had to rethink the experiential possibilities of epilepsy conditions. Indeed, Gastaut felt that he needed to rethink precisely what kind of epilepsy affected Dostoevsky. His paper sparked a minor debate on the nature of epileptic experience.

Gastaut's work raises important points about the relationship between medical discourse and cultural narratives. He freely acknowledges the importance of literary imagery and patient narratives about the subjective aspects of temporal lobe activity to medical understanding of the phenomena. He also contends that the stories folk tell about their temporal lobe experiences will be shaped by a range of philosophical, cultural, social and historical factors. Both Persinger and Khoshbin argue that their temporal lobe stories will provide preferable, if not 'easy' or 'pat', explanations for those with temporal lobe epilepsy and the implication is that the medical story will obviate the need for any further considerations; that these medical explanations will fit unproblematically into a patient's cultural identity, symbolic world, life narrative.

Despite these researchers' confidence in their narratives, there seems to be something missing from the medical temporal lobe story for Reen Carter. While she accepts the medical explanation that her vision of Jesus was a temporal lobe seizure, she keeps hoping that something of the richness of that event, and of her spiritual life in general prior to her conversion to the medical model, 'will come back'. The sense of longing for spirituality lost threaded through her story hardly seems compensated by her medical treatment. This sense of loss is underscored by the scientific acquisitiveness in the stories told by Khoshbin and Persinger: both want, in some form or other, what she has or had. In *Brain Story*, the narrative play between the medical and personal stories of temporal lobe epilepsy and spirituality becomes an allegory of loss and envy. Khoshbin strives to 'see' what fuels van Gogh's creativity and Reen Carter's spirituality; Persinger wants to make these 'talents' available to the many rather than just the 'privileged few'.

IV

It may seem odd and possibly even simplistic at this point, but in light of Gastaut's recantation it is necessary to ask the question: what *is* epilepsy? Epilepsy has a consistent presence in the annals of western medical writing from the time when physicians first began to regulate thinking about the condition in the Hippocratic text *On the Sacred Disease* to the present day. Just as consistently, it has generated hotly contested debate about precisely what it is, what it means and what it entails, for roughly the same period. According to *Blakiston's New Gould Medical Dictionary*, the term 'epilepsy' is derived from the Greek word *epilepsia*, meaning seizure, and is defined as:

> A disorder of the brain characterized by a recurring excessive neuronal discharge, manifested by transient episodes of motor, sensory, or psychic dysfunction, with or without unconsciousness or convulsive movements. The seizure is associated with marked changes in recorded electrical brain activity.[22]

This concise and seemingly clear-cut definition is followed by a further page and a half of refining categories and sub-categories. Invariably, these further explanations of epilepsy are organised around manifestations of the seizure.

On closer scrutiny it becomes evident that the term 'seizure' and the type of event it describes are both, in fact, quite elastic, even as they are confined within the parameters of a medical signifying system. Seizure may entail the dramatic and catastrophic *grand mal* episode, which is characterised by 'sudden loss of consciousness, tonic convulsion, cyanosis, and dilated pupils, followed by a clonic spasm of all voluntary muscles, with the eyes rotated upward, the head extended, a frothing at the mouth, and, frequently, incontinence of urine'. However, the term 'seizure' can also refer to states of transient psychic disturbance without loss of consciousness. Khoshbin talks about van Gogh's 'seizure of ideas' in his temporal lobe story. To further compound the possibility of confusion when trying to understand what it means when someone is said to 'have seizures', a seizure may be no more than localised, spasmodic muscular contractions, with full retention of consciousness. Some of these seizure states are the consequence of underlying disease, but most are not. So-called idiopathic epilepsy, for example, is defined as a convulsive disorder not attributable to any known or specific brain disease. What becomes clear through a close reading of these definitions is that the neurological category 'epilepsy' is by no means a finitely demarcated concept.

Even the term 'seizure' has not been used consistently across English-speaking cultures to describe these types of paroxysmal states: 'fit' and 'attack' also enjoyed regular usage until very recently. 'Attack' is suggestive of the physiological violence of some forms of paroxysmal episodes and harks back to ancient beliefs that the seizure marked some sort of hostile assault from external forces. Its use also encodes vestiges of the Greek *epilambanein*, meaning seize or attack, a stem of the word epilepsy.

In nineteenth- and early twentieth-century British, American and Australian medical journals the term 'fit' saw common usage, as it did and does in other cultural contexts. According to the *Oxford English Dictionary*, 'fit' can refer to 'A sudden and somewhat severe but transitory attack (of illness, or of some specified ailment)'. In this sense, its place in the medical language of epilepsy again seems perfectly straightforward. However, even here there is no guarantee against slippage and on further investigation 'fit' proves to be a satisfyingly ambiguous term. It also signifies a sense of excitement and danger, which can be either pleasant or painful. As Reen Carter's story suggests, not all of the sensory experiences associated with those cerebral paroxysms known as epilepsy *are* unpleasant. In fact, the nineteenth-century British neurologist John Hughlings Jackson (the so-called 'Father' of British neurology) expressed concern that some patients found the phenomena 'positively agreeable' and failed to report them to their doctors.[23]

Suggestively, though, the etymology of the word 'fit' also connects it to ideas of conflict and struggle, and this is where the term can be used to deconstruct a diagnostic and therapeutic opposition between 'illness' and 'well-being'. It alludes to ideas of administrative power, as when it refers to the process of making a person fit for something: 'To make fit or suitable; to adapt the object in view.... To render (a person) competent or qualified'. In the linguistic register of biology it means possessing or conferring the ability to survive and reproduce in a particular environment. Also included in the list of meanings for 'fit' in the *Oxford English Dictionary* are 'angry, desperate, exhausted' and, in one sense, 'conflict, struggle; a position of danger; ... a mortal crisis'. These latter meanings have relevance to some of the more aggressive medical responses to folk with epilepsy discussed in Chapters 2 and 3, and are evocative of the linguistic and category instabilities still haunting epilepsy discourse. Fit. A small yet complex word. To fit; to be fit; to be made fit; to be made *to* fit.

In relationship to what is being observed and recorded, this taxonomic uncertainty presents problems for epilepsy narratives. Debates around whether some forms of convulsion owe their origins to disturbances in the cosmos, the psyche or the synapses, and what the differences might mean to medical interpretations of cerebral paroxysm, have maintained momentum from Hippocratic times through to the present day. A perceived instability of meaning prompted Hughlings Jackson to proclaim in the closing decades of the nineteenth century that the term 'epilepsy' was, in some sense, obsolete and that physicians should more appropriately use the term 'epilepsies' to describe the diverse range of signs and symptoms that had by then become associated with the condition. Just over a century later the American neurologist Joel Reiter worried that the changing medical terminology used to classify epileptic symptoms risked miscommunication with his patients.[24] We similarly get a sense of the instability of meaning circulating around the epilepsies from the stories told by Khoshbin and Persinger.

As Gastaut's work confirms, supplementing its medical signification, epilepsy has acquired a range of historical, social and symbolic meanings through cultural representations, and medical culture is not immune to these representations. When recording his ideas on 'dreamy state' or reminiscence – that pre-seizure state described so evocatively by Dostoevsky – Hughlings Jackson followed a patient's lead and deferred to the words of Dickens to try to capture the sensory experience associated with the state. Charcot called on Shakespeare to infuse drama into one of his presentations on ambulatory automatism associated with epilepsy:

> In *Macbeth* there is a very significant observation on somnambulism. The doctor sees Lady Macbeth get up and begin her somnambulic activity; he turns to the other characters on the stage and, supposing them better informed than they are in fact, exclaims: 'Look, her eyes are open.' Indeed in some somnambulism whether the eyes are open or closed is the most important question.[25]

The twentieth-century American neurologist William Lennox favoured militaristic tropes to write about what he dubbed western medicine's 'war against man's ancient enemy'.[26] In the closing years of the twentieth century an American physician described his entry into an emergency room where a young patient was being treated for *status epilepticus*[27] as being 'like something out of *The Exorcist*'.[28] His description of the scene suggests the *unheimlich* effect of the seizing body on medical sensibilities. His reference to the film to convey his initial subjective response to this kind of emergency also suggests the limitations of the medical register to tell his story of the episode.

V

At the outset, I declared my interest in the kinds of stories we tell about epilepsy and those affected by the condition in light of a long and complex history of representation. Throughout this history there have been cultural and medical stories which have worked against the grain of a narrative tradition that casts 'the epileptic' as disordered 'other'. That these stories are too often backgrounded by the dominant tradition suggests the hold that narrative associations between epilepsy, social disorder, excessive spirituality, divine possession, tainted bloodlines, sexual deviance and criminality have on the collective imagination. In an attempt to break the hold of these established 'language games' on the production of epilepsy narratives, throughout the following chapters I read biographical and personal stories about what epilepsy means to cultural identity and narrative autonomy in relationship to concurrent cultural and medical systems of representation. This play of personal stories against the backdrop of cultural and medical narratives provides further critical perspective and reveals the restrictions on the free trade economy introduced above. With notable exceptions – Dostoevsky, for example – it is rare indeed to find counter-narratives from those with epilepsy given purchase in the dominant representational systems.

I have chosen this approach for several reasons; not least because, regardless of cultural context, the search for meaning is often viewed as a central endeavour of human experience. Hamlet's dying request, 'To tell my story', reflects the centrality of personal narratives to claims for identity and cultural presence. The importance of personal narratives to psychological and social health is now well recognised in the field of psychotherapy. As Hall argues, we understand what things *mean* (socially and culturally) 'through the words we use about them, the stories we tell about them, the images of them we produce',[29] as well as through the sorts of emotions that we associate with different meanings. For Hall, as for other scholars working in this area of cultural identity, language – both spoken and written – is a primary medium through which 'we make sense of things [and] in which meaning is produced and exchanged'.[30] We conceive and understand our identities as cultural subjects in narrative terms. These are the tools we use to tell our stories about who we are, our lives and our experiences.

Over and above personal identity stories, each culture also has its keynote stories. These stories circulate cultural ideas (and ideals) about what it 'means' to be female, to be male, to be a parent, to be of particular ethnicity or cultural background, to be from the working class, to be educated, to be rich or poor, to be disabled – indeed, to be human – within specific cultural contexts. As cultural subjects, we attach ourselves to particular types of stories because we understand them as providing our lives with social meaning: 'Aaah!' we think, '*This* is what it means to be…'. What happens, though, when our personal life story – the story we *want* to tell about who we are and how we see ourselves fitting into the scheme of things – crashes headlong into a keynote story of our identity in such a way that we find ourselves dislocated from all that gives meaning to our lives? In other words, what happens when we lose the rights to our own life story? It seems to me that more often than not this is what happens for those defined by a keynote disability story. For Reen Carter, this collision between her personal narrative of identity and medicine's keynote story of temporal lobe epilepsy has meant trying to find a new way of being as she lives in the borderlands between a pathologised sensory life and the hope that one day something of her personal spirituality story 'will come back' to her. It may be the case that cultural languages of creativity and spirituality offer a better rate of exchange than the medical languages of diagnosis and treatment for folk like van Gogh and Reen Carter.

The keynote stories of epilepsy have simultaneously produced a solidified picture of the condition and one that is oddly elusive to any sort of clear signification. Despite western medicine's considerable efforts over the last century or so to extricate epilepsy narratives from the signifying legacy of past centuries of representation, elements of the old stories remain stubbornly persistent. In this narrative economy, the epileptic body and, by extension, those who experience any one of the conditions become a palimpsest: the shadows of ancient inscriptions never completely erased from more recent writings. At the benign end of its signifying possibilities, this has led to an overdetermining of personality in relation to epilepsy. At this end of the scale, my experiences of temporal lobe epilepsy would be more or less interchangeable with those of Reen Carter, just as *Brain Story* overlays her experiences with those of Vincent van Gogh.

It may well be that comparative EEG readings of our brains, if that were possible, would show similarities in neuronal patterns. However, the empirical frameworks that provided each of us with reference points to navigate and make sense of our temporal lobe phenomena are presumably specific to our cultural and historical contexts. The religiosity that becomes the *leitmotiv* of *Brain Story*'s account of temporal lobe epilepsy via the experiences of van Gogh and Reen Carter is not a significant part of my story. My belief system organises around the secular rather than the spiritual. This is not to say that I do not experience dimensional visual phenomena on occasion or that I cannot be entranced by the colours of a sunset or transported by certain forms of music. My temporal lobe condition is the filter through which I perceive the world: its perceptual effects do not locate me beyond the world. But then, everybody filters sensory experiences through a conditioned temporal lobe, however that condition might be described and interpreted.

More problematically, in this complex and unstable signifying economy, epilepsy can be produced and manipulated. Persinger's manipulations of healthy brains to produce those sensory changes associated with temporal lobe epilepsy can be seen as a somewhat innocuous example of this type of brain mapping process. It is more difficult to clearly identify where the balance is in a cost–benefit assessment of Reen Carter's medicalised story. The drive behind the stories told by Khoshbin and Persinger is to reveal otherwise hidden epileptic potential in the brain and has antecedents in the brain mapping projects of the mid and late twentieth century. These projects saw twentieth-century neurologists develop a range of activating techniques to arouse those 'dormant abnormalities' not usually detectable: that is, to clinically diagnose epilepsy, by the 1950s western medicine had begun to find ways to artificially produce and visually record physiological states denoting epilepsy.

Medicine's visual culture began to gain momentum in the closing decades of the nineteenth century. In relation to epilepsy, there were numerous projects attempting to map and photographically record definitive catalogues of epileptic physiognomies and other physical features. Cesare Lombroso and Charcot are possibly the two most notable proponents from this time. Although the aetiology of epilepsy continued to elude medicine's grasp well into the next century, by the 1960s there was a scopic satisfaction and authority to be had in the ability to render epileptic disorder visible to scientific study via the medically provoked seizure. If medicine still could not decipher the epilepsies, it could now author them. Medical researchers had developed the wherewithal to produce their own epilepsy; and at will. In part, the scopic pleasures to be had from the body in seizure spiral from an artificial reinforcement of that boundary between the controlled (controlling), normalised, authoritative researcher and the pathologised otherness of epileptic identity, captured irrefutably by the outward signifier of seizure. This medical 'outing' of concealed epileptic potential, issues of passing in relationship to the syndrome and discussions of how dis-ease is encoded (and disavowed) in the practices identified above are subject to further analysis in later chapters.

By the 2000s, production of the signifiers and symptoms of epilepsy under laboratory conditions had become an accepted part of the diagnostic process and wrought some complex changes for the medical gaze. Increasingly, its attention was held by the effectiveness of the diagnostic tools to stimulate electronically recordable changes to brain wave patterns and provoke observable pathologised behaviours, rather than the consequences that these methods might have for immediate and long-term patient well-being. To recall Khoshbin's words about van Gogh for a moment: the medical gaze when it focused on epilepsy now 'saw the world differently'.

VI

The chapters that follow attempt to unravel the intimately entwined threads of meaning and narrative relationships that have given rise to and shaped the stories and practices explored in the preceding pages. There are three key touch points between the medical and wider cultural systems of representation engaged in the book. Early chapters examine a range of texts from the late nineteenth and early twentieth centuries, which are read against a background of contemporary social change and the developing discourses of degeneration and eugenics. Throughout these chapters I draw on popular fiction as well as *fin-de-siècle* narratives of deviancy to examine the emergent neurological discourse of epilepsy in Britain, France and the United States. I then examine the implications of cultural representational systems for the inception of the epileptic colony project. The following chapter focuses on the mid twentieth century, where I draw on cultural narratives, including film and televisual narratives, of science and fiction as well as technologies of control and subversion to engage contemporary medical systems of representation. Finally, I examine the representational legacy from these touch points for twenty-first-century medical concerns about epilepsy.

I argue that, in a sense, late nineteenth- and early twentieth-century medical stories of 'the epileptic' become allegories for wider social concerns and escalating anxieties about disorder and degeneration from within an ailing society. In this narrative economy, the figure of the 'epileptic' is inscribed with the political and social complexities of the age. The terms 'epileptic', 'epileptic body' and 'epileptic figure' are used at various times throughout the following chapters to draw attention to that type of textual construct that has come to stand for the subject affected by epilepsy. It seems to me that this idea of the 'figure' as it functions in literary theory yields a useful way of thinking about that space between what is written about 'the epileptic' and the lived experiences of those with an epilepsy condition. One of the claims that I explore in the following chapters is that literary medical–cultural constructions of the epileptic body become a dangerous supplement, a fetishised third term that conflates differences between the textual and corporeal. Furthermore, the iterability of these constructs perpetuates an orthodoxy of epilepsy that establishes irrefutable images of disruption, disorder and irresponsibility. Nineteenth-century neurology's discourse of epilepsy not only registered wider scientific and social concerns about the perceived escalation of social disorder, poverty and disease but, to a significant extent, it located the symptomatology of these social ills with the epileptic. Traces of this signifying legacy still permeate some of the more prevalent narratives today.

In some ways this book is a detecting story. In the following chapters I sift through the evidence of 150 years and more to find out how current systems of representation came into being. I also attempt to sort out the myth from the matter in an endeavour to reconfigure narrative possibilities for future epilepsy stories. It may well be that how well future stories of epilepsy are told will depend on recognition of the complex relationships between medical and cultural systems of representation. It cannot be said that what follows is an entirely unbiased process: I have picked over some of this ground before, trying to find myself in medical narratives that reshaped my identity after being diagnosed with temporal lobe epilepsy in 1971 as a consequence of provocative diagnosis, or medically induced seizure. This was my first *grand mal* seizure; it was by no means my last. Decades passed; time moved on; stories changed. Or so I thought. But then there was *Brain Story.*

Notes

1 *Brain Story.* Series prod. Sam Roberts. Written and presented by Professor Susan Greenfield. BBC Worldwide, 2001. Unless otherwise indicated, the quotations that follow are from this source.
2 Henri Gastaut. 'Vincent van Gogh's disease seen in the light of new concepts of psychomotor epilepsy'. *Annals of Medical Psychology (Paris)*, vol. 114, 1956, pp. 196–238.
3 Dietrich Blumer. 'The illness of Vincent van Gogh'. *American Journal of Psychiatry*, vol. 159, no. 4, April 2002, p. 522.
4 John R. Hughes. 'A reappraisal of the possible seizures of Vincent van Gogh'. *Epilepsy and Behaviour*, vol. 6, 2005, p. 508.
5 Richard Dawkins. Transcript, 'God on the brain'. *Horizon*, BBC 2, 17 April 2003. http://www.bbc.co.uk/science/horizon/2003/godonbraintrans.shtml.
6 Michael Persinger. Transcript, 'God on the brain'.
7 Stuart Hall. 'Introduction', in Stuart Hall, ed. *Representation: Cultural Representations and Signifying Practices*. London: Sage, 1997, p. 3.
8 Hall, 'Introduction', p. 3.
9 Peter Wolf. 'Epilepsy in literature'. *Epilepsia*, vol. 36, 1995, pp. 12–17.
10 Jennie F. Kerson, Toba Schwaber Kerson and Lawrence A. Kerson. 'The depiction of seizures in film'. *Epilepsia*, vol. 40, no. 8, 1999, pp. 1163–67.
11 Sallie Baxendale. 'Epilepsy at the movies: possession to presidential assassination'. *Lancet Neurology*, vol. 2, December 2003, p. 770.
12 See William Gordon Lennox. *Epilepsy and Related Disorders*. 2 vols. London: Churchill, 1960, vol. 1, p. 18.
13 William Shakespeare. *King Lear.* Ed. Ralph E. C. Houghton. Oxford: Clarendon Press, 1967.
14 'Homicidal epilepsy'. *Lancet*, 14 September 1889, p. 554.

15 S. Wilks, 'An address on some of the more unusual phenomena of epilepsy'. *British Medical Journal*, 2 January 1892, p. 3.
16 F. Norton Manning. 'The epileptic: his treatment and care'. *Australasian Medical Gazette*, 20 June 1900, p. 217.
17 W. R. Gowers. 'The Gulstonian lectures on epilepsy: lecture II – part II'. *Lancet*, 20 March 1880, p. 436.
18 See, generally, Joseph Ernest Renan. *History of the Origins of Christianity. Book 1: The Life of Jesus* and *Book 4: Saint Paul, The Antichrist*. London: Watts, 1864. http://www.infidels.org/library/historical/ernest_renan/life_of_jesus.html. Accessed 6 November 2007. Quotation from the King James Version of the Bible.
19 Michel Foucault. *The History of Sexuality, Volume I: An Introduction*. 1976. Trans. Robert Hurley. London: Penguin Books, 1990, p. 44.
20 Henri Gastaut. 'Fyodor Mikhailovitch Dostoevsky's involuntary contribution to the symptomatology and prognosis of epilepsy'. *Epilepsia*, vol. 19, 1978, p. 186.
21 Gastaut, 'Fyodor Mikhailovitch Dostoevsky's involuntary contribution', p. 197.
22 Alfonso R. Gennaro, *et al*., eds. *Blakiston's New Gould Medical Dictionary: Illustrated*. 4th edition. New York: McGraw-Hill, 1983.
23 John Hughlings Jackson. 'On a particular variety of epilepsy ("intellectual aura"), one case with symptoms of organic brain disease', 1888, in James Taylor, ed. *Selected Writings of John Hughlings Jackson*. 2 vols. London: Hodder and Stoughton, 1932, vol. 1, p. 388.
24 Adrienne Richard and Joel Reiter. *Epilepsy: A New Approach*. 2nd edition. New York: Walker, 1995, p. 27.
25 Jean-Martin Charcot. 'Ambulatory automatisms: a diagnosis of epilepsy: January 31, 1888'. In *Charcot the Clinician: The Tuesday Lessons*. Trans. and commentary Christopher G. Goetz. New York: Raven, 1987, p. 39.
26 Frederic A. Gibbs. 'William Gordon Lennox: 1884–1960'. *Epilepsia*, vol. 2, 1961, p. 1.
27 This is an acute neuronal event that entails multiple tonic/clonic or *grand mal* seizures occurring in rapid succession, with the patient not regaining consciousness between episodes. *Status epilepticus* is extremely difficult to treat. Unchecked, the condition can be fatal.
28 Anne Fadiman. *The Spirit Catches You and You Fall Down: A Hmong Child, Her American Doctors, and the Clash of Two Cultures*. 1997. New York: Noonday Press, 1999, p. 143.
29 Hall, 'Introduction', p. 3.
30 Hall, 'Introduction', p. 1.

CHAPTER 1

From Hippocrates to Shakespeare and Dickens: epilepsy's entry into 'the circuit of culture'

If I wished to show a student the difficulties of getting a truth from medical experience I would give him the history of epilepsy to read. (Oliver Wendell Holmes, 'Currents and counter-currents in medical science', 1911)

I

At the dawn of medicine's engagement with seizure conditions, Aretaeus proclaimed 'Epilepsy is an illness of various shapes and horrible'.[1] Over 2,000 years later, the medical descendants of Hippocrates and Aretaeus shouldered the task of trying to understand this most puzzling of chronic neurological conditions with renewed vigour. The closing decades of the nineteenth century saw the emergence of neurology as a specialist medical discourse. Committed to moving beyond the rather bleak epilepsy stories bequeathed them by their predecessors, these latter-day physicians determined to cultivate an innovative system of representation specific to their areas of concern. The hope was that a formalised and technical system of representation would allow them to modernise epilepsy and create stories that would bring it into a new scientific age.

By the 1880s the profession had gone some way in the quest to develop a contemporary lexicon to describe and record patients' symptoms so that they accorded with a range of evolving neurological taxonomies. Medical practitioners were encouraged to use standardised forms to record the outward signs of epileptic seizures, recovery times, post-seizure mental states, vital signs, reflexes and so on.[2] Nevertheless, the project to develop a clear and concise medical language to describe and thus anchor the condition within a neurological paradigm remained haunted by the legacy of ancient significations. Owsei Temkin's 1971 comprehensive and minutely detailed chronicle of epilepsy is still regarded as the most meticulous account of the condition's cultural and medical history. Inevitably, more recent texts engaging with the historical origins of the epilepsies – this one included – draw on his work as their most consistent historical reference. He provides a valuable starting point to begin an examination of epilepsy's representational history from Hippocrates and Aretaeus through to that late nineteenth-century struggle to re/present the condition.

The detecting work of this chapter traverses complex and diverse textual terrain. It involves consideration of the medical–cultural languages of epilepsy from Hippocrates through to William Shakespeare, William Gowers and Charles Dickens. Along the way, we will consider the textual play between different narrative genres. We are looking for the origins of the 'circuit of culture' that produced and set into circulation some of the stock meanings that have come to be associated with seizure conditions and linger with such disturbing effect in the neuroscientific endeavours of the late nineteenth century. Discussion will range across the writings of historians, authors of literature, physicians, social reformers, theorists and biographers. It seems to me that only through this kind of archaeology can it become possible to understand the entrenched signifying relationships between the figure of the epileptic as cultural artefact and the medicalised epileptic.

II

Medical historians acknowledge that recorded histories of epilepsy long preceded Hippocrates' seminal text,[3] *On the Sacred Disease*, produced around 400 BCE. However, it is as part of the Hippocratic corpus that western civilisation first received a systematic account of the diagnosis and prognosis of the condition. It was an area of medical research that captured the attention of ancient physicians for various reasons, not least because of the superstitions and social biases that adulterated understanding of seizure disorders. In 1960 William Lennox observed that proportionately more of the Hippocratic writings were devoted to the diagnosis and treatment of epilepsy than is the case in any modern neurological textbook. He noted that 2.6 per cent of the Hippocratic writings were about epilepsy and 3.4 per cent of the writings of Aretaeus dealt with the subject.[4]

In rejecting established belief systems that epilepsy was divine or sacred, visited on mortals by gods, demons or spirits, Hippocratic physicians argued that the disorder, like other diseases of the body, was hereditary. This insistence on the hereditary nature of epilepsy formed part of the Hippocratic dialectic against beliefs in magic and superstition. Furthermore, these physicians insisted, epilepsy emanated from the brain and was caused by profound disturbances to the humours or vapours. The Hippocratic physicians regarded epilepsy as a sort of softening of the brain; cold phlegm (*pituita*) was thought to be the primary culprit in the genesis of the disorder, depriving the veins of air as it passes into the warm blood, where it then 'congeals and stops the blood'.[5] Hippocratic theories of epilepsy owed at least some of their conceptualisation to animal models and empirical observation was substantiated by autopsies on goats and sheep because those animals were thought to be particularly vulnerable to seizure. This aspect of ancient medical research, coupled with a rhetorical linking of physical aspects of the human seizure to goats, birds and horses, established a pervasive imagery.

As Henri Gastaut and his colleagues were to do in the latter decades of the twentieth century (see Introduction), the Hippocratic physicians fell prey to the 'demon of analogy and the desire for symmetry'. We are told in *On the Sacred Disease*:

> men being in want of the means of life, invent many and various things, and devise many contrivances for all other things, and for this disease, in every phase of the disease, assigning the cause to a god. Nor do they remember the same things once, but frequently. For, if [epileptics] imitate a goat, or grind their teeth, or if their right side be convulsed, they say that the Mother of the Gods is the cause. But if they speak in a sharper and more intense tone, they resemble this state to a horse, and say that Poseidon is the cause. Or if any excrement be passed, which is often the case, owing to the violence of the disease, the appellation of Enodia is adhibited; or, if it be passed in smaller and denser masses, like bird's, it is said to be from Apollo Nomius. But if foam be emitted by the mouth, and the patient kick with his feet, Ares then gets the blame. But terrors which happen during the night, and fevers, and delirium, and jumpings out of bed, and frightful apparitions, and fleeing away – all of these things, they say, are attacks by Hecate and assaults by the Heroes; they make use of expiations and enchantments, and in my opinion, at least, they create a divine power that is most wicked and impious.

Although the Hippocratic physicians were attempting to move beyond these ways of describing various manifestations of epilepsy and to bring it out of the realms of the gods and into the natural world, the web of animalistic and abject associations continued to haunt epilepsy narratives well into the nineteenth century.

The language used by the Hippocratic physicians to rebut the disorder's 'sacred' origins provided the foundations for a later interdependent economy of metaphors, bestial imagery and mythic potential that continued to frame articulations of what seizures looked like for medical and non-medical observers alike. To be sure, the ancient physicians had not set out to refute those associations that linked human epilepsy with the animalistic as such. Rather, they were set on removing its treatment from the sphere of 'magicians' and 'averters of evil'. William Heidel wrote of the Hippocratic corpus that 'Medicine, whether regarded as an art or as a science, is inevitably the product of the thought of the age; and Hippocratic medicine, in particular, reflects and shares the virtues and limitations of contemporary science'.[6] Even so, the Hippocratic tradition provided a rich rhetorical economy that was to survive well beyond the age of its production and prove seductively compelling for later writers.

In the millennia since the Hippocratic writings, physicians and healers managed to produce a considerable body of literature on the subject. Yet for all this intense scrutiny and hypothesising, advances in medical thinking about epilepsy were often accompanied by relapses into cultural superstition. Perhaps not surprisingly, at least some of these cultural superstitions have their origins in the legends of the ancients, and some in later cultural formations. It has been argued, for example, that the myth of Hercules suggests he killed his wife and children in an epileptic furore, thus occasioning the eponym 'the Herculean disease', or *Herculeus morbus*. While acknowledging the link other historians have made between the legend of Hercules' killing of his family and epilepsy, Temkin maintains that the evidence supporting this association between maniac frenzy and the condition is open to debate. Still, the idea of mythic and potentially murderous epileptic rage exercises a powerful grip on the cultural imagination. Seneca's *Hercules Furens*, written in the first century CE, provides a dramatic accounting of the furore in which Hercules murders Megara and their sons. In Shakespeare's *Othello*, the protagonist's epilepsy is implicated in the murder of Desdemona.

Illness and disease were very much part of the public spectacle in ancient times and diseases that were somehow written on the body generated both suspicion and fear. Lepers were driven from the centre of healthy society in most cultures and forced to wander the less travelled roads proclaiming their unclean state so that the uninfected knew to stay clear. Pox and plague lesions were on display in the crowded streets of the cities where the mad, the sad and the physically disabled scrabbled for survival along with the wider population. Those diseases and disabilities deemed incurable held a particular dread; they made that struggle for survival even more tenuous and like as not condemned the sufferer to life on the fringes of society. It is therefore not surprising that some of these conditions made it into popular vernacular as curses. Nor is it surprising that, centuries after Seneca, Shakespeare was to feature them so strongly in his plays. For Elizabethan audiences, as for audiences in ages past, visible signs of disease and disability both reflected life's less desirable realities and added a shiver of excitement and fear to the action on stage. Demonstrating awareness of his audiences' tastes, Shakespeare used the trope of epilepsy to heighten a sense of the dramatic or herald the encroachment of tragedy. In *King Lear* it is hurled at Oswald as a curse for ambitions beyond his class and for his duplicity. In *Julius Caesar* and *Othello* it marks the protagonists for a fall from grace.

Julius Caesar's epilepsy functions dramatically as a device of transition in plot development. In the first act, as he is being offered the crown of the Empire in perpetuity, he has the seizure that irrevocably changes the course of his life. In conversation with Cassius and Brutus, Casca blames the 'stinking breath' of the crowds for almost choking Caesar so that 'He fell down in the market-place and foamed at mouth and was speechless' (1.2.253).[7] Casca struggles to avoid laughing when Caesar falls, worrying that if he opens his mouth he too will become stricken. Brutus's explanation that it is 'very likely' the 'falling sickness' that stops Caesar's hand rather than the stink of the crowd or an insulting refusal to accept the honour being afforded him by the people of Rome is not enough to forestall ensuing events and Caesar is ultimately assassinated.

Shakespearian craft notwithstanding, Julius Caesar's fate is dictated by history. Othello's story, however, is determined by the possibilities and limitations of contemporary representational systems. By the time the Shakespearian plays first began appearing on the London stage, epilepsy's metaphorical value for denoting breaches in the boundaries of social and moral propriety had become established in both popular and medical imaginations. In part, this semiotic value was seeded in the Hippocratic tradition and in time the bid to locate epilepsy in the natural rather than supernatural world was to result in some unforeseen resonances across the culture/nature divide.

Robert Miola explores the influences of the Hercules myth on the creation of Othello's character in his examination of Seneca's *Hercules Furens*. Drawing on what Rolf Soellner calls the '*Hercules furens* convention – raging madness followed by a palliative sleep',[8] Miola argues that the structural and thematic import of Seneca's dramatic archetype in *Othello* transforms the play from melodrama to profound tragedy. Furthermore, he concludes that reading the Moor from the perspective of classical tragedy transforms him from malleable dupe to hero through association with an ancient metaphysical economy. Othello's murder of Desdemona is presaged by fugue states associated with epilepsy: the *Hercules furens* convention. Othello's epilepsy symptoms become ever more apparent as Iago drips virulence into his psyche and his seizure states come to function as visual manifestations of an increasingly disordered mind. That Othello *is* murderously seized, whether by Iago's psychological vitriol or his epilepsy condition, is suggested in Desdemona's plea for her life: 'And yet I fear you, for you're fatal then when your eyes roll so' (5.2.37).[9]

The influences of Hippocratic imagery are discernible in Shakespeare's rendering of Othello's epilepsy in the way the character is associated with both nature and the animalistic. When Iago begins planting seeds of doubt in his general's mind about Cassio's fidelity and Desdemona's love, Othello exclaims: 'Exchange me for a goat/When I shall turn the business of my soul/To such exsufflicate and blown surmises' (3.3.183–85). He initially rejects Iago's insinuations and insists that without proof of the double betrayal there can be no doubt or jealousy. It is a key moment in the dramatic progression of the play. Othello's invocation and rejection of the goat imagery is also a rejection, albeit a temporary one, of the cuckold role being crafted on him by Iago. However, the semiotic play of the image reverberates with Iago's earlier efforts to locate the Moor beyond the boundaries of Venetian civilisation. To Brabantio, Iago compares Othello to 'an old black ram' (1.1.88) and a 'Barbary horse' (1.1.111). These metaphors suggest a bestial sexuality and are crucial to the developing theme of Othello's essential otherness, an otherness that locates him in the natural world rather than the civilised society of his adopted culture. Othello is cast by Iago as being of a 'free and open nature/... And will as tenderly be led by th'nose/As asses are' (1.3.387–91). Miola argues that Iago's insults have rightly attracted analyses of the racism evident throughout the text. He also suggests that there is more going on here than racism. I agree.

Othello's likening of himself to a goat signals a threshold crossed in the play. Stepping across this threshold, Othello quickly moves from rejecting all ideas of infidelity without proof to entertaining the possibility of truth in Iago's insinuations. Read from the perspective of a Hippocratic representational economy, the goat imagery foreshadows his epilepsy. The Hippocratic physicians conducted much of their research on goats because they were deemed particularly susceptible to seizures. The image also foreshadows the tragedy to come; the term 'tragedy' itself derives from the Greek *tragōidiā*, literally meaning 'goat song'. In a sense, Othello becomes epileptic at the moment he succumbs to Iago's manipulations. Within the context of this reading, Iago becomes both the trigger for the onset of Othello's epilepsy and his diagnostician. It is he who first names Othello's altered states 'epilepsy' when he tells Cassio 'My lord is fallen into an epilepsy' (4.1.46). With this pronouncement, Iago consigns Othello to the netherworld beyond the boundaries of mainstream society and rationality. Semiotically, this netherworld comprises the negative axis in the culture/nature dichotomy.

Soon after the encounter with Iago where he likens himself to a goat, Desdemona notes that Othello speaks faintly and looks unwell. He tells her: 'I have a pain upon my forehead, here' (3.3.287). Having stepped across the threshold into the altered reality crafted by Iago, Othello's increasingly florid symptomatology gradually erodes those qualities and capabilities that allowed him to gain the respect of civil Venetian society and to win the love of the civilised Desdemona. He is no longer the man that Iago describes early in the play as being 'of a constant, loving, noble nature' (2.1.280). Driven to the edges of jealous suspicion, he begins to exhibit a growing sense of dislocation from the ordered thinking that graces his character in the earlier scenes and takes to referring to himself in the third person at times of extreme stress. This growing dislocation echoes in his words to Iago: 'Farewell! Othello's occupation's gone' (3.3.359). Like so much of the language and imagery in Shakespeare's plays, the pronouncement is inflected with multiple meanings. Othello's proclamation gestures to a perceived loss of sexual occupation in Desdemona's bed; it also evokes the diminishment of his psychological autonomy. Finally understanding the profundity of his crime against Desdemona and confronted by Lodovico's question 'Where is this rash and most unfortunate man?' (5.2.281), Othello acknowledges the deep and irremediable schism within in his response: 'That's he that was Othello: here I am' (5.2.282).

Medical historians applaud the closeness of Shakespeare's representations to the medical theories of his day and have debated how he might have acquired this knowledge. Some have argued that he was able to draw on the assistance of his son-in-law, John Hall, a physician and herbalist who obtained his degree from Cambridge University in 1597. The counter-view points to the richness of his representations of disease and infirmity before Hall came into his circle of family and friends. Whatever the sources were for Shakespeare's medical turns, most agree that Galen's work would have provided at least some grist for the creative mill. Five hundred years after the Hippocratic School, this Greek physician from Pergamum was to take the medical project on epilepsy a step further. Galen remained faithful to the representational economy established by his predecessors and while agreeing with Hippocrates in principle – that seizures emanated from the brain – went on to expand medical thinking about the part external factors might play in the process. His ideas were still very much at the centre of sixteenth- and seventeenth-century medical and cultural understanding of epilepsy and it is reasonable to argue that at least some of these ideas make it into the dramatic representation of the aetiology, progression and resolution of Othello's seizures.

III

Like the Hippocratic physicians, Galen (129–200 CE) relied on animal models to develop his thinking about epilepsy. Proceeding from a theory of nervous disorders based on both anatomical knowledge and traditional speculation, he nevertheless attempted to cultivate a more technically sophisticated understanding of seizure conditions. He began to describe epilepsies rather than a single entity, epilepsy, and divided the symptoms into three categories. The first he called idiopathic, claiming that the cause here was 'dyscrasia of the humours of the brain, brought on by cold'.[10] The second category of epilepsy, he claimed, was due to the brain's efforts to repel irritating substances transmitted to it from other locations in the body. This category he called sympathetic epilepsy. In the third category, a pathological humour was thought to form in an extremity and extend to the head. This last description was a precursor of the seizure form described by Hughlings Jackson in the late nineteenth century and named for him.

Galen is credited with being one of the first physicians to explicitly augment his interpretation of what a seizure looked like with a patient's description of what a seizure, or at least the preliminary to a seizure, felt like. Near the beginning of his career, he evidently visited a young male patient who, when asked to describe what his seizures felt like, told his physician that the sensations started in his lower leg. These sensations, which usually preceded seizure, 'felt like a cold breeze' as they climbed up through his body to his head. 'Aura', taken from the Greek word meaning 'breeze', passed into medical terminology to describe those phenomena signalling the onset of some seizure forms.

Despite efforts to rid epilepsy stories of metaphysical import, the seizure retained some of the mythic (and mystical) signification eschewed by the Hippocratic physicians and in Christian theology became a privileged code, along with leprosy, blindness and death, denoting Christ's power. According to St Luke, the salient confrontation between Jesus and the falling sickness took place in the mountains near Bethsaida:

> Master, I beseech thee, look upon my son: for he is mine only child. And, lo, a spirit taketh him, and he suddenly crieth out; and it teareth him that he foameth again, and bruising him hardly departeth from him. And I besought thy disciples to cast him out; and they could not. And Jesus answering said, O faithless and perverse generation, how long shall I be with you, and suffer you? Bring thy son hither. And as he was yet a coming, the devil threw him down, and tare him. And Jesus rebuked the unclean spirit, and healed the child, and delivered him again to his father. (Luke 9:38–42)[11]

With somewhat more success in dealing with intractable epilepsy than Hippocrates or Galen, Jesus heals the convulsing youth. The distraught father whose story is recounted in the Gospels of Luke and Matthew tells Jesus that he has already approached the disciples to beg surcease for his son's affliction and they could not help him. Jesus rebukes his disciples for their failure to deliver the youth from his disorder – from the 'unclean' origins of his seizure states: 'O faithless and perverse generation, how long shall I be with you, and suffer you?'

Within this powerful cultural text, the lines of demarcation between the afflicted, unclean (fallen) and the healed, clean (upright) body are unequivocally drawn and the disciples instructed to deliver the afflicted from their impurities. The disciples are called upon to exercise sovereignty over the stricken body in Christ's name, 'casting out devils'. Failure to quell the disorder is flagged as 'perverse'. It is a narrative of encounter and mythic conflict, with the pressure of victory placed squarely on the shoulders of the healer. This image of the diseased, afflicted or fallen body delivered from the corruption of epileptic disorder has enormous symbolic resonance within western medical culture. The physician's authority over the patient is founded on beliefs that medical knowledge will provide the keys to health and longevity. Failure to curtail the machinations of convulsion in these symbolic and narrative economies constitutes not only lack of knowledge but also lack of faith.

Within Hippocratic and Galenic traditions, both the exhalations and the exudations of the epileptic body were seen as potential sites of contamination. It was believed that to share eating and drinking utensils with those suffering from epilepsy risked contagion. By the thirteenth century, not much had changed. Berthold of Regensburg was insisting that epilepsy, like leprosy, could not be cured and as such was to be feared:

> And when he falls down, lies on the ground, and froths – beware of him if you value your life! Let nobody go near him, for such a terrible breath comes forth from his mouth that the person into whose mouth this breath enters may acquire the same disease. Beware then lest you approach him when he is seized by the disease![12]

The fifteenth century saw Siegmund Albich issue a warning to his contemporaries that the mere breath of folk with epilepsy will infect. Therefore, he advised, 'neither talk nor bathe with them'.[13] In churches, those defined as 'epileptic' were often refused access to the Eucharist because it was believed that they could infect communion cups and plates.

By 1520 Theophrastus Aurelus Bombastus von Hohenheim, to be known as Paracelsus, had begun to make contributions to the field of knowledge about epilepsy and included a chapter on the condition in his collection of essays. Five years later he wrote about epilepsy from a psychiatric perspective and around 1530 produced two books on the 'Falling Evil'. Paracelsus' view that the solution to epilepsy was to be found in hermetic medicine became a basis for the iatrochemists of the sixteenth and early seventeenth centuries. Johann Weyer, a contemporary of Paracelsus, rejected the physician's philosophies and accused the Paracelsians of being 'special slaves of arrogance, self-love, and vainglory'.[14] Weyer's views aside, Temkin notes that Paracelsus' later writings on epilepsy accuse doctors of a lack of compassion for their patients. Paracelsus insisted that compassion be maintained as the very foundation stone of medical practice. The accusation levelled by the physician at his colleagues was to become a recurring lesion on the surface of medical discourse.

IV

The link between healing and faith established by the theological celebration of Christ's curing of those afflicted with epilepsy became a crucial factor in western medical responses to the condition. The drive to medicalise epilepsy and the impulse to retain its metaphysical significance were to combine to provide at least some of the fuel for debates sparked by the convulsive episodes manifested by a London adolescent in 1602. Reminiscent of the Hippocratic struggles with the temple priests of ancient Greece for the pre-eminence of knowledge claims about the seizure-prone body, a dawning seventeenth century saw contestations for knowledge and power coalesce around 'Mary Glovers late woeful case, together with her joyfull deliverance'.[15]

Mary Glover was the fourteen-year-old daughter of a London shopkeeper. After a confrontation with an older woman, Elizabeth Jackson, Mary began experiencing 'fits' of illness variously manifesting as problems with swallowing, apparent unconscious states, convulsions and other bodily contortions. Evidently Mary had accused the older woman of fraud, an accusation that was to rile Jackson's not inconsiderable temper. She first confronted Mary alone, railing at her for gross dishonesty, raining curses down on her head and finally sending her on her way with the grim statement 'my daughter shall have clothes when thou art dead and rotten'.[16] Three days later Elizabeth Jackson was to follow up this first confrontation with a visit to Mary's home to see the girl's mother. It was after this second visit that Mary began complaining of an inability to swallow. Soon after, she was also struck dumb and blind. Her condition deteriorated over the next few weeks and, despite her physicians' best efforts, her illness remained resistant to any form of medical therapy. Rather worryingly for Jackson, as Mary's fits became more complex and dramatic, the barely audible words 'hang her' seemed to come from her nostrils.

Fairly quickly, the case was to come to the attention of the College of Physicians, at that time beset by its own internal conflicts. The College was in the process of consolidating and policing its hold over knowledge production in medical matters and showed no qualms in actively silencing or discrediting those who posed any sort of threat to its disciplinary aspirations. Various doctors associated with the College were to see Mary over the course of her illness but none was able to settle on a definitive diagnosis or, more importantly, find a cure for her woeful case. Robert Shereman, the first physician to consult with the family, eventually opted for at least the possibility of some supernatural cause when Mary failed to respond to treatment. Thomas Moundeford, President of the College, insisted, despite his failure to cure the young woman, that her ailments were due to some natural cause. The ensuing debates about the aetiology of Mary's condition were to split along ideological, religious and political lines as physicians, churchmen and magistrates tried to decide whether Mary was ill from 'som naturall cause', suffering from a flux of 'hystericall passions'[17] or had, in fact, been bewitched by Elizabeth Jackson.

Eventually Elizabeth Jackson was brought to trial. Edward Jorden presented evidence on her behalf for the natural origins of Mary's afflictions, arguing that they were manifestations of some sort of hysterical disorder. Although the magistrate was dismissive of Jorden's claims, reason was to eventually hold sway. Initially found guilty of witchcraft – and of being an ill-tempered and bad-tongued woman – support for the rationalist cause she represented, rather than for the woman herself, was such that Elizabeth quickly stepped free of incarceration and further punishment. Mary was subjected to trial by ordeal as her body was tested for the authenticity and natural origins of her malady. In the court she was loudly and repeatedly accused of counterfeiting her condition while her hand was being burned over an open flame. She continued to suffer from her episodes until finally given surcease via an exorcism conducted by a group of 'Puritan divines and godly laymen'.

Both Elizabeth Jackson and Mary Glover were but pawns in a much grander and more dangerous quest for power. Although there seems to have been no doubt that Mary's affliction was not due to epilepsy, the liminal place the disorder still held in discourses of the physical (natural) world and a metaphysical or supernatural unknown were called upon to argue the possibility that her paroxysmal episodes denoted bewitchment. Battle lines were drawn between a dissenting Protestantism and the state-ratified power of the Church of England. As Michael MacDonald points out, Mary's case became the focus in a 'bitter and protracted struggle between the church hierarchy and its Catholic and Puritan opponents'.[18] He argues that the ultimate triumph of reasoned argument based on medical understanding of the body over the metaphysical belief systems of the day marked a turning point in charges of witchcraft. However, in refuting Edward Jorden's claim for a natural aetiology arising from a form of psychosomatic disorder called 'suffocation of the mother' or 'Green sickness', Stephen Bradwell stubbornly refused to desert the metaphysical cause and argued that even though certain diseases *seemed* of natural origin, '*Sathan* the Ocean sea of subtleties, can ... hide his own ougly shape, under leaves of ordinary symptomes'.[19] He posited biblical proof for his contention, for, after all, did not Christ cast out the evil spirits that cause epilepsy?

Bradwell's arguments for at least the diabolical potential of epilepsy accorded with the belief systems of other players in the politics of witchcraft and demonic possession. Citing the Hippocratic corpus, Weyer's 1583 account of classical medicine's references to the syndrome had continued to locate its metaphorical associations with the bestial, although he was unwilling to completely cede its metaphysical possibilities. Like the Hippocratic physicians before him, however, he sought to rid cultural and medical understandings of epilepsy of those fanciful allusions drawn upon by 'mountebanks' and 'arrogant individuals' to serve their own ends. In agreement with Levinus Lemnius, Weyer argued for the potential diabolical significance of epilepsy, hysteria and melancholy. Although, like many of his contemporaries, Weyer believed in witches and witchcraft, his was a dissident voice in that he also argued that witch hunters made the diagnosis of bewitchment all too readily.

Thomas Szasz suggests that Weyer's stance against the legal definitions of witchcraft foundered – as did Edward Jorden's, to a point – on a shortfall in the language and conceptual models available to capture that which seemed inexplicable in the contemporary terms of natural disorders. Weyer, it seems, was especially critical of fellow physicians who wilfully remained 'uninformed and unskilled': they 'relegate all of the incurable diseases, or all of the diseases the remedy for which they overlook, to witchcraft'. Szasz goes on to conclude that 'they, the physicians themselves are thus the real malefactors'.[20]

Over and above the symbolic and political baggage accumulated on the syndrome's journey from Hippocrates' Cos to seventeenth-century London, this regressive loop in thinking about epilepsy so long after the ancient physicians had tried to lever it from the morass of superstition can be understood through consideration of two further factors. First, medicine's ongoing uncertainty as to the cause of and cure for epilepsy combined with the sometimes strange outward manifestations of the disorder to perpetuate confusion. Surgeon and physician Fabricius Hildanus wrote to a colleague in the early seventeenth century: 'I agree with you in declaring that something divine can be observed in epileptics, since experience has not seldom taught me this. For very often something lies hidden in the bodies of epileptics which is above our power of comprehension.'[21] The second point I want to take on board is from MacDonald's analysis of the political, cultural and symbolic systems framing the debates around Mary Glover's malady.[22]

MacDonald aptly demonstrates the way that medical thinking is always embedded in a wider cultural context, the politics of which will shape, at least to a degree, in what ways, and what directions, the knowledge system can develop. Accordingly, he argues that Edward Jorden's celebrated, if brief, treatise on the psychosomatic effects of hysteria[23] must be understood as a reaction to and product of the socio-political exigencies of the time as much as any breakthrough in medical thinking about the body. In examining the relations between science and social context in Britain from 1865 through to 1930, Donald MacKenzie notes that 'Science should not be bound off *a priori* as an intellectual activity to be studied in isolation. Both the social organisation of science itself and that of society at large can affect scientific thought and activity.'[24] That there is or can be a science, or indeed a medicine, unaffected by ideology and social context is a concept that has been increasingly opened to scrutiny.

V

The Hippocratic tradition of representation, leavened with a theologically ratified brief to heal at all costs, infused medical responses to epilepsy throughout the seventeenth century and beyond with a curiously heroic element. Despite the Paracelsian dictum on compassion, its lack remained evident in some of the more aggressive medical practices visited on the seizing body. This kind of medical response to seizures was cautioned against by Thomas Willis, a physician, who wrote in 1684:

> I say this kind of practice is often too roughly instituted or ordained; because after this manner is double-trouble put upon nature, to wit, one from the disease, and the other not lighter from the standers by, and helpers, when it were much better, for the fit to be suffered to pass over after its own manner, and the sick to endure one trouble only.[25]

Similarly in the nineteenth century, and concomitant with descriptions of heroic medicine in the medical journals, are calls from within the profession for compassion and a rethinking of contemporary medical attitudes to the epileptic. In 1854 Joseph Williams stated at the beginning of his *Lancet* paper 'Practical observations on the cure of epilepsy':

> There is no known specific for the cure of epilepsy, and in all human probability none will ever be found, inasmuch as this disease depends upon causes very varied; consequently those medicinal agents which may be prophylactic and even remedial under some circumstances, may under other conditions not only mitigate, but positively only aggravate every symptom.[26]

In criticising the trend towards aggressive therapeutic responses to epilepsy syndromes, Williams argued that the violence and futility of this type of medicine were forcefully illustrated for him through encounters with several patients who had presented to his care after having exhausted – and been exhausted by – the therapeutic efforts of numerous other physicians. Not only had these patients not benefited from medical attention, but it seemed that their original symptoms had been exacerbated.

Williams framed his concerns through a lengthy recounting of the case history of a male patient: the married, thirty-seven-year-old 'Mr. P—'. After experiencing his first seizure on 11 June 1847, Mr P—, then aged thirty-two, began his sojourn as an epileptic patient. He was to experience recurring attacks between that initial episode in 1847 and his coming to the attention of Dr Williams on 2 November 1852. Over the intervening time, the unfortunate Mr P— had been bled frequently and copiously, leeched, cupped, had a seton in his leg for five weeks and was subjected to 'severe antiphlogistic treatment; ... blisters to the nape of the neck, with severe purgation'. Both the patient and his wife informed Williams, as they had told treating physicians before him, that Mr P—'s episodes seemed to be aggravated rather than alleviated by these interventions.

Although Mr P— managed to survive his encounters with heroic physical medicine, he was also treated with a polypharmacy of increasingly unsystematic dosages and combinations of drugs and anodynes. His condition continued to deteriorate. By the time the patient was seen by Williams, not only was his seizure disorder worse than it had been when he first presented himself for medical attention, but his general bodily and psychological health had also broken down. His 'fits' had come to conform to the latter meanings of the term explored in the introduction to this book: he was 'desperate, exhausted' and in 'mortal crisis'. The totality of this bodily failure was judged by Williams to be as much due to the ministrations of medicine as to the processes of epilepsy. By 1852 Mr P— was 'pale, bloated, and bilious', depressed, tearful and generally weak. Williams had no miracle response to his patient's condition. He merely took on board Mr P—'s concerns about the possibility that the medical treatments were implicated in this ongoing deterioration. He then strategically backed away from the systematic overkill that had brought the man to his sorry state of affairs and gradually implemented a single regime of treatment at a time, beginning with diet, exercise and increased attention to the patient's general state of poor health. By June 1853, Mr P— had been seizure free since October 1852, and was active and happy, 'his gait erect and firm; his eye intelligent'.

Williams was by no means the only nineteenth-century physician expressing concern about medical treatments of those with epilepsy. In 1872, also in the *Lancet*, Dr J. Thompson Dickson, from Guy's Hospital in London, reported seeing patients blistered round the neck and the length of the spine 'till the exhaustion produced by the raw surfaces was far greater than that resulting from epilepsy'.[27] He criticised the practices of blistering and bleeding, and levelled the 'strongest condemnation' at a reactionary recourse to wildly varying dosages of calomel in the face of persistent seizure episodes. Of blistering, he wrote of seeing a patient who had developed albuminuria as a result of the practice, 'which had not only aggravated her epilepsy, but produced strangury', a painful urinary tract condition that results in urine being voided drop by drop. He argued that bleeding as it was currently practised 'is certainly fatal'. The following year, again in the *Lancet*, Dr D. de Berdt Hovell was moved to describe those more florid responses to intractable seizure conditions as medical '*morbus hystericus*', 'mental perversity' and punitive 'moral obliquity'.[28] In this 1873 article on hysteria and hystero-epilepsy, de Berdt Hovell reinflected Christ's charges of an apostolic perversity, arguing that his medical colleagues too often held their patients responsible when the limits of medical knowledge and skill were exposed by a persistence to seize despite therapeutic ministrations.

As extreme as these responses to the syndrome appear, they nevertheless kept faith with Hippocratic tradition, which advised the need for drastic measures against epilepsy. At the same time, they ran somewhat counter to the first tenet of the Hippocratic oath, which counsels the physician, above all else, to do no harm. The Paracelsian dictum on the necessity of medical compassion also seems to be missing from these models of therapeutic intervention. We could argue that the cases recounted by Williams and Dickson merely refer to examples of accumulative bad medicine. And, indeed, there is a sense in which this is true. However, taking a line from Miola's work, I want to suggest that there is more going on here than just 'bad' medicine.

The keys to understanding at least some aspects of the signifying relationships that result in the kind of practices criticised by the likes of Williams and Dickson are to be found in journal articles and news items published in late nineteenth-century editions of the *Lancet* and the *British Medical Journal*. In the stories that physicians share with each other in these journals about what constitutes epileptic disorder and what counts as appropriate medical response, they frequently invoke a cultural language that remains encoded with historical biases and fears. They use words such as terrible, taint, defective, degenerate, dangerous, irresponsible, violent, imbecile, genius, unfortunate, hopeful, malicious, decadent, irritable, riotous, greedy, ingenious, creative, duplicitous, unreliable, murderous, lazy and wilful to weave epilepsy narratives that sit uncomfortably with calls to provide compassionate healing. The struggle to develop a neuroscientific discourse of epilepsy from 2,000 years and more of superstition is fought with some vigour and more than a little blood letting, literally and metaphorically, through the pages of these journals. It is worth taking a closer look at the relationships between this kind of language and the practices it inspires.

Above, I indicated that this chapter is in part an archaeology of those signifying systems and narrative relationships that have come together over time to inscribe epilepsy with meaning within western medical–cultural systems. I want now to set out how this idea of archaeology takes shape from the work of Michel Foucault. Rather characteristically, Foucault is somewhat ambiguous in delimiting his thinking on the parameters of 'archaeology' as he uses it in his own work. He claims it is an appropriate methodology for the analysis of local discursivities and a heuristic device for the reclamation and examination of subjugated knowledges, the tactical component of which is a genealogy.[29] Hubert Dreyfus and Paul Rabinow argue that it is this genealogy-driven analysis that leads Foucault to his position of *déchiffrement*. This notion of *déchiffrement*, they suggest, facilitates comprehending the intelligibility of social practices in ways that are radically different from the understandings available to the actors.[30] Foucault has argued for the value of archaeologically inflected analyses in uncovering a level of unconsciousness embedded in scientific discourse, an unconsciousness that eludes the perception of the scientist. In the spirit of Foucauldian archaeology, I enlist the concept of double consciousness to explore and decipher the sub-text, or textual unconscious, of the medical texts discussed here and in later chapters.

In an early-developing neurological discourse, the use of terms such as malicious, decadent, irritable, duplicitous and so on to describe 'the epileptic' are concomitant with an increasingly standardised technical language of neurophysiology. The two strands of linguistic register remain separated only by a thin membrane of disciplinary aspiration to medicalise knowledge of cerebral paroxysm. The simultaneity of the two identified modes of signification in late nineteenth-century medical texts suggests a threshold between what Foucault identified as *langue* and *langage*.[31] I argue that it is an unstable threshold, subject to rupture and vulnerable to a return of what has been repressed. From this perspective, the repressed language of social and cultural disaffection can be said to function as a sort of waking dream at the dawn of neurology's efforts to slough off the stagnation of past signification, to slough off the metaphors, metonymy and symbolism of over 2,000 years of unscientific inscription. These historically entrenched units of signification (*langue*) become the *a priori* value-laden trace in the terminology (*langage*) of medical discourse. The evocative shadows of these signifiers remain discernible beneath the smooth and supposedly neutral surfaces of medical knowledge.

Foucault cautions against the naïveté of chronologies and the limitations of lexical analyses in relation to discourse. Yet he also acknowledges that these are not necessarily illegitimate points from which to at least begin the critical process. Eventually, though, any critical engagement with discourse must move beyond 'treating discourses as groups of signs (signifying elements referring to contents of representations)'. The task of analysis, he insists, should entail consideration of discourse as a set of practices 'that systematically form the objects of which they speak'.[32] Bearing these precautions in mind, I examine the signifying elements of neurological discourse in order to better understand it *as* a set of practices. Cultural and medical perceptions of what it means to experience epilepsy will often hinge on how the condition is represented. From this analytical perspective, the rhetorical vision of epileptic bestiality inadvertently set in play by the Hippocratic tradition is illuminated by an unpacking and examination of some of the *languages* of medicine as they define 'the epileptic'. Medical journals are particularly useful in this type of archaeology because they provide a window into the *langue* used when physicians communicate with each other via the correspondence section and published minutes of medical meetings in a forum beyond the more technically mediated and disembodied modes of expression usually found in medical textbooks.

VI

While notions of the elusive *pituita* may well have lost attraction in late nineteenth-century brain research, the evocative images produced by the Hippocratic writers continued to hold sway. By the late nineteenth century and into the early decades of the twentieth century the 'something divine' noted by Hildanus was to be once again contained by a medical rhetoric of bestiality. In the latter decades of the nineteenth century, the English physician William Gowers records a description of epileptic seizure forms eerily similar to the Hippocratic description. He collects and modifies to a more urbanised scale the bestial images identified by Hippocrates, dubbing this category of behaviours theriomimicry (from the Greek *therion*, meaning wild animal):

> The noises and actions of animals are strangely imitated. The patient mews like a cat, or, much more frequently, barks like a dog. This is evidently in part mimetic, although some patients who present the symptoms are, in the intervals between the attacks, as far as possible removed from any absurdity. But it seems to be, in part also, the

> manifestation of some strange animal instinct which we possess in a latent or modified condition, like our canine teeth. A frequent characteristic is the tendency to bite, which may exist apart from any other imitation of animals. It renders the task of attending to these patients in the attacks not wholly devoid of danger. Not only do they bite, they do so in a curiously animal manner. I have seen a lad of sixteen take the corner of his pillow between his teeth, and shake it exactly as a cat does a mouse, or as a lion shook Livingstone.[33]

We may well ask: what was Gowers looking at? Even more importantly, what was he seeing? Are the outward signs of epilepsy captured by his observations here a seamless continuation of the Hippocratic project or is this vision merely a refraction in the rhetorical spectrum of medical discourse?

The importance, in a medical context, of the act of seeing – 'the gaze' – forms a primary concern in Foucault's *The Birth of the Clinic*. He opens the text with a description of a cure for hysteria implemented by a French physician, Pomme, on a patient in the mid eighteenth century. Pomme evidently treated his patient by making her take baths for 'ten or twelve hours a day, for ten whole months'. As a result of this treatment, Pomme reports:

> membranous tissues like pieces of damp parchment ... peel away with some slight discomfort, and these were passed daily with the urine; the right ureter also peeled away and came out whole in the same way. The same thing occurred with the intestines, which at another stage, peeled off their internal tunics, which we saw emerge from the rectum. The oesophagus, the arterial trachea, and the tongue also peeled in due course; and the patient had rejected different pieces either by vomiting or by expectoration.[34]

The description reads as a quaint and somewhat amusing example of a medical fantasy from a bygone age but as Foucault asks: how can we be sure that Pomme was *not* seeing what he describes?

The idea being so incisively demonstrated by Foucault with this strategy, and elaborated further throughout *The Birth of the Clinic*, is that the organisation and articulation of medical description (at any given time) will be governed by 'codes of knowledge'. And it is worth noting that Heidel is saying much the same about the Hippocratic writings as is Szasz about Weyer's theories. Foucault argues that it is not the conception of disease that changes first, to be later followed by modes of recognition. Nor is it a linear progression from symptom to theory. Rather, the relation between disease and the medical gaze is mutually constitutive. One can only understand the relations between theory and experience, methods and results, by making visible and examining the field that binds disease and the gaze in a shared signifying (political, cultural, symbolic) economy. The gaze will see what it is codified to see and the observer will articulate what is seen according to prevailing linguistic conventions and signifying possibilities. Byron Good neatly encapsulates this idea with his point that medical language is not merely reflective of illness or disease processes but rather is constituted by 'a rich *cultural language*, linked to a highly specialised version of reality and system of social relations'.[35]

If his colleague Hughlings Jackson ever saw bestial symptoms of the type recorded so vividly by Gowers, it did not make it into any of his writings. Yet these two physicians did share the same codes of knowledge. Gowers completed a significant part of his neurological training under Jackson's tutelage. Both were at the forefront of the project to modernise epilepsy and create medical narratives that would bring it into a new scientific age. Both were writing around the same period in nineteenth-century neuroscience, although Jackson was senior, beginning his medical career around the middle of the century. Both men are cited as figures of eminence in twentieth- and twenty-first-century neurological texts. At one stage in their respective careers, they were co-researchers at the National Hospital for the Paralysed and Epileptic, Queen Square, in London. They were part of a group researching and developing a map of the human brain organised around theories of localisation. Although localisation theories were being worked on in other countries at this time, it was at Queen Square that this work developed in its most widely propagated form.

Like their Hippocratic predecessors, the neurologists engaged in brain research at Queen Square were trying to discover a model of human nervous function by reproducing human disease conditions in healthy laboratory animals. The limitation of this mode of knowledge production prompted Gowers' observation that 'No symptoms have been observed in man corresponding to the functional centres that you often see marked on those convolutions in diagrams of the human brain, to which they have been transferred from the brains of monkeys'.[36] Clearly, an interspecies model of neuronal function was proving to be an unsatisfactory way of trying to advance scientific knowledge of human neurology for Gowers. Yet, in a rhetorical economy at least, some of his epileptic patients mew like cats and bark like dogs.

Despite their shared codes of knowledge and a shared socio-cultural framework, Gowers and Jackson see and register significantly different versions of the epileptic. Somewhat mystified about what could have caused them to record such variant images of those with an epilepsy disorder, I looked to their biographies to try to better understand the perspectives from which they levelled their gaze upon the seizing body. Macdonald Critchley has written biographical accounts of both men and refers to Gowers' many tributes to his senior colleague, whom the younger neurologist acknowledged as 'one of the most benevolent and noble-minded, as well as one of the most able physicians of the day'.[37] While Critchley's biography of Gowers records a career that is prolific in terms of the contributions made to neurophysiological research, he notes the 'peculiar difficulties' in obtaining wider objective material about his subject and is compelled to limit his study primarily to Gowers' medical writings. 'Gowers', he writes, 'was not a man with a wide circle of professional friends and correspondents. He was reserved and apparently difficult to know. Warmness and conviviality were foreign to him and he remained among his colleagues a lonely and unapproachable figure, admired but not understood.'[38] The neurologist was evidently noted for his coldness and caustic speech, his aloof manner keeping all but the very few at a distance.

Where Gowers was perceived as intolerant, harshly spoken and difficult, Jackson was deemed easygoing and warm-hearted, if rather shy. Gowers' professional persona was often unfavourably compared with that of Jackson. Nevertheless, the two men held each other in mutual respect. Gowers, not noted for his overt interaction with the published work of his contemporaries, warmly engaged with Jackson's writings on aphasia and went on to adopt his phraseology in his own work. Jackson was always grateful for the way that Gowers took up and further expounded his theories of brain function. In his writing, Jackson makes repeated references to his younger colleague's expertise with the ophthalmoscope and concise articulation of the neurophysiological theories that claimed their mutual attention. In crucial ways Gowers and Jackson can be said to embody and enact disparate, yet nonetheless coexistent, strands extant in Victorian intellectual and medical development.

Jackson appears to have reflexively aspired to Cartesian ideals of neutral observation, both in theory and in practice. Throughout his writings he describes in minute detail the external effects of excessive, sudden and abrupt electrical cerebral discharge, yet he refrains from ascribing value judgements to the resulting behavioural disturbances.

Critchley notes of Gowers' approach to neurological research that the physician's 'concern was with the bricks and mortar of the subject, and he set out patiently to observe phenomena and to collect facts, rather than to weave speculative webs'.[39] But of course Gowers did weave webs, in that he speculated in specific ways on what he perceived to be the behavioural consequences of epilepsy conditions; his views on therio-mimicry, for example, made a distinctive contribution to the web of signification begun in Hippocratic times.

Like Jackson, Gowers was meticulous in his clinical observations of neurophysiology. However, in his descriptions and statements about the consequences of epilepsy for the patient, Gowers repeatedly extended his statistical analyses to hypothesise a range of prognostic social limits based on his clinical observations. What gets left out of these prognostications are those multiple social, cultural and economic factors that have immediate and secondary effects on the subjectivity of his patients and directly inform individual response to illness. Gowers' primary focus was very much on the big picture of the disorder. He based many of his theories about epilepsy on observations made of the relatively large number of cases he saw at the National Hospital. Strobing across Gowers' emphasis on the big picture is Jackson's concern that medical students be routinely taught 'to study cases as the symptoms show *approaches* to certain clinical standards, and not as they show departures from healthy states'.[40]

Both of these medical men demonstrated the will to knowledge, the will to unlock neurological mysteries about brain function and facilitate understanding of the neuronal conditions precipitating epilepsy. Even so, where Jackson seemed only to want to better understand the organic causes of the epilepsies in order to help his patients deal more effectively with their disorder, Gowers extended this project to include social and moral control of 'the epileptic'. Jackson was fastidious in maintaining the boundaries between pathological affect and social supposition, sometimes to the point of protracted repetition. He was routinely criticised by his peers for the discursiveness of his arguments, while applauded for their intellectual content. In keeping with the dominant biomedical practice of this era, Gowers had a tendency to conflate these concepts. Too often the patient with epilepsy was reduced to the sum total of pathological possibility in his stories of epileptic limitations. The presumptive bedrock of Gowers' representations of epileptic disorder is best summed up in his own oft-repeated philosophy that, along with an ambiguous epileptic irritability, 'there is [also] often defective moral control'.[41]

In the latter decades of the nineteenth century a range of so-called 'epileptic' behaviours increasingly came under medical scrutiny. The evaluative medical gaze extended beyond changes in behaviour observable immediately pre- and post-seizure to take in the possibility of a generalised 'epileptic character'. Within this biomedical economy Gowers was relatively succinct on the nature of the 'epileptic character'. In spite of this relative brevity, however, he effectively and authoritatively captured the essence of the dominant discursive productions of his day. He expanded his ideas of an essentialised epileptic defective moral control by adding that: 'Mischievous restlessness and irritability in childhood may develop into vicious and even criminal tendencies in adult life'. For Gowers, representations of the epileptic, if not the epilepsies, remained encoded with notions of defective, degenerate and dangerous. From his position of medical authority, he spins back into the circuit of culture the belief that neuronal incontinence necessarily equates with social and moral incontinence.

Gowers' work was orchestrated, at least to a degree, by specific philosophical models relevant to his time. The anxieties he expresses about the social disorder associated with 'the epileptic' reflect wider issues of class structure, economic progress and national physical fitness. In the lead-up to the dawn of a new century, the national mood in Britain, as in the United States, was very much about 'cleaning house'. This meant identifying and excising sites of disorder, both real and potential.

Gowers saw himself as a central contributor to the coming age. In both his medical and his non-medical life he enthusiastically embraced the technologies of modernity. His off-duty interests reflect a love of order and precision. During his time away from clinical practice and research he developed his talents as an artist, favouring the technical skill required to reproduce the minute and precise detail of plants, architecture and human anatomy rather than more abstract modes of expression. It has been said of his etchings that they demonstrate considerable control and mastery of technique while adhering faithfully to the strict artistic conventions of his day. His preferences were also evident in a fondness for minutely detailed description, whether applied to his study of botany – he was said to be an authority on mosses – or his scrutiny of the human body. His landmark two-volume text *Manual of Diseases of the Nervous System* not only primarily comprised all his own case-note and clinical observations but also illustrations he drew himself. A propensity for order extended to his engagement with music and he once initiated correspondence with the journal *Musical News* to plead for an improved and more scientifically rational designation of musical notes. The disorder represented by the epileptic body appeared both to compel Gowers' attention and to profoundly offend what his biographer describes as his 'finicking' eye. He seems to have abhorred excess in any form.

When Jackson began writing on the syndrome, epilepsy was still being responded to as primarily a social disorder. One of his contemporaries, Edward Sieveking, advised the biomedical fraternity that 'We should regard the fit as the flower of a noxious weed'.[42]

Although Jackson repeatedly marked the referential importance of existing and coming philosophical models to his own work, he deviated quite eccentrically from the dominant interpretative models of epilepsy. Rather remarkably, he refrained from making any moral diagnoses about those affected by the syndrome.

This is not to say that Jackson refrained from recommending certain lifestyle changes to bring about for his patients better control over their symptoms. For example, although he argued that those with epilepsy (he claimed to use this word generically) 'must be content to live on a lower level', Jackson took pains to point out that he intended this in the sense that they needed to take more care with diet, exercise and the maintenance of general health than those not vulnerable to the syndrome:

> In cases of epilepsy the patient should 'avoid excitement'. But in young people we may err in being too strict; we may narrow a young epileptic girl's life too much by forbidding the amusements proper to her age. If she have a fit soon after a hearty game or a dance, it is, I think, only the premature development of a fit nearly due.[43]

It may well be that at least some aspects of Jackson's approach to patient care can be attributed to his familiarity with the day-to-day distresses and social anguish that can arise from living with a seizure condition. His wife of eleven years, Elizabeth Dade Jackson, had experienced repeated occurrences of those symptoms associated with temporal lobe epilepsy for some time before her death from a stroke just before her fortieth birthday.

As her congenital cerebral vascular condition deteriorated, she experienced tremors progressing up one side of her body (a sign that would become known as the Jacksonian march after Hughlings Jackson described it in relation to his later work on epilepsy syndromes) and episodes of 'dreamy' state lasting several minutes at a time.[44] The literature suggests that Jackson cared deeply for his wife.[45] He is quoted as confiding to a friend shortly after her death: 'There was nothing in the world to compare with domestic happiness'.[46] Although he was to live another thirty-five years after his wife's death, he never remarried.

Sifting through the biographical details of their lives and the recorded observations of their peers, it becomes apparent that the two physicians brought very different inclinations to their work. Undoubtedly, their respective medical gazes were inflected through a shared code of neurological knowledge. However, there is also evidence that these shared codes of knowledge were not enough to shade their respective medical gazes from differing empirical perspectives.

Whereas Jackson's recorded responses to his patients' epilepsy conditions suggest a knowledge impulse driven by an intellectual desire to restore wellness, Gowers' clinical responses are organised according to a more orthodox concept of disorder, and by extension a quest to recuperate that which has been lost – order.

Tensions between the project to modernise epilepsy as a neurological entity and frustrations with the intractability of the disorder to medical definition and control manifest in the language of Gowers and other physicians of the age as a type of 'double consciousness'. The notion of double consciousness suggests the capacity to simultaneously accommodate mutually exclusive ideas. Expanding on this idea, I take my meaning of double consciousness here from Jackson, who in turn appropriates it from Arthur Myers, his patient and also a physician with epilepsy. Jackson uses the concept to describe a state of ideational and cognitive splitting. He suggests that this double consciousness or 'mental diplopia' (from the Greek *diploos* and *opsis* meaning double vision, that is, one object being seen as two) represents a disruption to consciousness of present surroundings or intellectual context. It combines a heightened awareness of both current conditions and a consciousness of former surroundings or intellectual states. Kenneth Dewhurst notes that, for Jackson, disturbance to consciousness of present surroundings suggested diminished *object* consciousness, while increased 'reminiscence' of past surroundings and past mental states suggested increased *subject* consciousness.[47] Jackson uses the concept to describe a particular state of mind that precedes some seizure forms. At various times he also refers to this state as 'bemazement'. For those who experience it as part of their epilepsy condition, bemazement marks that volatile moment between ideational control and the possibility of synaptic overload. For the argument that I am progressing here, it manifests at the conceptual borders of medical–cultural representations of epilepsy when physicians find themselves 'bemazed' by the intractability of patients to medical control.

VII

Given the crisis of language haunting late nineteenth-century neurologists, it is not surprising that they sometimes looked outwards for representational inspiration. And in Britain, where better to look than the literature of the day? As Shakespeare had before him, Charles Dickens reflected, commented on and, at times, parodied the society of his era, and in doing so constructed characters astutely drawn from observations of his cultural environment. His work as a journalist took him to some of the larger psychiatric institutions and J. E. Cosnett notes with approval the degree to which Dickens' observations extended to medical conditions.[48]

Cosnett argues that Dickens wrote particularly well about neuropsychiatric conditions, dystonias and sleep disorders. It has been suggested that the author constructed the underpinnings of his more symptomatic characterisations from contemporary medical writing, with the work of Gowers as a favoured source. However, inspiration was not a one-way process. Medical writers also looked to Dickens when naming symptoms. The most well known example of this sort of free trade is Pickwickian syndrome: a condition characterised by hypoventilation, somnolence and carbon dioxide retention. The naming of this complication of extreme obesity owes its origins to Dickens' graphic description of Joe, an immensely overweight youth in *The Posthumous Papers of the Pickwick Club*, who had a tendency to fall asleep on his feet at odd and unpredictable moments.

Dickens' descriptions of medical conditions and the significance of particular symptoms in a social context extended to epilepsy, particularly seizures, which he commonly refers to as 'fits' in his works. In the novels *The Life and Adventures of Martin Chuzzlewit*, *The Old Curiosity Shop* and *David Copperfield*, he uses the fit as a plot device: a convulsive moment that seizes a strand of the narrative and signals transition from one state to another in plot development. It is a convention that Shakespeare uses to effect in *Julius Caesar* and *Othello*.

In *Oliver Twist*, Dickens mounts an attack on the workhouse system. He also draws on the medical models of his day to create the criminal underclass. The novel delves into issues of class and heredity, primarily through the characterisations of Oliver and his half-brother, Edward Leeford (also known as Monks among his criminal cohort). We are told at the outset of the narrative that Oliver survives the circumstances of his illegitimate birth in a workhouse because 'Oliver and Nature fought out the point between them'.[49] This early triumph over nature suggests the boy's rightful place in culture. The rightness of his 'true' place in civilised society is further reinforced by civilised society's repeated recognition of his worth. The recognition is mutual. Mr Brownlow registers something in the boy's face that touches him and invokes ideas of innocence, although their first meeting is in court, where Oliver stands accused of theft. Oliver responds powerfully to the portrait of Agnes Fleming hanging in Brownlow's home, not yet knowing that she is his mother. He tells Mrs Bedwin it is as though the image wanted to speak to him but could not.

After being shot during an ill-fated burglary and abandoned to die by Bill Sikes, Oliver inadvertently finds his way back to the scene of the crime and is taken in to recover from his injuries. There is an elemental recognition of his genetic origins when Rose (who turns out to be his maternal aunt) first sits beside the bed where he lays unconscious. As her tears fall on his face:

> The boy stirred, and smiled in his sleep, as though these marks of pity and compassion had awakened some pleasant dream of a love and affection he had never known. Thus, a strain of gentle music, or the rippling of water in a silent place, or the odour of a flower, or the mention of a familiar word, will sometimes call up sudden dim remembrances of scenes that never were, in this life; which vanish like a breath; which some brief memory of a happier existence, long gone by, would seem to have awakened; which no voluntary exertion of the mind can ever recall.[50]

But of course Dickens' novel is also a story of the triumph of nature over nurture. Despite his beginnings, Oliver remains immune to any blight from those early years in the workhouse and later resists the call to criminality offered by Fagin because he is coded with the 'right stuff'. Fagin tells Monks: 'I saw it was not easy to train him to the business, ... he was not like other boys in the same circumstances'.[51]

The class hierarchy of the novel reinforces an already established framework of what constitutes normality: an innate impulse to bourgeois respectability and a native moral fibre. Because of his maternal connections to the middle class, Oliver's hereditary legacy ensures reinstatement to his rightful place in the social strata despite the impoverished conditions of his early life. In the social realist novel of the nineteenth century, nature inevitably wins out over nurture. 'Oliver will always be normal', Lennard Davis points out, 'even in abnormal circumstances'.[52]

The defining boundaries of normality are demarcated by abnormality: just as Oliver is indelibly marked by heredity, so too is Monks. If Oliver carries the genetic legacy of his mother's inherent middle-class decency, Monks inherits, undiluted, the impulse to moral laxity of both parents. His father, Edwin Leeford, seduces Oliver's mother, Agnes, promising her marriage, while he is still married to Edward's mother. Edward's mother, Elizabeth, is 'wholly given up to continental frivolities', leaving her marriage vows behind. She tears up Edwin's will, so depriving Agnes and Oliver of their inheritance. Because of her machinations, Rose, like Oliver, is also dislocated – if not disconnected – from her rightful place in middle-class society. The parentally corrupted (abnormal) Monks is castigated by Mr Brownlow thus:

> you, who from your cradle were gall and bitterness to your own father's heart, and in whom all evil passions, vice, and profligacy, festered, till they found a vent in a hideous disease which has made your face an *index* even to your mind.[53]

Brownlow's description begs the question: why was Monks 'gall and bitterness' to his father's heart, even in those cradle days? Because he is issue of a forced and unhappy marriage or because he has epilepsy? In other words, is his villainy the product of his seizure condition or paternal rejection?

Just as Oliver's 'rightness' is discernible at a glance, so too is Monks' 'wrongness' clearly written on the body and amenable to exegesis. Dickens' view that the face can serve as a reliable index of moral character is rooted in nineteenth-century scientific and medical belief systems. Despite Mr Losberne's musings to Rose that 'Vice ... takes up her abode in many temples; and who can say that a fair outside shall not enshrine her?',[54] Dickens is orthodox in his representations of the criminal character. The notion that inner corruption is always somehow visible to the discerning eye is evident in his construction of the criminal classes. Jack Dawkins is 'one of the queerest-looking boys that Oliver had ever seen'. He is 'flat-browed' with 'little, sharp, ugly eyes'. Fagin is 'hideous' with a 'repulsive face'. But Monks' impulse to criminality far exceeds the mundane larcenies and murderous endeavours of his colleagues; he is prepared to engineer his half-brother's induction into the criminal classes to gain his ends, even if this results in Oliver's death. Dickens uses epilepsy to denote the more extreme depths of the character's moral dissolution and his 'unclean spirit'. The conflation of Monks' vicious criminal tendencies and his epilepsy foreshadows Gowers' theories about the 'epileptic character' sketched above.

Although Monks shares his half-brother's class background, he cannot transcend the 'natural' state imposed by his seizure condition. He is associated with darkness and storms. He is 'a dark figure' emerging from 'deep shadow' to discuss Fagin's progress with Oliver's criminalisation. He is the 'tall man wrapped in a black cloak' who rains curses on Oliver's head before falling to the ground in a seizure. He is described as 'withered and haggard' and having 'a lurking walk'. In his meeting with the Bumbles, the forces of nature momentarily overcome him. As the lowering storm shakes their meeting venue, Monks' epileptic nature resonates with the elements:

> 'Hear it!' he cried, shrinking back. 'Hear it! Rolling and crashing on as if it echoed through a thousand caverns where the devils were hiding from it. Fire the sound! I hate it!' He remained silent for a few moments; and then, removing his hands suddenly from his face, showed, to the

> unspeakable discomposure of Mr Bumble, that it was much distorted, and discoloured. 'These fits come over me, now and then,' said Monks, observing his alarm; 'and thunder sometimes brings them on. Don't mind me now, it's all over for this once'.[55]

Part of the attractiveness of Dickens' styling for physicians here is his valid rendering of the sensitivity to flashing light and sudden sound manifest in some forms of seizure conditions. Ancient civilisations understood that flickering light sometimes provoked seizures. Prospective slave purchasers used to rotate a wagon wheel in front of a flame to test their 'stock' for epilepsy. Since the latter decades of the twentieth century and beyond, neurologists have used flashing light to provoke seizure as part of a provocative diagnostic process. Of course, being sensitive to sound and light to the point of seizing does not necessarily equate with desires to have your half-brother transported to the colonies or killed so that you can inherit the family wealth. Although Gowers might disagree.

There can be no doubt that Dickens shrewdly captures what was to become a resurgent preoccupation with hereditary taint in his exploration of the biological links between Oliver and Monks. He also perpetuates an image of the morally lax, violent epileptic that keeps returning to the centre of scientifically inclined discourse. Monks' epileptic potential to inspire fear and loathing in outsiders is manifest in the self-inflicted stigmata of his inner neuronal storms. Nancy describes him as having 'lips [that] are often discoloured and disfigured with the marks of teeth; for he has desperate fits, and sometimes even bites his hands and covers them with wounds'.[56]

Evocative of the biting epileptic given fictional presence by Dickens and medical validation by Gowers in his thoughts on therio-mimicry, in January 1884 there appeared in the editorial section of the *Lancet* an item titled 'Bite of an epileptic'.[57] Through a series of rhetorical flourishes, readers were informed that a young man died three days after being bitten by a woman. The young man had 'assisted a woman who had fallen in a fit and was convulsively biting everything within reach'. Readers were reassured that, despite the demise of the unfortunate young man post-bite, 'There is no poison in the bite of a person in a fit, as there is in the bite of a rabid dog. Many scores of attendants on epileptics are bitten and nothing comes of it.' Even with a tone of ostensible reassurance, the writer of this news piece creates a vivid picture of teeth-gnashing epileptics indiscriminately biting the hands that help.

At first glance, the hyperbolic style of the item suggests its function is as a curiosity or colour piece: of some interest because of its reliance on more ancient superstitions, but of spurious medical value. Nevertheless, a week later the writer was moved to defend the claim that the bite of an epileptic is *not* poisonous. It seems that the editorial writers for the *Lancet* had been accused by an unpublished correspondent of ignoring the work of M. Gautier, which provided evidence to the contrary. The journal responded to this unpublished criticism with some righteous indignation, claiming that the work of M. Gautier *had* been considered but was deemed irrelevant to the incident reported. In a somewhat extraordinary attempt at further reassurance, the writer concluded this defence of the earlier item by declaring:

> There is neither rage or rabies [in the bite of an epileptic]. The bite of a bestial man in a paroxysm of rage may be as bad as that of an infuriated rat; but, as we have said, that is a different matter, and we would certainly advise that such persons should be kept at a safe distance.[58]

The language (*langue*) used to record both items associates the epileptic with the bestial, evoking images of mindless and random danger for any altruistic bystander incautious enough to offer assistance to the one stricken. The item faithfully reproduces a signifying economy put into play by Hippocrates and given new life by Dickens' fictive creation and Gowers' medicalised images. The words of the *Lancet* contributor written in the latter part of the nineteenth century echo Berthold of Regensburg from the thirteenth century and leave the darkness of this earlier superstition unilluminated and undisturbed: 'And when he falls down, lies on the ground, and froths – beware of him if you value your life!'

VIII

By the late nineteenth century, the medical–cultural languages of epilepsy still relied on much the same signifying economy and systems of understanding established by writers in ages past. Despite concerted efforts to move the medical project to a new level of scientific understanding, few physicians would find fault with those words recorded by Aretaeus near the very beginning of medicine's engagement with the syndromes: 'Epilepsy is an illness of various shapes and horrible'. From the 1820s, contributors to the *Lancet* and the *British Medical Journal* occasionally revisited Hippocratic theories in attempts to develop further consensus on the precise location of epileptic disorder and it is evident that Galen's ideas continued to shape the medical imagination. In an 1826 paper on diseases of the nervous system published in the *Lancet,* a Dr Clutterbuck began his remarks on epilepsy with a degree of qualification that suggested the work still to be done in developing the defining boundaries for a medical model: 'There may be a single fit only, without repetition; as is often the case in infants. Or fits may recur daily or oftener, or weekly, or monthly, or at still longer intervals.'[59] Dr Marshall Hall argued in 1838 in the same journal that in 'eccentric epilepsy' the 'encephalon' suffers only as an effect of convulsive attacks in other parts of the body.[60] In Samuel Solly's view, nineteenth-century physicians were as much in the dark about the epilepsies as their Hippocratic predecessors.[61]

In his work on nineteenth-century psychiatric discourse, Foucault identifies as one of his points of intervention 'the establishment at the beginning of the century of a new mode of exclusion and confinement of the madman in a psychiatric hospital'.[62] During this time of institutional expansion, the madman, the imbecile, the feeble-minded, the morally insane and the epileptic become undifferentiated components in a homogenous mass to be contained and administered within the regimes of the asylum. But even in the early years of the century, those with epilepsy were beginning to draw particular attention. The French psychiatrist Étienne Esquirol was arguing against the placement of epileptics in asylums. He insisted that the disruptive nature of the disorder placed undue and insupportable pressure on the insane. The reasoning of his argument appealed to common sense: if witnessing an epileptic seizure was enough to risk acquired epilepsy in a healthy person, how much more vulnerable was the deranged individual?

Despite Esquirol's arguments, it is not until the latter half of the nineteenth century that 'the epileptic' begins to really emerge from this wider category of exclusion as an object of specific biomedical, institutional and legal inquiry. By the end of the century in Britain, folk with epilepsy were seen as a problem not only for the asylum: they were also presenting an increasing dilemma for the state as destitution forced them into the workhouses. Scrutiny of their living conditions was not due to any particular concern for those with epilepsy as such, but rather a growing preoccupation with the perceived threat of disorder that the syndrome posed for working-class communities. The impulse to protect the working classes from the threat of internal disorder had profound implications for what happens next to epileptic populations in industrial societies and I will discuss these matters at length in Chapter 4.

In relation to psychopathology, Foucault argues that efforts to locate 'the unity of the object of madness' must necessarily founder within the discontinuities and overlays of multiple discursive formations. He suggests two reasons why this might be the case. Firstly, he claims:

> mental illness was constituted by all that was said in all the statements that named it, divided it up, described it, explained it, traced its developments, indicated its various correlations, judged it, and possibly gave it speech by articulating, in its name, discourses that were to be taken as its own. Moreover, this group of statements is far from referring to a single object, formed once and for all, and to preserving it indefinitely as its horizon of inexhaustible ideality; the object presented as their correlative by medical statements of the seventeenth or eighteenth century is not identical with the object that emerges in legal sentences or police action....[63]

He then suggests that changes to nineteenth-century medical discourse in matters of style, form, types of connection, modes of representation and shared presuppositions about pathology in relation to the visible space of the body further undermine the possibility of a stable and definitive object. Quite simply, the madmen of the seventeenth, eighteenth and nineteenth centuries are not the same madmen because of profound changes in definitions of madness and categorisation.

There are some notable similarities between this accounting of the discursive formations of madness and productions of epilepsy. Temkin has argued that epilepsy has always been considered a disease and, while I take his point, I think that in some ways it is also profoundly compromised by ideational shifts and confusions about precisely what symptomatology constitutes epilepsy. The idea of disorder, if not disease, holds, but what the concept contains remains unstable. Convulsive episodes were once thought to signify attention from the gods rather than pathology. In moving beyond this metaphysical explanation, Hippocrates claimed that it was due to a superfluity of phlegm suddenly released into warm blood so impeding circulation to the brain. The Gospels of Luke and Matthew attribute the 'epileptick' attack to demonic possession. Seneca, Shakespeare and Dickens provide dramatic accounts of the various ways epileptics can be murderously dangerous. Shakespeare and Dickens create representations that rhetorically locate those with epilepsy in a disordered nature beyond the boundaries of social and cultural order. By the early nineteenth century, the defining boundaries of epilepsy included convulsive episodes that were to be later attributed to eclampsia, uraemia and febrile states.

By the late nineteenth century, epilepsy came to include the phenomenon of 'bemazement' or intellectual aura, with Jackson the one to finally acknowledge the possibility that the term had reached its use-by date in medical discourse. He argued that many medical men still subscribed to but one type or model of epilepsy – that entailing 'loss of consciousness with severe universal convulsion' – and went on to claim that this picture was profoundly complicated by the variety of symptoms and effects attributable to sudden neuronal discharge.[64]

In accord with Foucault, I argue that 'the epileptics' produced through these genealogies are not the same epileptics. Whatever referent existed beyond the limits of the text has been swallowed up by the multiplicity of statements, descriptions, interpretations, cultural correlations and political conditions that have constituted its articulation. Nevertheless, by the end of the nineteenth century there is still something intransigently familiar in the conflation of neurological process, visible loss of bodily control and the potential for mythic violence, as well as social and sexual excess; in some salient still-to-be-defined way, there *is* a historically persistent 'epileptic'.

Notes

1 Owsei Temkin. *The Falling Sickness: A History of Epilepsy from the Greeks to the Beginnings of Modern Neurology*. 2nd edition, revised. Baltimore, MD: Johns Hopkins University Press, 1971, p. 36.
2 Susan Leigh Star. *Regions of the Mind: Brain Research and the Quest for Scientific Certainty*. Stanford, CA: Stanford University Press, 1989, p. 52.
3 See Temkin, *The Falling Sickness*. Also William Gordon Lennox. *Epilepsy and Related Disorders*. 2 vols. London: Churchill, 1960, vol. 1; D. F. Scott, *The History of Epileptic Therapy: An Account of How Medication Was Developed*. Nashville, TN: Parthenon, 1993.
4 Lennox, *Epilepsy and Related Disorders*, vol. 1, p. 13.
5 Hippocrates. *On the Sacred Disease* (*c*. 400 BCE). Trans. Francis Adams. http://classics.mit.edu/Hippocrates/sacred.html. Accessed 12 August 2007. Unless otherwise indicated, all Hippocratic quotes below are from this text. See also G. E. R. Lloyd, ed. *Hippocratic Writings*. 1978. Trans. J. Chadwick and D. Mann. Harmondsworth: Penguin,1983.
6 William Arthur Heidel. *Hippocratic Medicine: Its Spirit and Method*. New York: Columbia University Press, 1941, p. 18.
7 William Shakespeare. *Julius Caesar*. Ed. John Dover Wilson. Cambridge: Cambridge University Press, 1968.
8 Robert S. Miola. 'Othello *furens*'. *Shakespeare Quarterly*, vol. 41, 1990, p. 51.
9 William Shakespeare. *Othello*. Ed. Kenneth Muir. Harmondsworth: Penguin, 1968.
10 Quoted in Lennox, *Epilepsy and Related Disorders*, vol. 1, p. 14.
11 All biblical quotations are from the King James Version.
12 Quoted in Temkin, *The Falling Sickness*, p. 115.
13 Quoted in Lennox, *Epilepsy and Related Disorders*, vol. 1, p. 18.
14 Johann Weyer. *De praestigiis daemonum*. 1583. *Witches, Devils, and Doctors in the Renaissance*. Ed. George Mora. Trans. John Shea. Binghamton, NY: Medieval and Renaissance Texts and Studies, 1991, p. 153.
15 Edward Jorden. 'A briefe discourse of a disease called the suffocation of the

mother'. London, 1603. John Swan. 'A true and briefe report of Mary Glovers vexation, and of her deliverance by fastings and prayer'. 1603. Stephen Bradwell. 'Mary Glovers late woeful case, together with her joyfull deliverance'. 1603. All pamphlets reprinted in Michael MacDonald. *Witchcraft and Hysteria in Elizabethan London: Edward Jorden and the Mary Glover Case*. London: Tavistock/Routledge, 1991. Unless otherwise indicated, all quotes from Jorden, Swan and Bradwell are taken from these reprinted pamphlets.

16 Bradwell, 'Mary Glover's late woeful case', p. 3.

17 Robert Shereman, quoted in MacDonald, *Witchcraft and Hysteria*, p. xii.

18 MacDonald, *Witchcraft and Hysteria*, p. viii.

19 Bradwell, 'Mary Glover's late woeful case', p. 60.

20 Thomas S. Szasz. *The Manufacture of Madness: A Comparative Study of the Inquisition and the Mental Health Movement*. 1973. London: Paladin Granada, 1977. Weyer quoted in Szasz, pp. 38–39.

21 Quoted in Temkin, *The Falling Sickness*, p.142.

22 MacDonald, *Witchcraft and Hysteria*.

23 Jorden, 'A briefe discourse of a disease called the suffocation of the mother'.

24 Donald A. MacKenzie. *Statistics in Britain 1865–1930: The Social Construction of Scientific Knowledge*. Edinburgh: Edinburgh University Press, 1981, p. 3.

25 Quoted in Lennox, *Epilepsy and Related Disorders*, vol. 1, p. 25.

26 Joseph Williams. 'Practical observations on the cure of epilepsy'. *Lancet*, vol. i, 1854, p. 128.

27 J. Thompson Dickson. 'On the nature of the condition called epilepsy'. *Lancet*, 24 August 1872, pp. 251–52; 31 August 1872, pp. 290–91. Quote from p. 290.

28 D. de Berdt Hovell. 'Hysteria simplified and explained'. *Lancet*, 20 December 1873, pp. 872–74. Quote at p. 873.

29 Michel Foucault. 'Two lectures', 1976, in Colin Gordon, ed. *Power/Knowledge: Selected Interviews and Other Writings 1972–1977*. Trans. Colin Gordon, Leo Marshall, John Mepham and Kate Soper. New York: Harvester Wheatsheaf, 1980, pp. 78–108.

30 Hubert L. Dreyfus and Paul Rabinow. *Michel Foucault: Beyond Structuralism and Hermeneutics*. New York: Harvester Wheatsheaf, 1982, p. xxiii.

31 Michel Foucault. *The Archaeology of Knowledge and the Discourse on Language*. 1969. Trans. A. M. Sheridan Smith. New York: Pantheon, 1972.

32 Foucault, *The Archaeology of Knowledge*, p. 49.

33 W. R. Gowers. 'The Gulstonian lectures on epilepsy: lecture II – part II'. *Lancet*, 20 March 1880, p. 436.

34 Michel Foucault. *The Birth of the Clinic: An Archaeology of Medical Perception*. 1963. Trans. A. M. Sheridan. London: Routledge, 1991, p. ix.

35 Byron J. Good. *Medicine, Rationality, and Experience: An Anthropological Perspective*. Cambridge: Cambridge University Press, 1994, p. 5 (original italics).

36 Quoted in Star. *Regions of the Mind*, p. 69.

37 Macdonald Critchley. *Sir William Gowers 1845–1915: A Biographical Appreciation*. London: Heinemann, 1949, p. 91.

38 Critchley, *Sir William Gowers*, p. vi.

39 Critchley, *Sir William Gowers*, p. 27.

40 John Hughlings Jackson. 'Observations on the localisation of movements in the cerebral hemisphere, as revealed in cases of convulsion, chorea, and "aphasia"', 1873, in James Taylor, ed. *Selected Writings of John Hughlings Jackson*. 2 vols. London: Hodder and Stoughton, 1932, vol. 1, p. 79.

41 W. R. Gowers. *A Manual of Diseases of the Nervous System*. 2nd edition. 2 vols. London: Churchill, 1893, vol. 2, p. 748.

42 Quoted in Macdonald Critchley and Eileen A. Critchley. *John Hughlings Jackson: Father of English Neurology.* Oxford: Oxford University Press, 1998, p. 61.
43 John Hughlings Jackson. 'Remarks on the diagnosis and treatment of diseases of the brain', 1888, in James Taylor, ed. *Selected Writings of John Hughlings Jackson.* 2 vols. London: Hodder and Stoughton, 1932, vol. 2, p. 392.
44 Neurologist Michael Trimble identifies Elizabeth Jackson's condition as thrombophlebitis of the brain complicated by a form of partial epilepsy. Michael R. Trimble. 'Neuropsychiatry or behavioural neurology'. *Neuropsychiatry, Neuropsychology, and Behavioural Neurology: A Journal of Clinical Neuroscience*, vol. 6, no. 1, 1993, p. 61.
45 Critchley and Critchley, *John Hughlings Jackson.* See also Eve LaPlante. *Seized.* New York: HarperCollins, 1993.
46 Critchley and Critchley, *John Hughlings Jackson*, p. 173.
47 Kenneth Dewhurst. *Hughlings Jackson on Psychiatry.* Oxford: Sandford, 1982, pp. 81–82.
48 J. E. Cosnett. 'Charles Dickens and epilepsy'. *Epilepsia*, vol. 35, no. 4, 1994, pp. 903–5.
49 Charles Dickens. *Oliver Twist.* 1837–39. London: Octopus Books, 1983, p. 18.
50 Dickens, *Oliver Twist*, pp. 155–56.
51 Dickens, *Oliver Twist*, p. 141
52 Lennard J. Davis. *Enforcing Normalcy: Disability, Deafness and the Body*. New York: Verso, 1995, p. 42.
53 Dickens, *Oliver Twist*, p. 262 (italics added).
54 Dickens, *Oliver Twist*, p. 156.
55 Dickens, *Oliver Twist*, p. 198.
56 Dickens, *Oliver Twist*, p. 245.
57 'Bite of an epileptic'. *Lancet*, 12 January 1884, p. 82.
58 'No poison in the bite of an epileptic'. *Lancet*, 19 January 1884, p. 131.
59 Dr Clutterbuck. 'Lectures on the diseases of the nervous system: lecture XVI'. *Lancet*, 23 June 1826–27, p. 355.
60 Marshall Hall. 'Lectures on the theory and practice of medicine'. *Lancet*, vol. ii, 14 April 1838, p. 66.
61 Samuel Solly. 'A clinical lecture on epilepsy following injury to the cranium'. *Lancet*, 5 January 1850, p. 9.
62 Foucault, *The Archaeology of Knowledge*, p. 40.
63 Foucault, *The Archaeology of Knowledge*, p. 32.
64 Jackson, 'Remarks on the diagnosis and treatment of diseases of the brain', p. 370.

CHAPTER 2

Hystericity and hauntings: the female and the feminised

Life is short, science is long; opportunity is elusive, experiment is dangerous, judgement is difficult. It is not enough for the physician to do what is necessary, but the patient and the attendants must do their part as well and circumstances must be favourable.
(Hippocratic aphorism, 400 BCE)

I

The Hippocratic physicians insisted that epilepsy was a physical disease rather than a metaphysical mutation. This way of thinking about the disorder circulated beyond Cos and into a new millennium: Galen developed his theories about the disorder from similar principles. Nevertheless, fear that epilepsy signified spiritual contagion from possession was to play a part in discriminatory and stigmatising processes in biblical narratives. That fear reappeared in the political propaganda circulated in early seventeenth-century debates about witchcraft, religious faith and knowledge boundaries. By the eighteenth century, the notion that epilepsy was contagious had been more or less refuted, only to be replaced by a widely held conviction that exposure to the convulsing body could excite disorder in the sensitive and vulnerable bystander and the sight of a *grand mal* seizure was enough to contaminate the foetus of a pregnant woman.

To a significant extent, and despite some progress in modernising medical models of epilepsy, this stream of beliefs continued to hold some sway over medical thinking through the latter decades of the nineteenth century and into the twentieth. Whereas in earlier times in the syndrome's history the problem for the physician and priest had been to differentiate between epilepsy and possession, nineteenth-century medical practitioners became increasingly concerned about locating the boundaries between 'true' epilepsy, symptomatic epilepsy and hysteria. Most British physicians admitted that precise differentiation between epilepsy and hysteria was difficult and not always possible. To privilege the diagnosis of hystero-epilepsy over epilepsy could, at best, risk mistreatment and at worst, death for the patient. Furthermore, although it was now believed that the primary mode of transferral for the syndrome was through the hereditary taint of blood, anxiety was still being voiced about the seductively inciting potential of the convulsing body.

By the 1860s the body prone to seizure was becoming a liminal figure, consigned to the 'borderlands' of normative society by both medical and literary narratives. Ideas of reliable boundaries that might delineate the potential for disorder and provide a notional space for safe containment had begun to fire the imagination of writers and became a recurring motif in the cultural circuit. As the century moved to a close, the 'borderlands' evolved into an enduring trope in medical and cultural systems of representation.

Within the context of the nineteenth-century social realist novel, seizures were often utilised to position characters at the margins of mainstream society such that their perspective both illuminated and reinforced the boundaries between normality and abnormality, between social orthodoxy and impropriety. Guster, Mr and Mrs Snagsby's maid servant in Charles Dickens' *Bleak House,* functions as both a barometer for the household's domestic climate and a cipher that links the middle-class mores of Victorian society with the desperate poverty of the unruly 'underclasses'. The seizures experienced by George Eliot's character Silas Marner are labelled catalepsy rather than epilepsy; nevertheless, his 'fits' consign him to the outskirts of Raveloe society. The transgressive sexuality of Lucette Le Sueur (Lucetta Templeman) in Thomas Hardy's *The Mayor of Casterbridge* becomes reified by the seizure – probably due to eclampsia – that ends her life and that of her unborn child. Fyodor Dostoevsky creates seizure-prone characters located at the brink of mainstream society. Although these characters often occupy complex narrative positions within his works, they nonetheless remain figures of liminality. The common feature linking these characters in both English and Russian nineteenth-century literatures, besides their vulnerability to seizure, is that none is allowed to procreate.

Concurrent with these fictional representations, physicians were debating possible links between epilepsy, sex, class, ethnicity and moral defectiveness. Just as urgently, they were trying to elucidate what, precisely, constituted epilepsy. For all the debate and conflicting ideas, however, a consistent theme had begun to emerge. Like their literary counterparts, medical writers were largely in accord about the undesirability of procreation for those with seizure conditions. They argued that it was still too difficult to differentiate 'true' epilepsy from other possible causes of seizure and thus it was best to err on the side of caution and advise against the risk of hereditary 'taint'.

In this chapter I examine systems of dispersal that operate between sites of definition and representation, locating the ways that these systems operate as discursive formations that conceptualise, define and promulgate medical, social and cultural understandings of 'the epileptic'. The borders, boundaries and lines of demarcation debated through the closing decades of the nineteenth century are as important to the refinement of what epilepsy *is* as they are in trying to decide what it *is not*. At the heart of these lines of demarcation and definition is the convulsive body. Nineteenth-century discursive strategies mobilise as much around the containment of this disruptive figure within the designated borders of abnormality as they do around the theorisation of brain function.

II

Writing in the 1870s, Andrew Wynter described the borderlands that had come to delineate deviation from the norm in general and epileptic identity in particular as treacherous space, littered with indefinable perils. It is a space where, sometimes, 'a passenger [can be] missed from the ever-ebbing stream of life, and none but the physician notes that he has dropped through the pitfall on the bridge and will never mix in the busy haunts of men again'.[1] In her study of nineteenth-century psychiatry and English culture, Elaine Showalter cites the English physician Mortimer Granville who dubbed the sub-territories of the borderlands – the uninhabitable zones of social life – 'Mazeland, Dazeland, and Driftland'. Granville argued that these were the zones 'where the degenerate lower classes and the effeminate upper classes filled an increasingly populous district'[2] as the latter decades of the nineteenth century progressed.

Drawing on theories of the nineteenth-century physician Henry Maudsley to support his own critique of degeneration at the *fin de siècle*, his contemporary Max Nordau confirms the view that 'the epileptic' is a 'borderland dweller' located with other degenerate figures 'on the borderland between reason and pronounced madness'.[3] William Gowers perpetuates the trope when, at the beginning of the new century, he affirms the significance of the borderlands as part of a medical rhetoric of containment for the epileptic in the preface to his 1907 publication *The Border-Land of Epilepsy*. He informs readers that his exploration of 'faints, vagal attacks, vertigo, migraine, and sleep symptoms' entails consulting a 'special list' assembled over many years 'of all cases which seemed to be in the border-land of epilepsy – near it, but not of it'.[4]

In the ongoing project to better map the boundaries defining the borderlands, physicians involved themselves in robust debates about what constituted 'true' epilepsy as opposed to symptomatic epilepsy, what symptomatology could be talked about as being epileptiform or epileptic equivalent, and whether hysteria and epilepsy were discrete conditions or somehow intimately linked. Conclusions about what the boundaries might be between hysteria and epilepsy often reflected wider tensions between English and French knowledge claims, as Gowers, among others, interrogated Jean-Martin Charcot's concept of mutually exclusive pathologies. Some modes of epilepsy were beginning to disappear because of an expanding and increasingly sophisticated body of knowledge, while others were emerging to fill the diagnostic space; this is probably not so surprising given the ever-changing contours of the terrain under scrutiny. Those convulsive states associated with infant dentition, eclampsia and febrile conditions had largely been reclassified as non-epileptic by the turn of the century, while 'psychic epilepsy' – an early name for psychomotor[5] or temporal lobe epilepsy, now called partial or complex partial epilepsy – began to appear in the spectrum of epileptic disorder.

The problems facing the physician worried about accurate diagnosis is highlighted in an anecdote related by Owsei Temkin about Étienne Esquirol, who claimed that it was always possible to discover any simulated case of epilepsy. Evidently, one of the French psychiatrist's male students suddenly fell before him, displaying all the typical signs of *grand mal* seizure. Esquirol was suitably concerned and sympathetic, only to discover that his student had in fact feigned the episode.[6] We are not told of the student's fate after this successful subversion of the master's dictum. Rudyard Kipling gives the feigned seizure a comic turn in 'The post that fitted' when, in order to jilt Miss Boffkin so he can wed his 'little Carrie', the inventive Sleary:

> ... started epileptic fits of an appalling kind.
> (Of his modus operandi only this much I could gather:–
> 'Pears's shaving sticks will give you little taste and lots of lather.')[7]

Many physicians, though, did not share Kipling's amused regard for the faked fit; nor did they share Esquirol's diagnostic confidence in being able to always accurately differentiate between *grand mal* seizures and feigned episodes. They worried that, at times, simulated seizures might be strategically used by those seeking to avoid unwanted duty, responsibility or criminal culpability. Cases of this particular type of malingering were deemed significant enough to be recorded in medical journals. In the 1870s, for example, thirty-three-year-old James Clegg became infamous with British police. He would feign a seizure in a public and preferably crowded place and, while the crowd were distracted by the spectacle, have his accomplices pick pockets. When the act wore thin and his notoriety became a liability, he relocated to North America, where he continued to confound physicians for some time to come.[8]

Debate also waged back and forth about which sex was more vulnerable to epilepsy. This was not an entirely new way of thinking about the disorder: Hippocratic physicians had attempted to understand which population sectors were most commonly affected and believed that epilepsy occurred more often in men than in women. Gowers concluded that females were more likely to be affected by idiopathic or primary epilepsy, while epilepsy traceable to some immediate cause (symptomatic or secondary) was more prevalent in males. He held the view that women were somehow more 'naturally' prone to the disorder because 'Mental emotion – fright, excitement, anxiety – is the most potent exciting cause of epilepsy',[9] and this therefore made women and children particularly susceptible.

Women were doubly implicated in this economy of biological predisposition. Gowers argued:

> When there is an inherited tendency, the females of a family are rather more likely to suffer than the males. This is due to two circumstances; the inheritance is rather more frequently from the mother's side than from the father's, and more females suffer when the heredity is maternal, more males when it is paternal.[10]

In North America, during the opening years of the new century, William Spratling was to articulate the gender divide more baldly. The epilepsies included for him male epilepsies and female epilepsies. In women, he claimed, paroxysmal potential was both innate and a sign of degeneration:

> More epilepsies occur in the 12th to 15th year than in any other period. This is especially true in women. At the Craig Colony we have performed much abdominal surgery in cases in which the seizures grouped themselves about the menstrual period. We have had some excellent results. We look for neurotic ancestry in such cases.[11]

Lisa Cartwright notes that Spratling (like Gowers) associated the male epilepsies with social factors, tagging alcohol, brain injury and illness as primary causative triggers; he also acknowledged the import of hereditary predisposition.[12]

The lower classes were another population sector being scrutinised for occurrences of epilepsy. In 1892, S. Wilks rather boldly declared in the *British Medical Journal* that 'The epileptic does not suffer from headache'.[13] This statement began the conclusion of a short discussion about the associations between migraine and epilepsy, and Wilks proceeded to offer evidence as to why migraine and epilepsy necessarily belonged to different classes of persons:

> If I wished to find epileptics, I should go to lunatic asylums or idiot asylums amongst the low and undeveloped; and, on the other hand, seek amongst the bright and intellectual for migraine; and if, moreover, I wanted to gain any information about the complaint, I should read the *Philosophical Transactions*, where are recorded the histories of many distinguished men who suffered from it.[14]

His argument hinges on the rather bizarre proposition that if 'soldiers, sailors, policemen, and engine-drivers' had migraines they would be incapacitated from their duties and he had never heard of a man being declared unfit for work because of a headache. Headache in this scenario is associated with the highly strung and evolved nervous system, whereas associations between epilepsy and the 'dull and stupid' necessarily preclude the epileptic from experiencing pain in 'his' head.

Concerns about the 'low and undeveloped' dangerous classes potentially contaminating the 'bright and intellectual' respectable classes were being further fuelled by evolutionary theory. Physicians in Britain, North America and Australia enthusiastically engaged with the implications of Charles Darwin's ideas and those of his cousin, Francis Galton, for medical research, policy and practice. John Hughlings Jackson was one of the many physicians of the day who defined themselves as evolutionists. In this aspect of his work, he repeatedly acknowledged his debt to the theories of the British philosopher Herbert Spencer, although some analysts insist that he gave too much credit to Spencer for his ideas. Jackson deployed what he called the principles of evolution and dissolution to set out the hierarchies of the nervous system as he understood them. This organisational paradigm was used to visualise an ascending scale of 'Lowest, Middle and Highest Level Fits', depending on the site of the discharging lesion and degree of cerebral involvement.

For Jackson, evolution in neurophysiological terms entailed passage from the most to the least organised cerebral centres:

> I say that the highest cerebral centres are the least organised (the 'most helpless centres'), although they are the most complex, whereas the lowest centres are the most organised, although the least complex. In other words, we may say that the evolutionary ascent is from the least to the most modifiable. If the highest centres were not modifiable, we should be very simple machines; we should make no new acquirements. If the lowest ('vital') centres were to become as modifiable as the highest are, life would cease.[15]

Jackson took some pains throughout his writings to emphasise that at this stage of his hypotheses there were no practical social purposes to be obtained from the doctrine of evolution but rather he advocated its value in clinical investigation. Nevertheless, at times he did allow himself to drift into a wider consideration of the applications of evolutionary theory, claiming that the model 'supplies us with a scientific measure, which ignores superior and inferior, as these terms are ordinarily used with regard to men's minds'. He wanted to talk about those 'races of men and adults [who] have the latest acquired faculties.... So that, instead of saying that a person is superior or inferior to most other men, we may say that he has more or less of the latest faculties of the race than most other men have'.[16] The careful, considered tones mark this as a rather typical Jackson statement; but it also suggests, I think, an underlying awareness of the evolutionary mood of the times and politics of representation.

His use of evolutionary models to expand his understanding of brain function was an undeniably productive component in his work. However, his view that the place of evolutionary theory in scientific thinking within the biosciences could be divorced from wider applications, while scholarly in focus, suggests a political naïveté about how evolutionism was being taken up in the circuits of culture that encompassed other areas of scientific and social debate. I think Jackson's work is genuinely free of the moral and social rectitude palpable in so many of the Victorian medical texts and have been unable to find any evidence in his *Selected Writings* or published journal articles that persuades me otherwise. His celebration in his writings of evolutionary theory seems not to extend beyond the ways that it facilitated his own thought processes in relationship to cerebral hierarchies and clinical analysis. Despite this reluctance to ascribe values of superior and inferior in his own work, it is difficult to gain any cogent sense of his views on the wider utilisation of evolutionary theory to inform ideas of sex, race and cultural hierarchies. However, his oft-repeated denial that his work could be used to facilitate this sort of prognostication seems to support the view that he was not unaware of the applications of evolutionist theory in social theory.

Nevertheless, as the century ticked on, class became an ever more compelling factor in the British medical project of mapping the borderlands. Jackson's case histories of 'two medical men'[17] who were in his care suggested that epilepsy was indifferent to class barriers. Yet evidence to the contrary notwithstanding, the general perception remained that epilepsy was more prevalent in the lower classes. This perception appears to have been supported by several factors. Firstly, occurrence in the British upper classes was more likely to be hidden because of both the social stigma attaching to the syndrome and the taint of heredity. This option was exercised by the British royal family during the early years of the new century when John (1905–19), the fifth son of King George V and Mary of Teck, was diagnosed with epilepsy at age six. News of his condition was suppressed and he was hidden from public view until his death at age fourteen. It is a factor also worth consideration in relation to Jackson's silence on the identity of his physician patient 'Dr Z', or 'Quaerens'. Both pseudonyms belonged to Arthur Myers and it is possible that Jackson's case histories of 'two medical men' actually represent aspects of Myers' medical history (a possibility discussed in more detail in the following chapter). Secondly, the lower classes were in the majority in terms of population numbers and increased population equals increased chances of occurrences of the syndrome. A third and obscured factor in associations between class and epilepsy concerns the impact of social stigma on the earning potential of those diagnosed with the condition, an effect that rendered even those from the middle classes or with artisan skills vulnerable to pauperism.

III

Associations between epilepsy, class and hereditary 'taint' had been firmly established in the public imagination by Dickens' rendering of the violent Monks (see Chapter 1). Imbued by blood with the moral laxity of both parents, the 'hideous disease' becomes an augmentation to his already considerable wickedness. Theories of degeneration developed by Cesare Lombroso some sixty years after Dickens' rendition of the criminal class in *Oliver Twist* medically formalise these fictional relationships between criminality and epilepsy. Lombroso argued that the two 'shared physiognomic signs, degenerative stigmata, and, above all, psychological traits. Epilepsy united the criminal and morally insane in one natural family'.[18] In his creation of Monks and the criminal class to which he belongs, Dickens is a key participant in a cultural circuit comprised of shared literary, medical and scientific representational systems. Jack Dawkins (the Artful Dodger) and Fagin have their class and criminality inscribed in their physiognomies, their faces a 'reliable index' of social status and 'natural' inclination. As I have suggested in the previous chapter, epilepsy is mobilised in *Oliver Twist* to signify the more extreme depths of Monks' moral dissolution and 'unclean spirit'. The character is a compelling distillation of all those inclinations to violence and moral turpitude ascribed to male epileptics in the medical journals of the latter half of the century. He is also curiously asexual.

Cultural associations between epilepsy, violence and, significantly, hereditary pollution from the maternal line were not limited to English literature or medicine. In *The Brothers Karamazov* (1880), Dostoevsky explores the more violent aspects of epileptic behaviours and links epilepsy with domestic disorder and parricide. Some fifty years after *The Brothers Karamazov* was published, in what might be deemed a case of medicine imitating art, potential links between Dostoevsky's own seizure condition and subconscious parricidal inclinations were discussed at length by Sigmund Freud in his essay 'Dostoevsky and parricide' (1927–28). Evidently, Dostoevsky's symptoms became overtly epileptic only at the age of eighteen and after the murder of his father. For Freud, the timing of this onset is suggestive of Dostoevsky's ambivalence about his parent and he argues that the writer's attraction in his literature to themes of violence, murderous impulses in otherwise law-abiding characters and egotism is a consequence of creative sublimation of those impulses in Dostoevsky's own psyche. He surmises that it is 'highly probable that [Dostoevsky's] so-called epilepsy was only a symptom of his neurosis and must accordingly be classified as hystero-epilepsy – that is, as severe hysteria'.[19] The writer's paroxysmal condition, Freud concludes, was most likely an expression of his mental life rather than an indication of organic disorder.[20] Freud's comments also reinforce the somewhat nebulous understandings of what constituted a 'seizure' and what a 'seizure' might mean for medical classification. Echoing John Hughlings Jackson (with whom he had corresponded at length as a young neurologist at the beginning of his career), Freud muses: 'It is no wonder ... that it has been found impossible to maintain that "epilepsy" is a single clinical entity'.[21]

In Dostoevsky's novel, the aetiology of Smerdyakov's epilepsy associates his seizure condition with his mother's idiocy, the fall which ends in her death and precipitates his birth, and his illegitimacy. He is raised by Marfa Ignatyevna and Grigory Vasilyevich, servants of Fyodor Pavlovich (father of the eponymous brothers), and is described as a 'strange boy', 'without any gratitude': 'In his childhood he had been very fond of stringing up cats and then giving them ceremonial burials'. Grigory tells Marfa that the boy is 'not human', but a 'cruel monster'.[22] Smerdyakov has his first seizure at twelve. Grigory slaps him after the boy argues about the significance of the religious teachings being conveyed to him by his foster parent. For several days thereafter, the child remains silent and withdrawn: 'Chance would have it that just one week later there became manifest in him, for the first time in his life, that falling sickness that was to remain with him for the rest of it'.[23] Smerdyakov's seizure condition brings about a positive change in Fyodor Pavlovich's attitude to him, although the older man (who is also most likely his biological father) still refers to him as 'fool' and 'Balaam's ass'. Smerdyakov eventually kills Pavlovich; his putative half-brothers, Ivan and Mitya, are also both implicated. Dostoevsky extends associations between organic and moral disorder in the text and Ivan's sense of remorse at his own murderous desires eventually brings him to a state of debilitation which his doctor diagnoses as 'something almost akin to a disorder of the brain'.[24]

N. M. Lary argues that 'The mark of Dickens is everywhere in Russian fiction' and points out that Dickens' work was translated and in circulation in Russia from 1840.[25] By 1847, with the Russian publication of the first instalments of *Dombey and Son*, Dickens' reputation with his Russian readership was well on the way to being established. In examining the direct influence of Dickens' work on Dostoevsky, Lary explores the very different visions represented in each writer's work and also locates their comparative positions in the tradition of nineteenth-century realist fiction. Both writers were caught up in societies that were in the throes of change and both sought to reflect in their respective works the fragmentation and reformation that necessarily accompany social upheaval. Both writers utilised signifiers that, by the late nineteenth century, had become associated with epilepsy symptomatology, and both drew on the dramatic possibilities suggested by the condition.

There are similarities in the ways that Dickens and Dostoevsky describe social conditions thought to contribute to epilepsy. There are also salient differences. In 1868, for example, Dostoevsky locates epilepsy with the character of Prince Myshkin in *The Idiot*. Myshkin marks a new development in literary representation of a character with epilepsy. Unlike previous epileptic figures in literature, he is a hero – if a flawed one – at the centre of the novel's plot development.

Dostoevsky's Prince is the end result of the writer's desire to 'depict a positively beautiful man'.[26] In pursuit of this idealised beauty, Dostoevsky acknowledged that Prince Myshkin was patterned in certain respects on Dickens' Pickwick.[27] The fate of this style of representation of the epileptic figure in the wider circuit of culture is discussed in further detail in the next chapter. However, and as Lary has argued, Myshkin was not always so beneficent. In the early planning stages for the novel, the 'Idiot' is a man of violent, unruly passions: an arsonist and rapist, more akin to Monks than Pickwick.

Between them, Dickens and Dostoevsky create representations that establish the figure of the epileptic as a stock literary device. Nevertheless, while drawing on medical models of epilepsy similar to those deployed by Dickens – including the extreme possibilities of so-called epileptic behaviour – Dostoevsky complicates these models somewhat by widening the range of social autonomy available to his afflicted characters. Consequently, the character with epilepsy in Dostoevsky's novels does more than patrol the fracture lines of social experience. Although he maintains links between the seizure and abjection, Dostoevsky does not close off the possibility of psychological recovery and the development of inter-seizure self-awareness and insight.

A little over a decade after Monks made his debut, Dickens again utilised epilepsy as a marker of class, if not moral turpitude, in *Bleak House*. Guster is 'a lean young woman from a workhouse (by some supposed to have been christened Augusta)' who 'has fits'.[28] Her disordered states have a metonymic function in the novel. They provide an embodied coda for the complex and dangerous currents that threaten the middle-class stability of Cook's Court, Cursitor Street, and, by extension, London society. During the night that marks the conclusion of the coroner's inquiry into the death of 'Nemo' (Captain Hawdon), Guster 'murders sleep' for the Snagsby household. Her nocturnal prolonged seizure episodes become a metaphor for the dis-ease that emanates from Hawdon's death and eventually infects the wider social milieu of the novel through the lurking machinations of Tulkinghorn.

On the night in question, Guster's seizures roll on 'out of one fit into twenty', so disturbing the household that, by the time a cock crows the break of a new day, Mr Snagsby comments to the bird: 'I thought you was dead, I am sure!'[29] The intensity and persistence of this episode is ascribed to Guster's 'tender heart', a causal diagnosis that prefigures Gowers' later argument (quoted above) that women are more prone to epilepsy because they are more prone to the 'mental emotion' that is 'the most potent exciting cause' of the condition. Guster's seizures have an emotional component and can be triggered by troublesome fluctuations in the dominant order. A visit to the Snagsby household from Lady Dredlock's maid, Hortense, with her 'fierce' foreign looks and 'grinding manner ... calculated to alarm a weak mind'[30] triggers another prolonged bout of seizures. The notion that women are generally more seizure prone than their male counterparts is further reinforced in *Bleak House* when Mrs Snagsby's suspicions about Jo's paternity seem to be confirmed by the loquacious Mr Chadband. On believing that she finally understands the 'Terewth' of the relationship between her husband and Jo, she delivers 'herself a prey to spasms'.[31]

In Dostoevsky's *The Insulted and Humiliated*, the fits experienced by Yelena (Nellie), like Guster's, have a strong psychological factor. In both characters, paroxysmal episodes are provoked by violently conflicting emotions or fear. For Yelena, psychological causative factors include: the realisation of her grandfather's death; response to the physical abuse of both herself and Vanya by Mistress Bubnov; and a sexual assault by one of the men at Bubnov's. Familiarity with medical models of epilepsy is also discernible in Dostoevsky's description of the epileptic cry that precedes some seizure states: Yelena's seizures are preceded by a sound described as a 'piercing inhuman scream'.[32] Gowers describes this sound as 'the epileptic cry' and suggests that it sometimes occurs at the onset of a seizure: 'It may be a harsh weird scream, but more often it is a sort of prolonged laryngeal groan, not very loud, but very characteristic'.[33] This 'pitiful scream', when Yelena is assaulted at the Bubnov house, associates aspects of her symptomatology with psycho-sexual trauma.

Guster's disorder is ultimately contained by middle-class patronage. And while her fits provide embodied barometric readings of the turbulent social and cultural climes within the text, her presence in the Snagsby household also affirms her moral worth to bourgeois society, albeit with some irony: 'she is a satisfaction to Mrs Snagsby, who can always find fault with her; she is a satisfaction to Mr Snagsby, who thinks it a charity to keep her'. Her position within the dominant milieu is further secured by her work ethic: 'except when she is found with her head in the pail, or the sink, or the copper, or the dinner, or anything else that happens to be near her at the time of her seizure, she is always at work'. Most importantly of all, though, Guster can in no way be considered a temptress. The physical toll exacted by the circumstances of her class and epilepsy is such that 'She is a satisfaction to the parents and guardians of the 'prentices, who feel that there is little danger of her inspiring tender emotions in the breast of youth'.[34]

For Guster, as for Oliver Twist, class is destiny. As indeed it is for her fellow orphans in *Bleak House*, Esther and Jo. Born in a workhouse but 'farmed or contracted for' by an 'amiable benefactor', Guster will never rise above her designated position in society. Although, in a sense, and despite her epilepsy, she does achieve some upward mobility because of her value to mainstream culture. Esther Summerson is also destined to find her right and proper place in the social hierarchy of the novel. Jo's fate is to always remain an unwanted outsider, to be constantly 'moved on' lest he offend the sensibilities of his betters. It is with Jo that Guster is most closely aligned. One of Guster's duties is to answer the door to her employers' middle-class home. She is the keeper at the threshold, literally patrolling the 'borderlands' between middle-class propriety and the unruly forces that threaten instability: to get to the Snagsbys, callers have to get past Guster. When she first ventures to speak with Jo directly, she offers him her supper at the kitchen door as he departs the Snagsby household after the meeting with the Chadbands. She is trying to suppress a seizure, and this time succeeds. For Guster, it is the first time she is able to share fellow feelings about her parentless state. For Jo, 'it is the first time in his life that any decent hand has been so laid upon him'.[35] Despite her proximity to the centre of bourgeois mores and her value in patrolling the borderlands that protect them, the encounter and fellow feeling shared with Jo in this moment underscore Guster's 'authentic' place in the class hierarchy of the novel.

Like Guster, George Eliot's character Silas Marner is also located in the borderlands of mainstream society. Eliot utilises Silas's seizure episodes as a transitional device within the narrative. His cultural identity in Lantern Yard is 'seized' by his condition and results in exile: from the community, as well as from all those social roles that he might have otherwise enjoyed as an appropriately acculturated – 'normal' – male subject. His first seizure establishes his 'otherness' in the religious environment of Lantern Yard; his second makes him vulnerable to William Dane's treachery and ends his engagement to Sarah. A later episode leaves him standing like a 'graven image', immobilised by 'the invisible wand of catalepsy' at the open door of his cottage and facilitates the entry of the lost child, Eppie, into his home and the centre of his life.[36] When he recovers from this episode he takes it upon himself to care for the child, assuming the role and responsibilities of sole parent. Like Guster, Silas also finds redemption in work and, significantly, it is work that serves the needs of his new host community. As a linen weaver, 'his handicraft made him a highly welcome settler to the richer housewives of the district, and even to the more provident cottagers, who had their little stock of yarn at the year's end'.[37] Silas recognises and accepts his place at the borders of

Raveloe and any potential for his condition to destabilise the social order of the community is ultimately contained by his compliant marginality and service to the dominant culture.

The aesthetics and politics of representation combine in *Silas Marner* to construct a character emasculated by his seizure condition. From being an active and valued participant in the social, intellectual and spiritual life of Lantern Yard, he becomes an ersatz 'wise woman' to Raveloe folk after successfully alleviating Sally Oates' 'dropsy' with herbal remedies. Silas's seizure condition locates him in the natural world rather than the cultural. He is 'both sane and honest, though, as with many honest and fervent men, culture had not defined any channels for his sense of mystery, and so it spread itself over the proper pathway of inquiry and knowledge'.[38] Rather than being the locus of masculine power and cultural authority, he manifests a hereditary 'natural' (feminised) wisdom and knowledge of medicinal herbs, charms and healing traceable to his mother. He eventually finds peace of mind in an Arcadian setting at the edges of a rural community.

His familiarity with the arcane mysteries of a nature that could be either curative or mischievously lethal serves to protect him 'from the persecution that his singularities might have [otherwise] drawn upon him'.[39] However, it is the uncompromising lack of any erotic potential whatsoever that definitively secures his acceptance within the community, despite his paroxysmal otherness. He is prematurely aged by the demands of his craft and his seizure condition. His physical appearance has the mark of the town about it: to the rural community of Raveloe, he is an 'alien-looking' man from a 'disinherited race'.[40] Reassuringly, his looks and general demeanour draw no admiring glances from the 'Raveloe lasses [and] he would never urge one of them to accept him against her will'.[41] Cultural emasculation of the character is reinforced when he assumes a maternal role in Eppie's life after the death of her biological mother.

In Silas Marner, Eliot creates an ambiguous figure, drawn from a range of possibilities in the representational spectrum. He is both saintly and venal: at home in the natural world far from 'the busy haunts of men', but at the same time in thrall to the gold he acquires and hoards beneath his loom. He is imbued with both a feminine and a masculine sensibility. His seizure episodes are similarly ambiguous and evoke possibilities of both a heightened spirituality and satanic visitation within the cultural framework of Lantern Yard:

> To have sought a medical explanation for this phenomenon would have been held by Silas himself, as well as by his minister and fellow-members,

> a wilful self-exclusion from the spiritual significance that might lie therein. Silas was evidently a brother selected for a peculiar discipline; and though the effort to interpret this discipline was discouraged by the absence, on his part, of any spiritual vision during his outward trance, yet it was believed by himself and others that its effect was seen in an accession of light and fervour.[42]

To the Raveloe villagers, Silas's seized states are utterly mysterious because they do not conform to the more familiar manifestations of 'stroke', which old Mr Macey, the parish clerk, insists is the underlying cause of all those fits that cause the sufferer to fall down with limbs jerking and flailing. The local poacher, Jem Rodney, tells the villagers of seeing Silas standing as though in a trance during one of his episodes.

In spite of his tendency to seize, observations made by various characters in the text ensure that Silas is *not* identified with epilepsy. This allows Eliot to involve him more diversely in plot and narrative development and he evolves as a hybrid figure. Despite exile from the urban Lantern Yard because of his seizure condition, he comes to enjoy a lucrative, if marginalised, status in rural Raveloe society. Significantly, and again in spite of his seizure condition, he is allowed to achieve a surrogate cultural capital unavailable to fictional counterparts with seizure conditions specifically identified as epilepsy. He may not be able to attain full cultural status in Raveloe society in his own right, but he is permitted to successfully raise a child: notably, a female child who grows into an appropriately decorous adult femininity.

As a narrative device, Eppie functions to endow cohesion on an otherwise fragmented Silas: she fills the void created by the theft of his gold; becomes a bridge to a wider and richer range of social engagement with his adopted community; and provides a context where both the feminine and masculine aspects of the character can integrate as a coherent and unified whole. She also becomes an appropriate repository for those maternal knowledges and female wisdoms that have been Silas's legacy, a legacy that had protected him from social persecution and neutered his masculinity. It is through Eppie that Silas's compliance with his earlier marginalisation in the dominant order is ultimately rewarded. At her wedding, she walked across the churchyard with one hand 'on her husband's arm, and with the other she clasped the hand of her father Silas'.[43] This image, near the end of the narrative, links Silas, through Eppie, to the socially and sexually viable masculinity represented by Aaron Winthrop, her new husband. It is a link that also restores Silas to a subject position akin to his rightful place in the symbolic order of the narrative. His 'strange history' notwithstanding, he had 'brought a blessing on himself by acting like a father to a lone motherless child'.[44]

Thomas Hardy's Lucette Le Sueur is quite another matter. She is middle class, physically and intellectually attractive, passionate, excitable, 'very' ambitious, and financially and sexually independent. Nonetheless, the character is drawn from the representational spectrum that produced Guster and Silas Marner. Lucette is prone to those excitabilities and moral 'defects' that Gowers and others will later formalise as precursors of female paroxysmal behaviours. This potential combines with her foreignness and transgressive femininity to consign her, at least notionally, to the borderlands of mainstream society. Unlike Guster and Silas, however, Lucette does not accept or comply with her marginalisation.

As Miss Lucetta Templeman, she moves into High-Place Hall, a residence that, despite its name and location so close to what is currently the centre of Casterbridge culture, is associated with the natural world. It has the 'characteristics of a country mansion' and is bedecked with fungi and damp nooks. The rear entrance to the hall is located in a back alley and marked by a 'queer old door' and a 'leering mask' that evoke the building's past associations with the forbidden. The alley links the respectable façade of Lucetta's residence with the underbelly of Casterbridge society:

> By the alley it had been possible to come unseen from all sorts of quarters in the town – the old play-house, the old bull-stake, the old cock-pit, the pool wherein nameless infants had been used to disappear. High-Place Hall could boast of its conveniences undoubtedly.[45]

Lucetta is unaware of the hall's back entrance, just as she is unaware of her 'proper' place in the symbolic order. She is a hybrid figure within the text, moving from the margins to the centre of Casterbridge society. She aspires to social and cultural legitimacy and within the representational logic of Hardy's *Casterbridge* this aspiration must prove fatal. Lucetta is, after all, a woman with a past and cannot be allowed to usurp the appropriately feminine Elizabeth-Jane Henchard's rightful place.

In *Casterbridge* Hardy deploys a narrative device used to effect by Dostoevsky in *The Idiot* and Robert Louis Stevenson in *The Strange Case of Dr Jekyll and Mr Hyde* (see Chapter 3): he creates a disjunctive doubling between two key characters and in so doing marks the boundaries between social order and illicit disruptiveness. Lucetta is semiotically coded as Elizabeth-Jane's negative image. She first appears in Casterbridge as a 'solitary dark figure', like Elizabeth-Jane, dressed in mourning garb, looking to be about the same general build and age:

'and might have been [Elizabeth's] wraith or double', except for the quality of dress and a certain 'flexuousness' in movement, deemed indicative of 'disposition'.[46] This disjunctive doubling – of appearance, of perception, of sensibility – becomes a recurring motif. From 'adjoining windows of the same room' the women strive to see from each other's perspective but their duality renders them unconscious of the other's true self. Lucetta remains unaware of Elizabeth-Jane's affection for Donald Farfrae as she pursues her own attraction to him; Elizabeth-Jane cannot see the truth of Lucetta's relationships with either Michael Henchard or Farfrae. Hardy represents both women as being somehow essentially fragmented by their respective pasts. Both are striving for integration into mainstream society; their survival depends on it. Unfortunately, both are competing for the same place.

Hardy casts Lucetta as the exotic 'other'. She is from Jersey, where, she tells Elizabeth-Jane:

> they speak French on one side of the street and English on the other, and a mixed tongue in the middle of the road. But it is a long time since I was there. Bath is where my people really belong to, though my ancestors in Jersey were as good as anybody in England.... But I don't value such past matters, and am quite an English person in my feelings and tastes.[47]

After her move to Casterbridge, Henchard reminds her of their shared liaison in her 'native Jersey' and she chides him, insisting that she is English. But despite her bids for English conformity, Lucetta's 'otherness' is written on her face and tongue: although she scrupulously avoids speaking French, lest her accent betray her, Elizabeth-Jane notes her foreign appearance as being of 'unmistakably French extraction on one side or the other'.[48] In direct comparison with Elizabeth-Jane's decorous – and English – stoicism in the face of emotional disappointment, Lucetta is excitable and prone to tempestuous outbursts. Indeed, when she realises her ploy of having Elizabeth-Jane as her live-in companion will not necessarily draw Henchard to her side, she bursts 'into hysterical sobs'.[49] She lacks Elizabeth-Jane's emotional constancy and compliance, and instead claims her rights to an essentially unfeminine impulse to ambition and to love as she chooses. Given the past relationship between Lucetta and Henchard, Elizabeth-Jane's father figure, the linking of the two women functions to further enhance and layer the impropriety located with the character.

Henchard and Lucetta become 'naturally intimate' during one of his visits to Jersey. Her reputation on the island is ruined by the scandal: a transgression that ensures her place beyond the boundaries of appropriate nineteenth-century English femininity. Henchard describes

Lucetta as a 'giddy girl' to Donald Farfrae and intimates that she is largely instrumental in her own downfall: 'She was terrible careless of appearances'.[50] He excuses his failure to protect her reputation as a consequence of illness and a generally 'dreary state'. After Henchard's remarriage to Susan, Lucetta writes begging him to keep their illicit liaison 'secret outside this isle'.[51] Her later insistence on innocence, despite appearances to the contrary and the ensuing social censure, is met by Henchard's observation: 'But it is not by what is, in this life, but by what appears, that you are judged'.[52] Her refusal to accept Henchard's belated proposal of marriage, and hence the chance to be reinstated to the dominant symbolic order, secures her place in the gender politics of the text as a disruptive element that must be contained if social order is to be restored.

In *Casterbridge*, as in several of his other novels, Hardy is interested in exploring that which is kept at bay by normative value systems, and which for him, as for many of his peers, continues to simmer at the borders of the decorous. Before becoming the respectable Mayor of Casterbridge, the young Henchard drank to excess and sold his wife Susan and their child to a stranger at a country fair. His new home, for all its social order, is merely a thin veneer of English values over the deeper reminders of foreign colonisation. The 'Ring', an ancient amphitheatre, is beyond the town's boundaries and is the point of convergence for its Roman antecedents and more recent English identity. It is also the favoured site for furtive meetings, intrigue and the unlawful. The town's subsoil is populated with the remains of Roman soldiers and their detritus, which at times resurface to an unfazed township. In Freudian terms, the Ring functions as the barely repressed subconscious of the town and the locus for all that remains 'improper'.

In nineteenth-century social realist fiction, female epileptic characters conform either to the disordered but domestically earnest characterisation of a Guster or to an eroticised convulsive femininity. After the incident with the man at Madam Bubovna's, Vanya takes Yelena back to his lodgings to care for her. He lays her on the sofa, unfastens the hooks of her dress and sprinkles her with water:

> Fever and delirium were setting in. I looked at her pale little face, at her colourless lips, at her black hair, tumbling down one side, though originally well brushed and pomaded, at her whole get-up, at the pink bows which still remained here and there on her dress – and I understood fully the whole of this hideous affair. Poor little thing! She grew worse and worse. I did not leave her, and I resolved not to go to Natasha's that evening. Now and then Yelena raised her long eyelashes and glanced up at me, and gazed long and intently as though she were recognizing me.[53]

Although there is no question in the scene of Vanya's propriety and genuine concern for Yelena, there is nevertheless an authorial recognition of her eroticisation, with the imagery of 'tumbling' black hair, her gazing 'long and intently' from her raised 'long eyelashes', her fever and delirium.

In *Bleak House, The Brothers Karamazov, The Insulted and Humiliated, Silas Marner* and *The Mayor of Casterbridge* the seizure-prone characters personify nineteenth-century concerns with notions of the fragmented self and social disintegration. In the nineteenth-century realist novel, these concerns are often located with the convulsive figure of the hybrid, a figure that evokes notions of cultural instability and fragmentation. Both Dickens and Dostoevsky played major parts in constituting and further developing the currency of the hybrid figure for twentieth-century literature. The hybrid figure also functions in opposition to the dominant real and social conventions, thus interrogating and destabilising those norms. It is only through reintegration or exorcism of the figure that any further threat to the status quo can be aborted and a superficial semblance of order recuperated. Smerdyakov is exorcised. His remorse at not being able to control his murderous desires leads him to hang himself. Yelena's convulsive vulnerability to the social and psychological traumas of life is compounded by her congenitally weak heart and she dies after making Vanya vow to marry the healthy and non-convulsive Natasha. Neither character has offspring.

In this literary climate, only those who do not threaten or undermine the dominant order survive. Guster 'survives' and can perhaps be best understood as a nineteenth-century version of the 'safe' epileptic. She has no ambitions beyond her station and is unlikely to contaminate the 'normal' gene pool. She is earnest in her service to the dominant order and compliant in her own marginalisation. Her seizures have symbolic value as manifestations of, and outlets for, all that cannot be expressed within the confines of bourgeois culture. In essence, she is the safety valve for the Snagsby household, venting what cannot be contained within the boundaries of respectability; her position in the household ensures the ultimate survival of its integrity. Her practical and symbolic utility within the aesthetics and politics of the novel also ensure her ongoing survival, if not complete integration into the dominant order.

Although Silas's seizures dis-integrate him from urban society, he, like Guster, accepts marginality and does not challenge social order. Nor does he seek to contaminate the 'normal' gene pool of Raveloe society with his paroxysmal tendencies. These factors, coupled with the ambiguity of his seizure condition, allow him to eventually achieve a reintegration of sorts as a surrogate parent to Eppie; and they also allow nineteenth-century readers to accept this reintegration as plausible.

Lucetta, on the other hand, embodies unruliness and must be excised from the healthy and decorous social body. She will not comply with her social and sexual marginalisation. Her potential for disturbing the protocols of public decorum cannot be contained within the borderlands demarcating and protecting respectable society: she usurps – albeit unwittingly – Elizabeth-Jane's position and marries Donald, the new Mayor of Casterbridge, so moving to the very heart of middle-class respectability. Moreover, her pregnancy threatens this middle-class respectability with hereditary disorder. Her seizures, when they finally occur in the advanced stages of her pregnancy, are the *sine qua non* of what has become, at this point in the narrative, an intractable impulse to transgression. Her death clears the way for a resumption of the relationship between Donald and Elizabeth-Jane and signals the restoration of 'respectable' femininity to the centre of the book's moral universe.

Although Lucetta's seizures are described as 'epileptic', their onset during pregnancy would seem to be indicative of eclampsia, a condition already recognised in the late nineteenth century as being due to some acute underlying cause. Nevertheless, symbolically and medically, the seizures are suggestive. In symbolic terms they affirm the incommensurability of her cultural identity with middle-class English mores. From a medical perspective, they suggest her potential as a carrier of hereditary 'taint'. Many physicians still believed in the late nineteenth century that eclampsia was a manifestation of acute and causally specific epilepsy. The seizures might resolve when the underlying cause was successfully treated, but the condition might also be the precursor to an 'epileptic habit' and result in a chronic impulse to seizure.

Transgressive sensuality, 'foreign' excitability and a vulnerability to seizure, traits deployed so effectively by Hardy to construct this incarnation of doomed femininity, also become markers of pathogenic sexuality in medical narratives of epilepsy. Although sex and spasm were not a new duo in the medical cosmos, the nineteenth-century medical gaze began to keenly reconsider the significance of its coupling for modern epileptology.

IV

Temkin reminds us that 'both Hippocrates and Democritus were credited with saying that "coitus is a slight epileptic attack"'.[54] In 'Dostoevsky and parricide' Freud reminds readers that 'the earliest physicians described coition as a minor epilepsy' and suggests that Dostoevsky's 'strong innate bisexual disposition' was perhaps implicated in his propensity to seize.[55] Michel Foucault notes the associations between the sexual act and the paroxysms of epilepsy recorded by Galen.[56] For Galen, the process of convulsion was the same as any other involuntary act. The seizures of epilepsy represent the body's efforts to rid the brain of an obstruction of 'thick humor', the agitation of epileptic seizures resembling 'the performance of the *aphrodisia*'. 'For in violent attacks of epilepsy', wrote Galen, 'semen is expelled because the whole body and with it the generative parts are strongly convulsed'.[57] Foucault – following Galen's lead – reads *aphrodisia* from an unreservedly male perspective, drawing connections between the thick humour obstructing healthy brain function and an accumulation of sperm in the testicles.

Echoing the views of Hippocrates, Democritus and Galen, in a somewhat breathless style, the nineteenth-century British physician Marshall Hall implies a forbidden eroticised potential located with the seizing body. At the same time, he also affirms its potential for criminality, by associating suspension of respiration in *grand mal* seizure with phenomena observed with death by hanging:

> I scarcely dare touch upon the phenomena presented by the generative system during strangulation by suspension. It is well known that those organs are excited, and that there are erection and emission of semen, in the male subject, and a uterine flow in the female. It is said that a recourse to a temporary suspension has been had by the sensualist. It is said that in this manner an unintentional suicide has been committed.[58]

In a more matter-of-fact tone, Gowers claims that:

> Masturbation in boys is undoubtedly an occasional cause, but the attacks which result from this influence are more frequently hysteroid than epileptic, or they present a hybrid character, so that it is difficult to say in which category they are to be placed.[59]

Along with many of his contemporaries, Gowers believed that circumcision was not inappropriate in cases of chronic youthful masturbation. Perhaps reflecting the irresolvable tensions in medical thinking about orgasmic and epileptic spasms – both, after all, disordered states – male epileptics were deemed to be violent and hyposexual, yet prone to the secret vice of onanism. Female epileptics were simultaneously eroticised and sexually negated by their problematically spasming bodies.

The erotic potential and seductiveness of the female convulsive body were identified, recorded and (re)presented by Charcot. With colleagues Paul Richer, Gilles de la Tourette and Albert Londe, he created a collection of images of these convulsive moments which eventually comprised the four-volume set *Nouvelle iconographie de La Salpêtrière*. His Tuesday lectures at La Salpêtrière drew both the medical fraternity and the intelligentsia of his day to view orchestrated performatives from the hysterical and hystero-epileptic patients under his care. In presenting a young woman to his Tuesday audience on 7 February 1888, the physician demonstrates a 'typical' case of what he called *la grande hystérie.* Rather dramatically, the young woman is brought into the amphitheatre on a stretcher. Charcot tells the audience that the woman has a 'hysterogenic point on her back, another under her left breast, and a third on her leg'[60] and that, for the purpose of the day's lesson, he will focus stimulation of the hysterogenic point on her leg.

For reasons unrecorded, when Charcot gives the signal for the lesson to commence, the attending intern touches the hysterogenic point beneath the young woman's left breast. The patient immediately begins those 'exotic movements' that the physician has identified as the signature of this particular form of disorder. As she moves through the various phases, Charcot provides commentary:

> Now, here we have the epileptoid phase. Remember this sequence – epileptoid phase, arched back, then vocalizations. The arched back that you see now is rather pronounced. Now here comes the phase of emotional outbursts, which fuses with the back arching, and now there is the contracture phase.[61]

The 'attack' is stimulated several times for the edification of the presumably all-male audience as Charcot continues with his commentary. At one point the young woman cries out 'Oh! Mother' and Charcot urges the audience to note the 'screams': 'You could say it is a lot of noise over nothing. True epilepsy is much more serious and also much more quiet.'[62]

Through the ages, historic and functional connections between sexual and cerebral paroxysms were to give rise to a group of therapeutic practices which included: imposing sexual abstinence; recommending 'unseasonable coition';[63] castration; clitoridectomy; and hystero-oophorectomy (the surgical removal of the uterus and both ovaries). In North America the last procedure was known as 'Battey's operation', named for the Professor of Obstetrics at Atlanta Medical College, Robert Battey, who first performed it in 1872.[64] Beliefs that sexual intercourse, sexual abstinence, sexual excess or sexual aberration could all exacerbate, or be exacerbated by, the symptoms of epilepsy persisted into the twentieth century.

Canadian psychoanalyst Ernest Jones informed delegates at a North American meeting of the National Association for the Study of Epilepsy in 1910 about the 'stronger and more imperious sexual desires' notable in those with chronic epilepsy.[65] It was generally believed by physicians around this time and beyond that epilepsy had a disinhibiting effect on the libido and those sexual drives normally held in check by socialisation and the conventions of propriety. This deviant eroticisation of the convulsing body assumes a somewhat ironic resonance when one recalls Temkin's observation that the patron saint of lovers *and* epileptics is St Valentine.[66]

Within the representational economies of late nineteenth-century British and American medical cultures, the more florid or overtly eroticised aspects of some seizure conditions were inevitably ascribed to Gallic or Latinate races: in other words, they were located more 'naturally' with the Lucette Le Sueurs of the world rather than the Elizabeth-Janes. Yet these eroticised qualities also remained as a barely expressible subtext in representations of the Anglo epileptic body.

In an echo of the Middle Ages, a *Lancet* editorial reported an outbreak of convulsive behaviour that began in January 1878 in the Tolmezzo district of Italy. This outbreak started in the local convent, with a spate of 'convulsive and clamorous attacks', and quickly spread to the surrounding districts.[67] The epidemic proved extremely obstinate, reportedly requiring intervention from the military to help stem its spread. It was pointed out by a Dr Franzolini that among the predisposing factors was a 'tendency to functional nervous diseases' among the general population of Tolmezzo. M. Colin argued that, due to the relative isolation of the district, 'Consanguineous marriages will be common ... and will contribute to the deterioration of the masses, and to the development of any common morbid predisposition'. It was further noted in the editorial that although such epidemics were now rare, the incident served as a reminder of the frequency of such events in ages past: 'Even in our own day, in some backward races, as of Norway and New Caledonia, similar outbreaks have been observed'.[68]

An item in the *British Medical Journal* claimed that evidence suggested male hysteria and hystero-epilepsy were frequent among semi-civilised nations.[69] In a discussion of hystero-epilepsy published on 16 February 1889, Dr Hughes Bennett observed that although rare (in males), some cases of the syndrome could be found 'abroad amongst men of the Latin races'.[70] A review of instances of hysteria and 'tremulousness' in males suggested that 'Frenchmen are far more subject to hysteria in adult life than Englishmen.... In a more excitable race, more acute nervous symptoms might be expected.'[71] Walter Friedlander recorded a very similar observation attributed to C. Mills in the 1886 medical textbook *A System of Practical Medicine by American Authors*; Mills went on to note that 'natives of more moderate or colder climes' are far less likely to be afflicted.[72] These rhetorical moves that located predisposition to convulsive disorder with women, the lower classes and beyond national boundaries were eventually to converge with growing concerns about racial and social degeneration.

Through the latter decades of the nineteenth century, medical frustration at the inability to control, if not eradicate, epilepsy found purchase in a range of extreme responses to the disorder. In a discussion of treatments, Marshall Hall in 1838 observed: 'Convulsion is frequently prevented for hours together by continuously watching the threatening of it, and dashing cold water on the face'.[73] As late as 1880, Gowers was advising in lectures that cold water over the head was often a successful antidote to convulsion: 'in severe attacks a moderate quantity only excites redoubled violence, while a second gallon is often more effectual than the first. This has the disadvantage of drenching the patient's head, and often giving cold.'[74] With what can only be unintended irony, Gowers informed his medical colleagues in 1893: 'Many epileptics die by drowning'.[75] Although he links his observation here to those occasions when one might fall into water at the moment of seizing, it cannot but resonate with a general advocacy for aggressive treatments that could and did result in death for the patient. Gowers' recommended use of a couple of gallons of cold water over the head of the violently seizing individual formed part of a rather desperate tradition of deflecting the threat of convulsion with counter-irritants. Setons, ligatures (thought to be particularly effective in Jacksonian epilepsy), blisters and, in some specific cases where a tender digital scar was thought to excite symptoms, amputation of the offending digit were all deployed in medicine's fight against stubborn disorder. Gowers suggested that in merely making a hole in the skull by trephining one might be said to be applying an 'energetic counter-irritation'.[76]

None of these medical responses to the syndrome was new or particularly original; most, if not all, along with much of the available pharmacopoeia, had been used by physicians for centuries. Earlier in Hall's article he acknowledged that washing the hands in cold water could induce an epileptic attack. Conflation of cures and causes was to become a controversial and continuing problem in epileptology. Working from the premise that convulsion was preceded by and contingent on 'closure of the larynx, forcible efforts of respiration, and general spasmodic contraction of the muscles', Dr Hall italicised the possibility (the 'singular idea') 'that *tracheotomy would effectively prevent the epileptic seizure*'.[77]

Trephining came back into fashion and, as I have indicated above, castration was to be joined by a developing trend towards hystero-oophorectomy. In 1887 a Dr Chiarleoni claimed that sham hystero-oophorectomy was as effective as surgical removal of the female organs of reproduction as long as the patient remained convinced of her own sterilisation. It was felt that the success of this type of intervention might obviate the need for actual 'spaying'.[78] Some months later Dr Francis Imlach related the success of hystero-oophorectomy in a forty-year-old woman with a twenty-year history of epileptic fits/hystero-epilepsy: 'Had this treatment been carried out years ago, the patient would probably have been a useful housewife, free from pain, and a fit companion to her husband, in place of a hopeless and expensive invalid'.[79] After recounting the death of a woman after oophorectomy to control her paroxysmal 'behaviours' in the *Australasian Medical Gazette*, J. D. Dunlop writes: 'It has been said that anaesthetising the patient and letting her believe on waking that some operation has been performed has been successful in curing the disease. I have not seen this tried.'[80] A physician relating two cases histories in a paper titled 'Clinical remarks on pseudo-peritonitis and epilepsy in hysteria' concluded, after the demise of one of his female patients, that the symptoms of epilepsy were often indistinguishable from hystero-epilepsy.[81]

Towards the end of the century an increasing number of physicians in Britain and the United States began to question ovarian involvement in hysteria and hystero-epilepsy conditions. Indeed, Gowers was unequivocal in his statement that: 'No case has come under my notice suggesting that uterine or ovarian disease can be regarded as a cause of epilepsy'.[82] Charcot was no less vocal about the issue – and his younger English colleague – telling one of his Tuesday audiences: 'In England there is a highly distinguished physician, Dr Gowers, who does not believe my descriptions. He sees things quite differently.... We are seeing the same thing and calling it by different names.'[83] The French physician insisted that ovarian involvement *was* a factor in some forms of convulsive disorder, if only for some patients: 'Clearly, all subjects are not ovarian'.[84] Despite his attachment to the ovarian theory, Charcot was adamant in his denouncement of the surgical operations being performed on convulsive women in America and elsewhere, and was furious that some American physicians cited his work in the medical rationale for hystero-oophorectomy.

Friedlander points out that there were prominent American physicians who viewed oophorectomy and hystero-oophorectomy with the 'severest condemnation' and argued that this 'unsexing' of women had no therapeutic value in the treatment of epilepsy. Nevertheless, a physician told his colleagues at a meeting of the New York Neurological Society in 1892: 'So far as unsexing an epileptic was concerned ... [I do] not understand how or why there was reason to feel compunction at such a suggestion.... [I can] hardly question the protective value to society not only of forbidding epileptics to marry, but of rendering them unable to procreate.'[85] Oophorectomy and hystero-oophorectomy continued to be performed on both sides of the Atlantic and in Australia for some time to come, and eugenicist arguments against procreation for those with epilepsy continued to amplify as the century drew to a close.

In an unusually cool and compassionate tone, D. de Berdt Hovell was to turn the defining medical gaze back on his colleagues when he suggested that, in matters of hysteria and hystero-epilepsy, doctors had lost sight of their purpose:

> Here it seems to me that the physicians – aye, and surgeons too – have frequently become the subjects of the 'morbus hystericus,' inasmuch as they have become the subjects of 'mental perversity,' and are not wholly free from a certain amount of 'moral obliquity'; for here, instead of being therapeutic and curative, the doctor has become vindictive, and desired to punish the patient whom his own want of skill has failed to relieve.[86]

The type of surgical interventions fostered by Battey, Chiarleoni and Imlach fall within the purview of de Berdt Hovell's diagnostic gaze, as do the treatment regimes critically identified by Joseph Williams and J. Thompson Dickson (see Chapter 1). At the end of his article, in relation to hysteria, de Berdt Hovell argues that mismanagement of paroxysmal disorders 'has, not in a few instances, gone on to the "bitter end" of the death of the patient'.[87]

Gowers attempted to cut through the entanglement of terminology and category instability haunting this aspect of the epilepsy debates by following a colleague's lead and deploying the term 'hysteroid' for those convulsive states obviously *not* epileptic. Nevertheless, he acknowledged that differentiation remained problematic. He was noted as a meticulous observer and analysed his clinical findings with systematic care, and this inability to definitively tease out salient differences between epileptic seizure and hysterical convulsion remained a source of frustration in his work. Gowers differed from Charcot in that he was prepared to allow that these convulsive disorders could present as a combined form, while Charcot maintained their status as separate paroxysmal processes. Charcot was as uncomfortable with the term 'hystero-epilepsy' as Gowers. He argued that what he was observing was basically an extreme form of hysteria – *la grande hystérie* – that presented with aspects of epileptoid symptomatology.

Gowers' dissatisfaction with Charcot's clinical observations provided some interesting subtext in his hypotheses on the subject. In a footnote to his section on epileptic and hysteroid symptomatology in *A Manual of Diseases of the Nervous System,* he takes an oblique swipe at his French counterpart: 'It is said that French hysterics bite their tongues during the attacks. In this country tongue-biting is practically confined to epilepsy.'[88] More explicitly, in the Gulstonian series of lectures on epilepsy published in 1880, Gowers refuted Charcot's thesis that by applying ovarian pressure a physician could either provoke or curtail an attack of hysteroid convulsion. This feature, it seemed, was the provenance of a more exotic female sexuality than that manifested by his female patients at Queen Square. Gowers claimed that another point of difference between his patient population and that written up by Charcot was that 'in the natives of this country, [hystero-epilepsy] is never, as far as I have seen, accompanied by any erotic manifestations'.[89] One might assume that if this racialised symptom did manifest itself, Gowers would draw on the treatment recommended above and throw a bucket or two of cold water over the doubly recalcitrant patient. North American physicians were equally steadfast in their insistence that women in the United States had ovaries that were made of tougher stuff than those of the more excitable French females and could withstand significant discomfort without succumbing to fits of hysteria.

Charcot refused to remain silent on the matter and told the audience at one of his Tuesday lectures that:

> It would seem by some accounts that hysteroepilepsy exists only in France; in fact, it has been said that it exists only at the Salpêtrière, as if I have created this condition by my own willpower. What a marvel this would be if I could, in fact, fabricate illnesses according to my whims and fantasies. But in fact all I am is a photographer. I describe what I see.[90]

Charcot's claim for a photographic eye that merely records and reflects back to medical science that which it focuses on is indicative of the interpretive power of the medical gaze. As I have argued in Chapter 1, the relation between disease and the medical gaze is mutually constitutive. Despite their many differences, Charcot and Gowers share a common trait: both physicians exhibit a sublime lack of awareness of their own constitutive functions. Where Charcot's gaze apprehends a particularly florid and eroticised convulsiveness in his female patients, Gowers perceives 'therio-mimicry' in epileptic patients who mew 'like a cat, or, much more frequently, [bark] like a dog'.[91] The two physicians were equally convinced of their own objective perceptiveness.

Charcot expressed complete confidence in his ability to differentiate between the paroxysms of genuine hysteria and a sham performance. He used hypnosis to induce trance and then measured his female patients' ability to maintain muscle posture while they held their arms at extension for prescribed periods of time. He argued that those with 'true' hysteria could sustain the pose without exhibiting any signs of undue stress in muscle or respiration, while those who were faking their condition quickly became fatigued. Nevertheless, he acknowledged: 'How sly, clever, and unexpectedly tenacious these women can be when in the midst of their mental disorder, they try to fool people, especially when the would-be victim is a doctor'.[92] When one of Charcot's more famous female hysterics, Blanche (Marie) Whittman, was asked by a physician at the end of her life whether at least some of the episodes made famous in the Tuesday lectures might have been simulated, she responded:

> None whatsoever.... We had these spells and were in these lethargic states because we could not do otherwise.... Simulation! Do you think it would have been easy to fool Dr. Charcot? Oh yes, lots of fakes tried; he gave them one look and said, 'Be still'.[93]

Blanche Whittman's convulsive episodes were eventually to cease a few years after Charcot's death. However, she did not completely abandon La Salpêtrière or her service to medical science: she became a radiology technician and was to eventually die of radiation-induced cancer.

Historically, the 'pinch method' had been a recommended strategy for differentiating between paroxysms of epilepsy and those associated with hysteria. The Hippocratic physicians suggested that three fingers were best for this procedure. The reasoning was that if the patient reacted, the episode was likely hysterical, but if the patient remained insensible, it was likely due to epilepsy. Gowers' biographer, Macdonald Critchley, claims that the neurologist had his own favoured response to paroxysms of questionable origin. In a gesture oddly Victorian in both its punitive puritanism and incontinent display (not to mention its latent misogynism – I find it difficult to imagine Gowers applying this method to his male patients), he was evidently prone to tugging vigorously on the pubic hair of the offending party and recommended this style of intervention to his junior colleagues.[94]

Gowers' scepticism about the applicability of Charcot's model to English paroxysmal behaviours aside, there were those who argued that the French writers (especially Charcot) had in fact recorded the more important description of hystero-epilepsy. Charcot's contributions to medical thinking on hysteria and hystero-epilepsy formed the basis of the discussion on hysterical anaesthesia. Although Gowers insisted on the absence of eroticism in English paroxysmal events, colleagues continued to record accounts that, while appearing to offer a counter-argument, nevertheless maintained the notion that paroxysmally related eroticism was somehow the consequence of some form of exoticism. Dr Sansom and Mr G. T. Stonham recount a case of hystero-epilepsy in a twenty-one-year-old, 'fairly intelligent' English woman, albeit one who was Roman Catholic and had lived in Canada from the age of thirteen to seventeen, 'with phases like those described by Charcot'.[95] In recording his agreement with Charcot's theories of an erotic component to hysterical convulsion, Wilfred Kingdon suggests that in the Anglo-Saxon race the disease is not infrequently traceable to over-education or improper education for women.[96]

Within this over-wrought environment of claim and counter-claim of what was and what was not epilepsy, the association of epilepsy with the inferior and feminised body became a constant. Men who were diagnosed with epilepsy, hystero-epilepsy, or the homologous hysteria/ hypochondria, had both their masculinity and racial antecedents thrown into question. In quoting Leslie Camhi's comments on 'the cadaverising gaze' of nineteenth-century medicine, Lisa Cartwright reproduces Camhi's point that there is 'a subtle encoding of feminized bodies in the pure materiality of epileptic movement and uncontrolled musculature of both male and female epileptics'.[97] Further, she argues, epilepsy manifesting in women was regarded by Spratling 'as innate, degenerate, and incurable – manageable only through the intervention of surgery', a philosophy he extended to a male patient identified as 'black' in his reports from the Craig Epileptic Colony.[98] For males, surgical intervention included testicular manipulation and surgical removal.

Apprehensions about hereditary transmission continued to gain ground and the notion of epilepsy as a primary hereditary pollutant or taint assumed greater conviction as nineteenth-century neurology developed. According to Temkin, statistics of the time suggested inheritance in about thirty per cent and Gowers considered hereditary a factor in about thirty-six per cent of all cases of primary epilepsy.

Gowers repeatedly deployed the idea of taint and inherited taint in writings and transcripts of his lectures. He insisted that the most effective treatment should begin with early detection where possible, before negative patterns were established; but it was prevention that would provide the most significant defence against the disorder. Although Dr Fletcher Beach, in a reported discussion of the subject that included Gowers and others, suggested 'that inheritance alone was not sufficient to produce epilepsy or insanity, but that many causes acting together produce the result',[99] he remained the dissenting voice of a minority. A developing literature of anxiety began to organise around the concept of hereditary taint; this anxiety found voice in the correspondence section of the *Lancet*.

Part of the problem of curtailing sexual reproduction in males with epilepsy syndromes was met by the widespread use of bromides. Bromide caused significant to complete suppression of sexual function. However, this did not resolve the issue of female reproduction; libido has never been necessary to conception. It was reported in January 1897 that Dr Gowers had laid down 'rules for guidance when the medical practitioner's opinion is sought respecting the marriage of an epileptic female':

> Dr. Gowers says that to the patient herself marriage and even pregnancy will make little difference, whilst the man who aspires to the hand of an epileptic lady must look to the severity of the disease and the extent to which it threatens mental powers, and must decide for himself whether he will inflict upon himself a wife with such an infirmity.[100]

Gowers argued that there were two aspects of the question to be considered: the possibility that marriage might 'involve deleterious sexual excess'; and the possibility of 'transmitted taint'.[101] If epilepsy was due to some secondary cause or lesion of the brain, he suggested, then one need not fear that future generations would be affected. However, he cautioned that the very great probability of hereditary taint was predictable if there was a traceable family history of epilepsy or insanity. His counsel was relatively conservative. Although he felt that the well-being of the community should preclude such marriages, he was reluctant at this stage to remove the ultimate decision from the individual. However, his claim that only those marked by true or idiopathic epilepsy would pass on the taint sparked a flurry of responses.

William G. Thistle became the main protagonist in a debate on the subject. He insisted that Gowers was being precipitate in his belief that not all epilepsy was hereditary.[102] This stance was quickly refuted by Edwin Ray Lankester, a respected Darwinian zoologist and author of *Degeneration: A Chapter in Darwinism* (1880), who defended Gowers' ideas with considerable anecdotal evidence.[103] Thistle responded by bringing in his own bevy of case histories and the evidence of a Dr Rolleston. He challenged his colleagues with the following reasoning:

> In the matter of epilepsy, we find traumatism, syphilis, alcohol, and the thousand other causes producing the disease *de novo* daily. How can we avoid the conclusion that the hereditary cases arose in a similar manner?

> If they did not, then from what did they arise? Did the creator plant a few original epileptics fully developed to disseminate the disease?[104]

James Adams pointed out that hereditary tendency was not always 'willingly acknowledged, endeavours to trace it are met by very circumstantial accounts of various injuries, and reasons'. He expanded on this position by arguing that 'perhaps in no form of cerebral disease is more ingenuity displayed than in accounting for the origin of epileptic fits'.[105]

The debate around hereditary probability and whether or not epileptics should be allowed to marry continued in the correspondence section of the journal into May 1897, but the defining word may be said to have gone to Mabel Anderson, Lady Superintendent of the Meath Home for Epileptics. Anderson's comments cut to the heart of the matter. For her, susceptibility to seizure – regardless of specific cause – must, for any right-thinking person, disqualify those affected from procreation. Any other conversation about the matter is therefore redundant. She tells the medical fraternity:

> Any one knowing much of epileptics – whether suffering from immediate traumatic epilepsy or transmitted or obscure epilepsy – must know that even the best of them are quite unfitted for responsibility. They may be abled up to certain points in music, art, literature, or manual work; but they are always subject to fits of more or less irresponsibility, they are always uncertain and not to be relied upon, and thus are quite unfit to have the training or hold the destinies of others in their hands.[106]

Anderson can only have applauded trends in literature that similarly represented those 'subject to fits' as 'unfitted for [parental] responsibility'. I wonder where she might have stood in relation to Silas Marner's fostering of Eppie?

Although issues of hereditary taint were to disappear from the correspondence section of the *Lancet* in the short term, they were not to disappear from medical, state or legal discourse. These concerns were soon to resurface in the pages of medical journals on both sides of the Atlantic, as well as Australia, *vis-à-vis* the burgeoning eugenics movement and an escalating interest in the possibilities of epileptic colonies and work farms as modes of containment.

V

The style of medical reportage explored here and in other chapters of this book became a recurring sub-genre in late nineteenth- and early twentieth-century medical journals and seemed to serve a particular type of function within newly developing discourses of epileptology. It provided a space where unscientific beliefs about the relations between epilepsy, social disorder and racial and cultural difference could be expressed safely beyond the borders of scientific rationalism. These items often entailed accounts of incidents occurring in foreign populations. This genre of medical writing also appeared to operate as some sort of conceptual hold-all for those cultural anxieties not yet re-articulated as biomedical truth.

Kathryn Montgomery Hunter marks the importance of the anecdote in the circulation of medical knowledge. On the one hand, she argues, the anecdotal ranks high in the list of pejoratives in western medicine; on the other, however, it persists in oral narrative as an important if neglected aspect of the way that medical knowledge is transmitted. 'The vehemence with which they [anecdotes] are condemned', she writes, 'suggests the collective pain of those moments in medical progress when the old understanding stood in the path of the new.'[107] Hunter argues that while the anecdote is perceived by some as a 'dangerous assertion of personality in a scientific field', it is nevertheless a necessary and intellectually healthy adjunct to the narrative development of medicine, functioning as a constant reminder of the uncertain and interpretative domain of medical inquiry.[108] Although late nineteenth-century journals were increasingly publishing extended analytical surveys of the type developed at Queen Square and other specialist hospitals, the anecdote of the single case that made or disturbed a taxonomic rule still seemed to hold some attraction for the Victorian readership of the *Lancet* and the *British Medical Journal*.

Throughout this textual repertoire it is also possible to discern the complexity of the medical project to comprehend epilepsy and 'the epileptic' as neurophysiological objects. The pursuit of biomedical knowledge about epilepsies repeatedly looped back to the establishment of medical control over perceived epileptic social and sexual intransigence. This doubling between medical and social models of epilepsy is examined further in the following chapter. For now, though, I want to suggest that these are not necessarily antithetical agendas. It has been argued that the will to knowledge can be traced back to the will to conquer and control.[109] If we accept that the connections between knowledge and power identified in western philosophy have valence, then it is possible to begin the task of examining the apparent contradictions in medicine's brief to heal – or at least to do no harm – in its encounters with this most troubling of bodies.

A waning in medical optimism about eradicating disorders amassed under the rubric of 'epilepsy' coincided with an escalation of social anxiety about the apparent corruption festering within the boundaries of western civilisations. As the nineteenth century drew to a close, western industrialised society seemed beset by a plethora of deviant bodies. Technologies of normalisation infused discourses of degeneration. Calls for urgent social reform became strident, and there was moral panic as social orthodoxies sought to identify and contain sites of internal contamination. Gareth Stedman Jones has emphasised the impact of an expanding poor and pauper population in the large city slums on late nineteenth-century social consciousness:

> The most characteristic image of the working class was that of increasingly prosperous and cohesive communities bound together by the chapel, the friendly society, and the co-op. Pitted against the dominant climate of moral and material improvement however was a minority of the still unregenerate poor: those who had turned their backs on progress, or had been rejected by it. This group was variously referred to as 'the dangerous class', the casual poor or most characteristically, as 'the residuum'.[110]

This upsurge of social anxiety about the price progress seemed to be exacting on the body politic sparked a flurry of commentary and investigations: 'Industry, capitalism and social mobility', notes Daniel Pick, 'appeared to produce a feverish political and physiological unrest'.[111]

Within this climate of somaphobia – a fear of the body deemed unmanaged or unmanageable – epilepsy was increasingly implicated in theories of mental, physical and social degeneration in biological evolutionary arguments central to discursive productions of the deviant body. By 1880, in Britain, Francis Galton had been working for nearly twenty years on what was to become the forerunner of statistical theories about regression and correlative factors. Suspected causal links between pathology – specifically epilepsy – and criminality had been theoretically consolidated by the turn of the century through the works of forensic specialists such as Cesare Lombroso and John Ferguson Nisbet. Lombroso was among those seeking the answers to society's problems in biological terms. His theories of social degeneracy placed those with epilepsy at the centre of a climate of increasing suspicion and rejection. The born criminal, the social deviant, the man of genius, he argued, were inscribed with the defining stigmata associated with 'the epileptic'. By the end of the century, the care taken by the likes of Hughlings Jackson to foreground a biomedical model of epilepsy was swamped by the recuperated figure of the demonised epileptic.

Foucault has argued that, in relation to psychiatric power, the asylum physician of the late nineteenth century 'is both the one who can tell the truth of the disease through the knowledge (*savoir*) he has of it and the one who can produce the disease in its truth and subdue it in its reality, through the power that his will exerts on the patient himself'.[112] He reads the relationships between disease and physician here through the work of the French scientist and bacteriologist Louis Pasteur, who uncovered the causal links between contagion and medical practice. Within this scenario, Foucault suggests that the physician not only produces through knowledge 'the disease "in its truth"' but in ignorance too often becomes an agent of propagation and dissemination.

Late nineteenth-century struggles to produce the biomedical truth of epilepsy and subdue this particular taxonomy of neurological disruption repeatedly foundered on a disaffection with the embodied subject of this therapeutic quest. Despite vigorous attempts to learn the limits of epilepsy syndromes, the epileptic body remained impervious to biomedicine's attempts to contain and administer its disorderliness well into the twentieth century. And despite prodigious efforts by the likes of Lombroso, Charcot and Hugh W. Diamond to map and visually record a definitive photographic and pictorial catalogue of epileptic physiognomies and physical features, the project to fix epileptic identity in a solution of corporeal characteristics, short of an epileptic equivalent of Nathaniel Hawthorne's scarlet letter to mark transgression, remained largely unfulfilled.

For a time, aggressive nineteenth-century treatments such as blistering and bleeding visually indexed the bodies of those with epilepsy as deviating from a healthy norm, but these therapeutic regimes were also used to treat conditions other than epilepsy. The florid acne-like rash often produced by long-term bromide use (a corporeal realisation of Hawthorne's stigma), with its accompanying torpidity and shambling gait, to some degree rendered the hitherto inaccessible visible to the medical gaze. By the turn of the century, and helped by the enthusiastic administration of bromides, epileptic sluggishness and lability had, to a point, materialised as reliable cues to identification. Nonetheless, as medical research moved into the new century, William Spratling was to reluctantly acknowledge that the causes of the syndrome had, in fact, eluded the medical gaze. Like Hughlings Jackson before him, Spratling had come to the conclusion that to speak of 'epilepsy' was erroneous: 'We must speak of the epilepsies', he asserted. Of the syndrome, he wrote:

> It is not a stable, fixed, definite, and, at this time, demonstrable cause that produces the convulsion, but something that comes and goes, that is most insidious – that is present to-day or this week, and absent to-morrow or the week after, and that often acts on an organism far below par.[113]

This apparent resignation to the elusiveness of his object did not dissuade Spratling from setting up and administering the 'Epilepsy Biographs', a series of cinematic case studies of his charges at the Craig colony (see Chapter 5). In doing so, he moved medicine's fascination with the visual signifiers of neurological difference a step further from the iconographies of Charcot towards the closed-circuit television monitoring of late twentieth-century electroencephalographic studies.

As I have been arguing, nineteenth-century medicine's escalating frustration with this state of affairs manifested with increasingly extreme therapeutic interventions, which resulted in the production of a body that came to epitomise its biomedical discursive formation. While symptoms of intellectual fragmentation, loss of motivation, physical and mental depression, apathy, irritability and recalcitrance affected some folk with epilepsy some of the time, systematic overuse of bromides dispersed these symptoms in epidemic proportions through epileptic populations not usually exhibiting them. Along with other side-effects, the bromides could also cause eruptions of an angry acne-like rash on the patient's skin, which, at the turn of the century, was often treated with arsenic. The arsenic then caused pigmentation loss. As the primary dispenser of these signs and symptoms, the physician became very much a part of the problem: both the site of contagion and the author of a visible and therefore medically knowable epileptic alterity.

Frustration at the intractability of the epileptic, if not the epilepsies, to medical intervention, despite being the focus of the best medical minds of the day, was foregrounded in the writings of Henry Maudsley, who veered towards prophylaxis rather than cure: 'It is a fact that a pathological evolution – or, more correctly, a pathological degeneration – of mind does take place through generations'.[114] In keeping with prevailing medical beliefs, he pointed out that, in the kinship web of nervous diseases and neurotic heritage, 'the most closely related ... are insanity and epilepsy; the descendant of an epileptic parent being almost if not quite as likely to become insane as to become epileptic, and one or other of the descendants of an insane parent not unfrequently suffering from epilepsy'.[115] Maudsley fluctuated between a profound pessimism in his accounts of an escalating degeneration observable in British society, arguing that it constituted a major counter-force to human evolution, and a belief that, in fact, the degenerate population represented a splintering malformation in human development. In line with the theories expounded by Bénédict Augustin Morel, he took comfort in the view that this deviating malformation would prove to be its own antidote, as degeneration would lead to sterility within a few generations. Although epilepsy was beginning to emerge as a distinct object for investigation, it was still usually referred to in conjunction with insanity, the two disorders often being represented as interchangeable within a milieu of medicalised deviant bodies.

Maudsley was a materialist and had garnered a reputation by the turn of the century for expressing his views on the subject of epilepsy in fairly extreme terms. The tone of his writing combines a stern pessimism about the inevitable degeneration of society with an oddly sentimental compassion for those deemed to be at the forefront of this decline. As Pick has argued, he both reflected and contributed to Victorian anxieties and debates about the proliferation of the deviant figure in the closing decades of the nineteenth century. Maudsley actively cultivated a religious, preaching persona in his texts, materially reinforcing this impression with his physical appearance in later life: 'his very appearance ... matched that image of the seer. A man with a straggling beard and piercing eyes, he wrote in a sombre and weighty style illuminated by vivid flashes of imagination.'[116] There are some notable similarities between the proselytising function of Maudsley's writing and that of William Lennox in the mid twentieth century (see Chapter 5). Both textually position themselves as being engaged in a morally elevated quest to rescue 'the epileptic' from a metaphorical pit of inexorable degradation.

Towards the end of the century these links between epilepsy and degeneration were taken up and extrapolated by Max Nordau in his work on the cultural dissemination of degenerative impulses. The book is dedicated to Lombroso and opens with a letter of gratitude to the physician and criminologist, lauding his work on identifying those pathological links between the degenerate, social transgression and crime. While praising the 'honoured Master's' efforts in pouring 'a veritable flood of light' onto the area of accurate identification of the degenerate, Nordau informs Lombroso of the work still to be done in tracking signs of deviance through 'a vast and important domain into which neither you nor your disciples have hitherto borne the torch of your method – the domain of art and literature'.[117] Nordau argued that the signs and symptoms of the degenerate proliferated in art, literature and society at the turn of the nineteenth century. In his social diagnosis of the decline of civilised and cultured society, he suggested that the closing decades of the century had produced a '*fin-de-siècle* state of mind'. This state of mind was marked by:

> practical emancipation from traditional discipline, which theoretically is still in force. To the voluptuary this means unbridled lewdness, the unchaining of the beast in man.... And to all, it means the end of

> an established order, which for thousands of years has satisfied logic, fettered depravity, and in every art matured something of beauty.[118]

Nordau's bleak view of society extended to fashion and home decor and he claimed that there was an increasing discordance between form and function.

By the end of the century, for Nordau, painting styles had become risible caricatures of art, music 'must continually promise, but never perform' and literature was just another site where human decadence postured as the norm:

> Mere sewage exhalations are played out. The filth of Zola's art and of his disciples in literary canal-dredging has been got over, and nothing remains for it but to turn to submerged peoples and social strata. The vanguard of civilization holds its nose at the pit of undiluted naturalism, and can only be brought to bend over it with sympathy and curiosity when, by cunning engineering, a drain from the boudoir and the sacristy has been turned into it.[119]

Nordau argued that the widespread rejection or even reversal of social and cultural standards of decorum and aesthetic norms associated with end-of-the-century disaffection could be located within the aetiology of degeneration.

To support this claim, he drew on biomedical discourses of degeneration and genetic taint. Nordau's interpretations of the noxious influences of the degenerate 'organism' on future generations were framed through the theories of Morel and developed through the works of Maudsley and Benjamin Ball, who had consigned the degenerate figure to the borders of mainstream society:

> Maudsley and Ball call them 'Borderland dwellers' – that is to say, dwellers on the borderland between reason and pronounced madness. Magnan gives to them the name of 'higher degenerates' ... and Lombroso speaks of 'mattoids' (from *matto*, the Italian for insane), and 'graphomaniacs,' under which he classifies those semi-insane persons who feel a strong impulse to write. In spite, however, of this variety of nomenclature, it is a question simply of one single species of individuals, who betray their fellowship by the similarity of their mental physiognomy.[120]

Nordau's text is unremittingly misanthropic; he writes like a man who has at last found his discursive milieu, the field where his deepest suspicions about society's ills can be finally articulated and resolved.

Structurally, the text locates itself within the field of bio(social) medicine, with lexical choices such as micro-organism, epidemic, morbidity, staphylococcus, streptococcus and bacilli, and sections titled 'Symptoms', 'Diagnosis', 'Prognosis' and 'Therapeutics'. Nordau positioned himself as the diagnostician and healer of an ailing society, marshalling theories of social Darwinism, forensic medicine and neurophysiology to support his thesis. These juxtapositions produce a grotesquely mutated curative in Nordau's closing arguments. In the final section, titled 'Therapeutics', Nordau exhorts the 'Mystics ... ego-maniacs, and filthy pseudo-realists' to be gone from the 'healthy organism' of civilised society: 'There is no place among us for the lusting beast of prey; and if you dare return to us, we will pitilessly beat you to death with clubs'.[121]

This kind of hate language is not easily dismissed. Obviously, though, it is an extreme example of its genre and its virulent prose is said to have inspired backlash productions such as the anonymous *Regeneration: A Reply* (1895) and George Bernard Shaw's *The Sanity of Art* (1908).[122] Nevertheless, throughout the pages of his text Nordau articulates many of the concerns and anxieties seeded in nineteenth-century productions of the epileptic. The undisciplined and undisciplinable epileptic body functions as a primary metaphor and embodied locus in turn-of-the-century tales of epidemic social fragmentation and decline. Nordau's reading of the degenerate, as lacking a sense of morality and of right and wrong, echoes Gowers' conviction that epileptics are often morally defective. Lombroso's work on the links between epilepsy, criminality and degeneracy form the cornerstone of Nordau's thesis in *Degeneration* and he insists that the degenerative spiral dragging civilised societies into the sewer must be curtailed at all costs. To this end, rigorous methods of identification of the disorder and then its containment or expulsion from the healthy organism were the recommended therapeutic response. This social therapeutic is realised to a degree with the inception of the colony movement for non-insane epileptics at the end of the century.

There were contemporaries of Nordau who strongly criticised this work. Pick argues that although there was a modicum of celebration of Nordau's theories for daring to frankly articulate that which had been dealt with a little more circumspectly hitherto, the work was also often dismissed as 'charlatanism'.[123] However, Pick adds to this observation that, while Nordau was taken to task for his generalisations and hysterical style of address, the validity of degeneration as a diagnostic category was not at stake in these criticisms. It is notable that *Degeneration* was translated from German into English, French, Spanish, Italian and Russian very soon after production. Although Freud, after meeting Nordau in Paris in 1886, dismissed him as 'vain and stupid',[124] his participation in and contributions to the discourses of degeneration cannot be simply jettisoned because his account of an ailing society's case history is couched in such florid terms. As Pick so cogently argues, Nordau's work demonstrates 'the crucial refraction' between medical and literary language; it also suggests the complexities of the intersections between the mythologies of culture and the intellectual development of western medicine. I will return to this point in later chapters.

As the 1890s ended, arguments for the benefits of segregation of 'the epileptic' from mainstream societies gained momentum in continental Europe, Britain, the United States and Australia, and, in a very short period of time, were translated into action. In keeping with a long history of complex and multiply inflected responses to the syndromes, this development was born out of a range of social, ideological and economic factors rather than a concerted focus on the health of those with epilepsy conditions. Mary Douglas's 1966 work *Purity and Danger* provides a useful platform from which to begin an examination of some of the deeper or subjugated influences underlying the 'feverish political and physiological unrest' later identified by Pick in relation to discourses of degeneration (see above). Over and above the latent threat of hereditary, psychic and cultural pollution, the epileptic body can be seen to violate those social constraints that maintain what Douglas calls the external boundaries between internally produced body fluids and the outside ordered environment of a community structured around rules of bodily containment and controlled permeability. She argues: 'The body is a model that can stand for any bounded system. Its boundaries can represent any boundaries which are threatened or precarious.'[125]

Transgressing the symbolic boundaries of social structure and corporeal containment that prevailed in western culture at the close of the nineteenth century, the body in *grand mal* seizure variously leaked spittle, blood, urine, faeces or sperm. Involuntary loss of control over those orifices both infantilises the adult body and contravenes those hallmarks of civilised subjectivity that hinge around socially constructed standards of self-discipline, cleanliness and order within dominant discursive regimes. Within these parameters, the loss of control represented by the seizing body necessarily signals a loss of subjectivity. Furthermore, the leaking human body challenges those privileged aesthetic values that define the symbolically clean and proper body. Douglas maps the various cultural meanings of dirt in European and primitive societies, working from the 'old definition' that 'dirt [is] matter out of place'. She argues that this proposal 'implies two conditions: a set of ordered relations and a contravention of that order'.[126]

Within the discursive environment of a late nineteenth-century British medical social economy, the figure of the epileptic represents embodied disorder. The leaking, jerking, uncontrolled body in *grand mal* seizure with its threat of hereditary pollution comes to epitomise 'matter out of place', a profound contravention and undermining of the social imperatives of an ordered and ordering culture. Preserving symbolic hygiene within this social and cultural environment is contingent on locating and identifying all sites of possible contamination, disorder and taint, then eliminating any threat of the unclean internal to the dominant system. Rather than being a negative response, this demonstrates, by Douglas's reckoning, a 'positive re-ordering' of the environment. The bounded system of nineteenth-century British society was represented and valorised through the white, middle-class, controlled, male body. This was the flesh and blood figure central to those discourses of normalisation circulating through both the intellectual aristocracy and the frameworks of capitalism. As the century drew to a close, the privilege of this authoritative norm was being threatened by upheavals in the socio-economic climate in Britain and an expanding working-class and pauper population. Feminism was being cited as a looming threat to the political and social status quo. The figure of the epileptic, with its concomitant class and gender associations, coupled with a growing belief that the epileptic could not function as a productive member of a society, indeed, could become a drain on that society's resources, became a locus for increasing social and cultural dis-ease.

By the end of the nineteenth century, efforts to reorder the environment by eliminating the disorder represented by the epileptic began to gain momentum, finding purchase in the growing debate around social Darwinism, eugenics, continued effective administration of the New Poor Law and a multinational development of colonies for non-insane epileptics. It was argued that placing non-insane epileptics in industrial villages or farming colonies, as they were variously called, was not only a humanitarian response to an intractable problem, but also nullified the danger that epileptics were reputed to represent to themselves and the general community. Having failed to contain the disorder from within, it was now time to excise it where possible from the healthy communal body. One of the conclusions that I want to draw from this chapter and explore further through the following pages is that, of all the voices that articulate epilepsy, the one that cannot register (with noted exceptions) within the discursive and symbolic systems under analysis is the voice of the subject with epilepsy.

Although specific signs, symptoms and behaviours coalesce through the decades bridging the nineteenth and twentieth centuries and become organised around medicalised theories of corporeality, this medicalised model neither is static nor completely displaces the rhetorical figure of the epileptic. This figure continues to be widely disseminated as a signifier of transgression and metaphysical menace in discourses of theology and superstition. Epilepsy and 'the epileptic' continue to be constituted through labyrinthine and shifting political, medical, social and cultural economies which often have little or nothing to do with those cerebral paroxysms defined as symptomatology.

Within this schema, the epileptic figure assumes the properties of an archive: multiple and layered significations accrete, each bearing traces of what has gone before. As the epileptic moves from religious signifier to literary device, to social pariah, to medical patient, shifts across multiple signifying possibilities are never linear, rarely sustained, never unambiguously demarcated. Because of this category instability, at various points in discursive histories the epileptic figure may bear the traces of all of these signifying economies, yet never be clearly defined by any single regime. The deployment of epilepsy in the debates sparked by Mary Glover's affliction is a case in point. Configured as a social, economic and moral problem, the epileptic has been the concern of both church and state. Defined as a particular type of threat to public health and safety or an overt manifestation of criminality, this figure becomes the object of a juridical discursive system. As a signifier of pathology, the figure becomes the object of biomedical inquiry and intervention. Within these discursive tangles and divergences, the markers of what constitutes epilepsy have expanded and contracted and expanded again, due to a combination of diagnostic ideology, technology and shifting defining boundaries. Despite conceptual (and categorical) fluctuations there is nevertheless a common thread through all of these discursive systems, regardless of boundary differences, that constructs the epileptic as a site of unruliness, disorder and abnormality.

Notes

1 Andrew Wynter. *The Borderlands of Insanity*. 2nd edition. London: Robert Hardwicke, 1875, p. 31.

2 Quoted in Elaine Showalter. *The Female Malady: Women, Madness and English Culture 1830–1980*. 1987. London: Virago, 1996, p. 105.

3 Max Nordau. *Degeneration*. London: Heinemann, 1895, p. 18.

4 W. R. Gowers. *The Border-Land of Epilepsy*. London: Churchill, 1907, preface, no page number.

5 The term 'psychomotor' had become part of the medical lexicon – albeit with limited circulation – by the early 1870s to describe a symptom that *may* be associated with some forms of epileptic seizure. It came into use to describe a particular form of epilepsy after the turn of century. See Owsei Temkin. *The Falling Sickness: A History of Epilepsy from the Greeks to the Beginnings of Modern Neurology*. 2nd edition, revised. Baltimore, MD: John Hopkins Press, 1971, p. 323.

6 Temkin, *The Falling Sickness*, p. 168.
7 Rudyard Kipling. 'The post that fitted'. 1886. *A Complete Collection of Poems by Rudyard Kipling*. http://www.poetryloverspage.com/poets/kipling/kipling_ind.html.
8 C. McDonald. 'Feigned epilepsy: case of James Clegg, *alias* James Lee, the "Dummy Chucker"'. *American Journal of Insanity*, vol. 37, 1880, pp. 1–22.
9 W. R. Gowers. *A Manual of Diseases of the Nervous System*. 2nd edition. 2 vols. London: Churchill, 1893, vol. 2, p. 732.
10 Gowers, *A Manual of Diseases*, vol. 2, p. 731.
11 Quoted in Lisa Cartwright. *Screening the Body: Tracing Medicine's Visual Culture*. 1995. MN: University of Minnesota Press, 1997, p. 66.
12 Cartwright, *Screening the Body*, p. 66.
13 S. Wilks. 'An address on some of the more unusual phenomena of epilepsy'. *British Medical Journal*, 2 January 1892, p. 5.
14 Wilks, 'An address', p. 5.
15 John Hughlings Jackson. 'On the comparative study of diseases of the nervous system (Leeds address)', 1889, in James Taylor, ed. *Selected Writings of John Hughlings Jackson*. 2 vols. London: Hodder and Stoughton, 1932, vol. 2, p. 395.
16 Jackson, 'On the comparative study of diseases of the nervous system', p. 398.
17 John Hughlings Jackson. 'On a particular variety of epilepsy ("intellectual aura"), one case with symptoms of organic brain disease', 1888, in James Taylor, ed. *Selected Writings of John Hughlings Jackson*. 2 vols. London: Hodder and Stoughton, 1932, vol. 1, pp. 386–91.
18 Temkin, *The Falling Sickness*, p. 366.
19 Sigmund Freud. 'Dostoevsky and parricide'. *Standard Edition of the Complete Psychological Works of Sigmund Freud*. Ed. and trans. James Strachey. Vol. 21 (1927–31). London: Hogarth Press, 1961, p. 179.
20 Freud, 'Dostoevsky and parricide', p. 181.
21 Freud, 'Dostoevsky and parricide', p. 180.
22 Fyodor Dostoyevsky. *The Brothers Karamazov*. 1880. Trans. and Introduction David McDuff. London: Penguin Classics, 1993, p. 141.
23 Dostoyevsky, *The Brothers Karamazov*, p. 142.
24 Dostoyevsky, *The Brothers Karamazov*, p. 732.
25 N. M. Lary. *Dostoevsky and Dickens: A Study of Literary Influence*. London: Routledge and Kegan Paul, 1973, p. ix.
26 Letter to Sonia Ivanova. Quoted in Lary, *Dostoevsky and Dickens*, p. 52.
27 Lary, *Dostoevsky and Dickens*, p. 67.
28 Charles Dickens. *Bleak House*. 1853. Ed. Norman Page. Introduction J. Hillis Miller. London: Penguin Classics, 1985, p. 180.
29 Dickens, *Bleak House*, pp. 201–2.
30 Dickens, *Bleak House*, p. 641.
31 Dickens, *Bleak House*, p. 416.
32 Fyodor Dostoyevsky. *The Insulted and Humiliated*. 1861. Trans. Olga Shartse. Foreword E. Starikova. Moscow: Progress Publishers, 1976, p. 145.
33 Gowers, *A Manual of Diseases*, vol. 2, p. 740.
34 Dickens, *Bleak House*, p. 180.
35 Dickens, *Bleak House*, p. 417.
36 George Eliot. *Silas Marner: The Weaver of Raveloe*. 1861. Ed. and Introduction Q. D. Leavis. Harmondsworth: Penguin, 1996, p. 110.
37 Eliot, *Silas Marner*, p. 9.
38 Eliot, *Silas Marner*, p. 10.
39 Eliot, *Silas Marner*, p. 9.

40 Eliot, *Silas Marner*, p. 5.
41 Eliot, *Silas Marner*, p. 8.
42 Eliot, *Silas Marner*, p. 10.
43 Eliot, *Silas Marner*, p. 181.
44 Eliot, *Silas Marner*, p. 182.
45 Thomas Hardy. *The Life and Death of the Mayor of Casterbridge: A Story of a Man of Character*. 1886. London: Macmillan, 1974, pp. 160–61.
46 Hardy, *The Mayor of Casterbridge*, p. 154.
47 Hardy, *The Mayor of Casterbridge*, p. 179.
48 Hardy, *The Mayor of Casterbridge*, p. 169.
49 Hardy, *The Mayor of Casterbridge*, p. 173.
50 Hardy, *The Mayor of Casterbridge*, p. 104.
51 Hardy, *The Mayor of Casterbridge*, p. 138.
52 Hardy, *The Mayor of Casterbridge*, p. 192.
53 Dostoyevsky, *The Insulted and Humiliated*, p. 168.
54 Temkin, *The Falling Sickness*, p. 32.
55 Freud, 'Dostoevsky and parricide', p. 180, p. 185.
56 Michel Foucault. *The History of Sexuality, Volume 3: The Care of Self.* 1984. Trans. Robert Hurley. New York: Pantheon, 1986, pp. 109–10.
57 Quoted in Foucault, *The History of Sexuality, Volume 3*, p. 110.
58 Marshall Hall. 'Lectures on the theory and practice of medicine'. *Lancet*, vol. ii, 14 April 1838, p. 68.
59 Gowers, *A Manual of Diseases*, vol. 2, p. 734.
60 Jean-Martin Charcot. 'Hysteroepilepsy: a young woman with a convulsive attack in the auditorium. February 7, 1888'. In *Charcot the Clinician: The Tuesday Lessons*. Trans. and commentary Christopher G. Goetz. New York: Raven, 1987, p. 103.
61 Charcot, 'Hysteroepilepsy', p. 104.
62 Charcot, 'Hysteroepilepsy', p. 106.
63 Temkin attributes this phrase to Aretaeus. Hippocrates and Democritus had argued that puberty was a key moment in sexual development that could resolve childhood seizures or set a lifelong epileptic pattern. Some physicians went on link pubertal cessation of seizures with sexual activity and recommended intercourse as a treatment. This practice prompted Aretaeus to observe that physicians who adopted this therapeutic practice did 'violence to the nature of children by unseasonable coition'. Temkin, *The Falling Sickness*, p. 32.
64 Walter J. Friedlander. *The History of Modern Epilepsy: The Beginning, 1865–1914*. London: Greenwood Press, 2001, p. 179.
65 Quoted in Friedlander, *The History of Modern Epilepsy*, p. 216.
66 Temkin, *The Falling Sickness*, p. 110.
67 'Epidemic of hystero-epilepsy'. *Lancet*, 16 October 1880, p. 625.
68 'Epidemic of hystero-epilepsy', p. 625.
69 'Hypochondria and hysteria in men and women'. *British Medical Journal*, 9 November 1889, p. 1054.
70 'Minutes from a meeting of the Clinical Society of London. Friday, February 8, 1889'. *British Medical Journal*, 16 February 1889, p. 358.
71 'Hysteria and tremulousness in males'. *British Medical Journal*, 18 July 1891, p. 136.
72 Friedlander, *The History of Modern Epilepsy*, p. 225.
73 Hall, 'Lectures on the theory and practice of medicine', p. 67.
74 W. R. Gowers. 'The Gulstonian lectures on epilepsy: lecture III – part III'. *Lancet*, 10 April 1880, p. 554.

75 Gowers, *A Manual of Diseases*, vol. 2, p. 760.
76 Gowers, *A Manual of Diseases*, vol. 2, p. 767.
77 Hall, 'Lectures on the theory and practice of medicine', p. 67 (original italics).
78 'Hystero-epilepsy cured by a sham operation'. *Lancet*, 8 October 1887, p. 726.
79 Francis Imlach. 'A case of hystero-epilepsy of twenty years' duration, treated by removal of the uterine appendages'. *British Medical Journal*, 7 April 1888, p. 740.
80 J. D. Dunlop. 'Two cases of hystero-epilepsy'. *Australasian Medical Gazette*, February 1883, p. 102.
81 John Syer Bristowe. 'Clinical remarks on pseudo-peritonitis and epilepsy in hysteria'. *British Medical Journal*, 22 February 1890, p. 403.
82 Gowers, *Manual of Diseases*, vol. 2, p. 734.
83 Charcot, 'Hysteroepilepsy', pp. 107–8.
84 Charcot, 'Hysteroepilepsy', p. 106.
85 J. Price quoted in Friedlander, *The History of Modern Epilepsy*, p. 180.
86 D. de Berdt Hovell. 'Hysteria simplified and explained'. *Lancet*, 20 December 1873, p. 873.
87 Hovell, 'Hysteria simplified and explained', p. 874.
88 Gowers, *Manual of Diseases*, vol. 2, p. 758.
89 W. R. Gowers. 'The Gulstonian lectures on epilepsy: lecture II – part II'. *Lancet*, 20 March 1880, p. 436.
90 Charcot, 'Hysteroepilepsy', p. 107.
91 Gowers, 'Lecture II – part II', p. 436.
92 Charcot quoted in Goetz's commentary, in *Charcot the Clinician*, p. 117.
93 Quoted in Goetz's commentary, in *Charcot the Clinician*, p. 121.
94 Macdonald Critchley. *Sir William Gowers 1845–1915: A Biographical Appreciation*. London: Heinemann, 1949, p. 41.
95 Dr Sansom and Mr G. T. Stonham. 'A mirror of hospital practice, British and foreign'. *Lancet*, 5 March 1881, pp. 369–70.
96 Wilfred R. Kingdon. 'The diagnosis of hystero-epilepsy from status epilepticus'. *Lancet*, 6 August 1898, p. 320.
97 Cartwright, *Screening the Body*, p. 65.
98 Cartwright, *Screening the Body*, pp. 66–67.
99 'Discussion on the relation of epilepsy and insanity'. Introduced by W. R. Gowers. *British Medical Journal*, 28 September 1895, p. 776.
100 'Marriage of female epileptics'. *Lancet*, 23 January 1897, p. 260.
101 Gowers, *Manual of Diseases*, vol. 2, p. 767.
102 William G. Thistle. 'Should epileptics marry?' *Lancet*, 13 February 1897, pp. 480–81.
103 E. Ray Lankester. 'Reply to letter from William G. Thistle, "Should epileptics marry?"' *Lancet*, 6 March 1897, p. 696.
104 William G. Thistle. 'Reply to letter from E. Ray Lankester, "Should epileptics marry?"' *Lancet*, 20 March 1897, p. 841.
105 James Adams. 'Should epileptics marry?' *Lancet*, 20 March 1897, p. 841.
106 Mabel Anderson. 'Should epileptics marry?' *Lancet*, 10 April 1897, p. 1053.
107 Kathryn Montgomery Hunter. *Doctors' Stories: The Narrative Structure of Medical Knowledge*. Princeton, MA: Princeton University Press, 1992, p. 72.
108 Hunter, *Doctors' Stories*, p. 82.
109 See, for example, Michel Foucault. *Ethics, Subjectivity and Truth*. Trans. Robert Hurley and others. Ed. Paul Rabinow. New York: New Press, 1997, vol. 1, pp. 13–14.
110 Gareth Stedman Jones. *Outcast London: A Study in the Relationship Between Classes in Victorian Society*. Oxford: Clarendon, 1971, pp. 10–11.

111 Daniel Pick. *Faces of Degeneration: A European Disorder, c. 1848–c. 1918*. Cambridge: Cambridge University Press, 1989, p. 11.
112 Foucault, *Ethics, Subjectivity and Truth*, p. 43.
113 Quoted in Cartwright, *Screening the Body*, p. 64.
114 Henry Maudsley. *Responsibility in Mental Disease*. London: C. Kegan Paul, 1876, p. 279.
115 Maudsley, *Responsibility in Mental Disease*, p. 41.
116 Pick, *Faces of Degeneration*, p. 204.
117 Nordau, *Degeneration*, p. vii.
118 Nordau, *Degeneration*, p. 5.
119 Nordau, *Degeneration*, p. 13.
120 Nordau, *Degeneration*, p. 18.
121 Nordau, *Degeneration*, p. 557.
122 See Pick, *Faces of Degeneration*, p. 25.
123 Pick, *Faces of Degeneration*, p.25.
124 Quoted in Pick, *Faces of Degeneration*, p. 24.
125 Mary Douglas. *Purity and Danger: An Analysis of Concepts of Pollution and Taboo*. 1966. London: Routledge and Kegan Paul, 1979, p. 115.
126 Douglas, *Purity and Danger*, p. 35.

CHAPTER 3

Notes from the borderlands: repressing the returned

I'm just a soul whose intentions are good.
Oh Lord! – Please don't let me be misunderstood.
(Gloria Caldwell, Bennie Benjamin and Sol Marcus,
'Don't let me be misunderstood', 1964)

I

In 1886, almost fifty years after Monks seized the reading public's imagination and his 'evil passions, vice, and profligacy' found expression in the 'hideous disease' that figured him epileptic, Robert Louis Stevenson published his novella *Strange Case of Dr Jekyll and Mr Hyde*. Through the character of the physician, Henry Jekyll, and his alter-ego, Edward Hyde, Stevenson explores nineteenth-century social and cultural conventions that seem to necessitate a double self. In doing so, he raises questions about identity, specifically in relation to the impossible yet necessary repressions entailed in constituting an identity that is both socially appropriate and seemingly integrated.

On 10 January 1894 a London physician, Arthur Thomas Myers, died at forty-two years of age. His untimely death continues to resonate through medical circles to the present day. Meteorological records indicate that Londoners experienced an unusually warm, damp January in the year Myers died, a fact referred to by one of the physicians involved in the deceased's autopsy. According to post-mortem findings, the cause of the physician's death was medical complications associated with his epilepsy, exacerbated by the narcotic medicine he took as part of the treatment for his condition. After extensive dissection and analysis, autopsy examination of his brain eventually identified what appeared to be a miniscule lesion in the uncinate region of the left hemisphere, thought by his treating physician to be the cause of some of his epilepsy symptoms. By the time the post-mortem examination could be carried out Myers had supposedly been dead for thirty hours. Yet the physician responsible for the necropsy of his brain worried that because 'the uncinate region became so soft and friable during the hardening process ... it was impossible to make satisfactory sections, and the microscope did not throw any further light on the cause of the lesion'.[1] The physician went on to record the advanced state of decomposition of the deceased's brain given the thirty-hour post-mortem time frame and suggested that this anomaly was perhaps due to the unusually warm, damp weather.

Monks; *The Strange Case of Dr Jekyll and Mr Hyde*; the untimely death of Arthur Myers: disparate ideas and disparate events, but bear with me as we travel the borders between these ideas and events. Monks, Stevenson's text and Myers' death are all part of the circuit of culture that shapes epilepsy narratives well into the twentieth century.

II

To begin with Dr Arthur Myers: why did he adopt the pseudonyms 'Dr Z' and 'Quaerens' (the Seeker)? And why do the circumstances surrounding his death still invoke so much interest for latter-day researchers? At least some of the answers to these questions can be found by examining the historical and cultural contexts in which he lived and struggled against the tide of contemporary keynote epilepsy narratives to reclaim/renegotiate the rights to his own life story.

Arthur was the youngest son of an intellectually prominent nineteenth-century English family. He, his grandfather, father and two brothers all appear in the *Oxford Dictionary of National Biography* and a collection of family papers is held at the Trinity College Library, Cambridge. Frederic, Arthur's oldest brother, was a respected published classical scholar and poet, most noted in this field for his work on Virgil. He also published a well received monograph on William Wordsworth. Yet it was his work in what was to become known as parapsychology that brought him notoriety in London's intellectual society. Along with the philosopher Henry Sidgwick and a small band of other like-minded researchers, he co-founded the Society for Psychical Research and set about exploring those phenomena that were thought to be manifestations of the spiritual or metaphysical world.

The middle son of the family, Ernest, was as adept scholastically as his older brother, if more politically conservative. He became a Fellow of Wadham College, Oxford, in 1868 and although called to the Bar, chose not to practise law. He achieved accolades for his skill as a translator of classical literature and acquired a reputation as a poet, publishing five volumes of verse throughout his life. Arthur demonstrated his intellectual capacities by obtaining a medical degree in 1881 and becoming a Fellow of the College of Physicians in 1893, shortly before his death.[2]

Arthur was very close to Frederic, whose interests in psychical research saw him cover some of the ground also being explored by the neurologists of the day. Both brothers made several trips to Europe to consult with Pierre Janet, Joseph Breuer and others, about research into mental states and hypnotism. They also visited Jean-Martin Charcot and attended some of his Tuesday lectures at La Salpêtrière to learn more about the subject. Arthur's interests in the possibilities of treating mental disorders with hypnotism placed him beyond the pale of contemporary trends in British medical research and his 1893 publication 'Mind-cure, faith-cure, and the miracles of Lourdes', co-written with Frederic, can only have compounded his intellectual marginality from the British medical fraternity.

Frederic's foremost work in this area of inquiry, *Human Personality and Its Survival of Bodily Death*, attempted to expand understanding of what he termed 'the problem of the hidden self' and its transgressive manifestations in lived experience. Extrapolating an evolving concept of double consciousness (shared to a point with John Hughlings Jackson), he argued that this sort of altered awareness represented simultaneity between the subliminal and supraliminal self. Not only are there points of cooperation between the subliminal and supraliminal, he argued, but there are 'also upheavals and alternations of personality of many kinds, so that what was once below the surface may for a time, or permanently, rise above it'.[3] Frederic hypothesised that this simultaneity constituted a breach in the threshold between otherwise discrete states. The subliminal self, he claimed, comprises those past experiences, thoughts and feelings that have been relegated to what would later become, in Freudian terms, the unconscious, while the supraliminal is situated above that threshold.

He identified a range of conditions that might cause a breach in the threshold between the supra- and subliminal self: sleep; waking into consciousness from sleep; hysteria; hypnotism; and so on. He argued that epilepsy is also one such condition. In many ways, Frederic's thinking on the supra- and subliminal self tracked Jackson's conceptualisation of the tiered levels of brain structure in relation to epilepsy. Jackson argued that the higher cortical levels of the brain controlled higher mental functions like thought and will; the middle level, voluntary muscular movements; and the lower level, basic functions like breathing and circulation. Using this model, one could hypothesise the location of a discharging lesion by noting the functions most affected by seizure states. For example, because one of the signs of Arthur's epilepsy was a tendency to make subtle tasting movements, Jackson theorised a lesion in the uncinate region of his brain before Colman's post-mortem confirmation.[4] For Frederic, though, this model fell short of providing a satisfactory explanation for the detail-rich altered states that accompanied some forms of epilepsy. Nor did it fully convey a qualitative sense of the simultaneity that defines double consciousness. It is at this point that Frederic's work saw him part company with British medical researchers and seek answers in the medical research being pursued in Europe and the possibilities offered by the Society for Psychical Research.

Investigation of the psychological possibilities suggested by the subliminal and supraliminal self was to hold Frederic's interest until his death on 17 January 1901 at fifty-eight years of age, seven years and seven days after that of his youngest brother. *Human Personality*, when first published posthumously in 1903, comprised a two-volume set, each volume approximately 700 pages in length. During his life, he published prodigiously, alone and with others – including Arthur. Frederic seemed to have hoped, at least for a time, that the altered states of consciousness accompanying Arthur's epilepsy would provide a key to understanding some of those mysteries of the mind that compelled his attention. It may well be that he also hoped his investigations would ultimately rescue Arthur's social and cultural identity from the one afforded by medicine.

III

Arthur's neurological symptoms began fairly innocuously while he was still a student at Cambridge. By the time they became disruptive enough to warrant medical advice, he was about to launch himself into his medical career. He turned to Hughlings Jackson for assistance. He also began to record his experiences of the condition, referring to it as his 'occasional epilepsy'. Significantly, he chose to publish these first-hand experiences under the pseudonyms 'Dr. Z' and 'Quaerens'.

Arthur's professional training gave him access to an increasingly rich medical lexicon to describe the sensory experiences associated with his epilepsy. Because of the project to modernise and standardise medical systems of representation, there was a growing movement to encourage those with epilepsy to speak of their symptoms in ways that made cerebral paroxysmal phenomena cogent to evolving taxonomies. He was very much part of this evolving system of representation, both through his position as a member of the medical profession and through the influences of Jackson, who was central to the medical reforms at the Queen Square hospital. Arthur also wrote for the leading medical journals of the day. Overall, however, he seems to have found the system of representation available to him as a medical writer and practitioner oddly inadequate to the task of recording his own case history, and so chose instead the language of literature to convey the qualitative aspects of his sensory experiences.

In his account of a 'Particular variety of epilepsy', Jackson quotes Arthur's self-written case history at length. In turn, Arthur draws on words penned by Charles Dickens in *David Copperfield* to describe his paroxysmal sensations of 'dreamy state' or reminiscence. With some pathos, given his ultimate fate, Arthur goes on to chide Samuel Coleridge, Alfred Tennyson and Dickens in this account for the ways their writings celebrate the sensory shift into reminiscence or *déjà vu*:

> whatever pretty suggestions [they] may make to account for it, and however universal its occurrence may be regarded ... it probably ought to be regarded as showing disturbance of brain function; and that, perhaps, its recognition and removal might sometimes prevent the development of a more important disorder.[5]

It must have bitterly taxed his sensibility that this expanded state, sought so assiduously by those engaged in the creative process, represented for him a precursor of neuronal dissolution and chaos. Jackson reports in musings on the subject: 'I have heard patients say that they used to "encourage" the feeling [of dreamy state and other pleasurable paroxysmal sensations], before they knew what it meant'. He goes on to relate an account passed on to him by a colleague, Dr James Anderson, of a patient who 'showed some reluctance to talk about the scene', that is, those pleasurable visual and sensory changes signalling some sort of paroxysmal event.[6]

Arthur appears to have been fairly open in discussing the various aspects of his condition with family, friends and trusted colleagues. Nevertheless, his awareness of the negative social and professional implications of being labelled 'epileptic' is suggested by his use of pseudonyms when writing about his epilepsy for a wider audience. Moreover, Frederic's activities in psychical research had begun to attract published ridicule from at least some of Arthur's medical colleagues. The import of these views in relation to his own condition cannot have been lost on Arthur. By all accounts the brothers enjoyed a warm and affectionate relationship and it is feasible that Arthur might have worried about the social consequences of his epilepsy for his sibling's already controversial reputation.

The scorn with which the medical fraternity viewed Frederic's work on psychical research was evident in the obituary for Arthur published in the *British Medical Journal* on 27 January 1894. The obituarist refers to Arthur's implicitly lamentable interests in those 'problems which the "psychical researchers" aspire to resolve'. Yet medical derision for Frederic's research group was more flagrantly vitriolic in an editorial item published in the *Lancet* some twelve years earlier:

> A Body [*sic*] calling itself 'The Society for Psychical Research' is addressing a series of what must surely be serio-comic interrogatories to the public in relation to 'hallucinations' and 'dreams.' An invitation is thrown out to all the weak-minded people who think they have seen 'ghosts' or 'spectres,' or been 'touched' by mysterious shades, and to all the dreamers who dream dreams of the nature of 'coincidences,' to state their experiences. Here is a grand opportunity for the mad folk outside Bedlam. If it were not for the trouble involved, we should like to peruse the mass of 'communications' these invitations will be certain to call forth. There are, however, two preliminary questions which ought to be asked. First, has any 'society' of presumably sane men a moral right to instigate the crazy public to formulate its 'mysterious' experiences! We know that the most disastrous consequences sometimes occur to weak brains from dwelling too intently on subjects of the nature of 'fixed ideas.' It is, therefore, doubtful whether this sort of thing ought to be allowed. No sober-minded person can doubt that all impressions of seeing, or hearing, or feeling spiritual manifestations must be morbid. Such things exist only in the imaginations of the persons who are subject to them.[7]

According to the meticulously researched account of the Myers family written by David Taylor and Susan Marsh, Frederic had a reputation for a certain flamboyance of character. He was evidently a man of self-confessed 'sensuous and emotional temperament and given to acts of swaggering folly':[8] personality traits that are at odds with nineteenth-century models of appropriate masculinity and traits that link him – at least conceptually – to developing medical models of male 'epileptic behaviours'. In an act of political commitment, Frederic resigned his university lectureship at Cambridge in 1869 to focus his talents on lobbying for the higher education of women. He is credited with coining the word 'telepathy', which he used in *Human Personality* to describe and explore the possibility of communication between minds. He argued that this capacity, where it existed, was at its most powerful at times of extreme danger or imminent death.

Despite the unameliorated disparagement directed at him by British medical writers of his day, in other circles Frederic enjoyed considerable respect as a researcher trying to grapple with some of the 'big' questions central to human experience. Two contemporaries, Oliver Lodge and William James (brother of Henry), note his philosophical grasp of the problems arising from discussions about those mental states that remain beyond the understanding and explanations available to either science or culture. James argued that Frederic's contributions to psychology could not be overstated. In his work Myers attempted to develop a research stratagem that would encompass psychological and parapsychological phenomena, bringing both into the realms of rational inquiry. While noting the conceptual and linguistic limits bearing on Frederic's work, James claimed that:

> Frederic Myers will always be remembered in psychology as the pioneer who staked out a vast track of mental wilderness and planted the flag of genuine science upon it. He was an enormous collector. He introduced for the first time comparison, classification, and serial order into the peculiar kind of fact which he collected. He was a genius at perceiving analogies; he was fertile in hypotheses; and as far as conditions allowed it in this meteoric region, he relied on verification.[9]

Frederic's work seems to have influenced at least some aspects of Freud's thinking in relation to psychoanalysis, a point I will return to later. If Arthur's epilepsy condition trapped him in the borderlands between life as an educated, professional, sensitive, kindly man and a representational system that figured him as degenerate, disorderly and morally insane, Frederic's personality traits and object of research, if not his method, combine to located him in the borderlands beyond British intellectual respectability.

IV

Almost a century after Arthur's death, Taylor and Marsh revisited the circumstances surrounding the event. They argue that, although in legal terms Arthur did not commit suicide, the possibility cannot be dismissed.[10] They point to those aspects of his life that connected with wider factors associated with suicide: the death of his father when he was only a few months old; his unmarried status; his chronic illness and its impact on his professional and social life; his deteriorating general health; the suicides of two people close to him; his left-handedness. Their examination of the available personal and medical histories of the deceased and their re-examination of the circumstances surrounding his death build a strong case for his self-termination, a claim that would seem to be validated by his treating physician's somewhat blunt statement in 1898 when reviewing a case history in *Brain*, a British medical journal. In what appears to be an oblique reference to Arthur, Jackson writes: 'The patient died, January 1894 from an overdose of chloral'.[11] Taylor and Marsh also suggest that by the time Myers came to the autopsy table he may well 'have been dead for rather more than 30 hours': an observation that would seem to be confirmed by the advanced state of brain decomposition noted in the autopsy findings.[12] There is no mention in available records of the unremittingly bleak epilepsy narratives circulating within the medical–cultural circuit in which Arthur lived his condition and died.

It is the possibility of Arthur's suicide that retroactively compels medical interest. Taylor and Marsh posit him as an early paradigm of temporal lobe epilepsy and it is now argued that this particular cerebral disorder carries with it a rate of suicide twenty-five times higher than that in the general population. They draw on statistics gleaned from a series of post-surgical patients with temporal lobe epilepsy at the Guy's/Maudsley Neurosurgical Unit in London to discuss this rather worrying aspect of the condition. The increased danger of suicide for those with temporal lobe syndromes has also been noted by other researchers,[13] who report a statistical spread of a five- to twenty-five-fold increase in this particular sector of the population. Several of these researchers note that the potential to suicide further increases in those who are also left-handed. The questions become for neurologists: *Why* do these patients kill themselves? Is the potential to suicide somehow encoded in temporal lobe epilepsy conditions? Or is it triggered by complex psychological reactions to social and/or therapeutic factors? The rather forlorn hope is that seeds to an answer might have been sown if Jackson had but revealed more about his patient's life beyond the boundaries of the doctor's consulting rooms.

Like Galen, Jackson explicitly incorporated patients' accounts of what epilepsy symptoms felt like into his record of what they looked like. His phrase 'dreamy state' to describe particular phenomena associated with paroxysmal neuronal discharge takes precedence for him over the more usual 'intellectual aura', because, he argued, this is how several of his patients described these sensations.[14] Despite Jackson repeatedly crediting his understanding of what those phenomena felt like to the descriptions made available to him by various patients, he has been criticised in later decades for not publishing more extensive and intimate biographical details of his most famous patient.

It has been argued that having a medically trained patient provide experiential data warranted a more expansive account of this patient's life than Jackson supplied. Taylor and Marsh claim:

> Jackson's account is totally mechanistic and lesion oriented. Despite his avowed interest in the 'organ of the mind' his separation from the interests of the asylum doctors is total. Thus a case placed at the frontier (and at the division) between neurology and psychiatry symbolises their subsequent parting to their mutual loss.[15]

While acknowledging Jackson's significant and valuable contributions to medical understanding of the epilepsies, the twentieth-century American neurologist William Lennox argues that Jackson's writings 'do not reflect a "human" interest in his patients' and Jackson himself displays 'little concern for the patient as a person'. He criticises Jackson for being more interested in the 'why' of epilepsy syndromes than the treatment, claiming that his observations 'offered little practical aid to the clinician busy with the diagnosis and treatment of patients'.[16] Another neurologist, Dietrich Blumer, when reviewing the case of Arthur Myers, writes: 'Although Jackson studied ictal and postictal mental disorders, he was not interested in understanding the whole epileptic patient'.[17]

These observations are open to closer analysis. While Jackson's published writings undoubtedly focus in minute detail on the structural and functional aspects of the brain, and he systematically worked to develop understanding of the connections between discharging cerebral lesions and subsequent disturbances to psychosocial and physiological function – the 'why' *and* 'how' of epilepsy syndromes – he consistently returns to the empirical accounts of his patients to supplement developing neurological models. Recurring comments in his writing gesture to concerns that too narrow a focus on the projected prognosis of a condition or disease entity not only risks missing significant aspects of the way disease develops in specific circumstances, but also obscures the relevance of symptomatology to the patient's healthy state. This impulse in his writing seems to suggest that he was at least moderately interested in ascertaining what that healthy state might be for the patient. His circumspection in revealing all aspects of his patients' lives to the full glare of the medical gaze, I argue, can also be read as acknowledgement that these folk were more than the sum total of their neurological conditions: that beyond the boundaries of the clinic, their epilepsy signified and was lived in a wider socio-cultural economy and a matrix of extended kinship relations. He cannot have been unaware of those various systems of representation circulating around his patients that figured the epileptic in uncompromisingly negative terms.

In the late 1880s, Arthur wrote with some dismay of prolonged and complex episodes of automatism, after which he would suddenly come into awareness dislocated from time and find himself in physical circumstances unfamiliar, unplanned and, at least once, according to Jackson, potentially scandalous. After reproducing Arthur's accounts of several of these automatisms, Taylor and Marsh observe: 'While these *amusing* episodes give clear evidence of his capacity to act apparently rationally and with intent whilst not fully subject to the monitoring process usually attributed to the self, ... they [the episodes] were not always benign'.[18] They go on to relate an incident reported by Jackson when, during a paroxysmal episode, Arthur retrieves a pin from the floor and attempts to 'playfully' prick the physician, and note also an unidentified potentially 'criminal' event referred to in Jackson's records. Without minimising the significance of these latter episodes, to summarise the earlier events recounted by Arthur as 'amusing' and 'benign' seems to misrecognise the profound psychosocial distress these sorts of spatio-temporal fractures present for the one experiencing them.

Taylor and Marsh attempt to recuperate those aspects of Arthur denied the medical gaze by Jackson through scrutinising his writing style in published articles and private letters to his family. Despite efforts to detect medically identified textual markers that might help define his epileptic character – hypergraphia, excessive philosophical interests, intellectual viscosity, perseverance, an obsessional preoccupation with seizure episodes – they conclude that his writing style, although sometimes 'dull' and 'routine', does not seem 'unduly verbose'.[19] In fact, they observe a certain elegance in some of his pieces. Of his personal letters they note that 'his graciousness, his warmth and his general tendency to trivialise his difficulty is everywhere apparent'. There is no evidence, they point out, to suggest either his temporal lobe symptomatology or any mental deterioration beyond the occasional hint of a 'less firm hand' in his letters to family. Their observations seem to perpetuate an ongoing concern of Jackson's, expressed a century earlier; that is, there is a medical tendency 'to study cases as the symptoms show *approaches* to certain clinical standards, and not as they show departures from healthy states'.[20]

These observations also raise questions when measured against wider comments on Jackson's writing style. The neurologist's written verbosity and obsessive preoccupation with the minutiae of seizure episodes were legendary, even among his most fervent admirers.

Although he was held in almost universal esteem by his successors and generated a palpable affection in his peers, Jackson has often drawn comment for his tendency to discursivity and an elaborately detailed philosophical engagement with his field of inquiry. Psychiatrist Sir George Savage claimed of the neurologist's published work:

> His whole frame of mind was so careful and exacting that he scarcely ever dares to make a definite statement without qualifying it in some way; so that in studying his writings one meets endless footnotes and parentheses, which are somewhat confusing.[21]

This tendency in Jackson's writing style makes any close reading of his work a necessarily unhurried occupation. For example, in the opening remarks to his paper 'On a particular variety of epilepsy ("intellectual aura"), one case with symptoms of organic brain disease', in a somewhat viscous turn, he uses the phrase 'dreamy state' seventeen times in the first two pages alone. Yet despite this tendency to circumlocution, his work remains celebrated in neurophysiology as marking a major step forward in medical thinking about brain function – and rightly so. In a mildly amusing twist, given the 'symptomatology' evident in his writing style, Jackson had a form of epilepsy named for him (at least for a time). We might wonder where the line *is* in the sort of textual diagnosis attempted by Taylor and Marsh between the potential (and pathologised) verbosity sought in Arthur's writing and the actual (deemed endearing) verbosity discernible in his physician's writings.

Both Jackson's circumspection in relation to his most famous patient and the criticism it has drawn cut to the heart of Arthur's life and death. He lived his condition in complicated times. The second half of the nineteenth century saw the growth of what has been called an 'intellectual aristocracy' in England, a powerfully influential group dominating the professions, the sciences, politics and literature; its members set and policed the standards of Arthur's day and his family history placed him at the centre of this elite class. Donald MacKenzie argues that by the mid nineteenth century this group was both tightly knit and well integrated into the ruling classes. He lists the family names of Galton, Darwin and Booth among its members. He goes on to argue that, initially, eugenics can be seen as 'the practice and experience of the intellectual aristocracy read onto nature'.[22] Given the associations already being made between epilepsy and hereditary taint, and in view of Francis Galton's up-and-coming work on eugenics and its implications for society, it can come as no surprise that Arthur might have sought to protect both himself and his family from the social stigma attached to his condition. What Arthur's seizures looked like within the clinical framework of Jackson's care and medical records was only one aspect of their signification. What it felt like for Arthur to suffer his prolonged automatisms in a climate that was increasingly linking epilepsy to discourses of degeneration, criminality and moral insanity can be surmised.

That Arthur trusted his physician to honour the self-defined boundaries of his privacy seems indicated by the fact that in the year prior to his death, and as his condition deteriorated, he chose to live next door to Jackson. This investment of trust and Jackson's honouring of that trust undermine Lennox's claim that Jackson was a physician who displayed little concern for the patient as a person and Blumer's conclusions that Jackson was uninterested in the 'whole' epileptic patient. Indeed, Jackson's reticence suggests a heightened sensitivity to the wider realities of Arthur's life. The laments recorded by Lennox, Blumer, Taylor and Marsh signal the insatiability of the medical gaze; there is a frank impulse to devour all aspects of Myers' life for the good of the medical cause. Yet in relation to his epilepsy, both Arthur and Jackson had written and published detailed accounts of the neurological and phenomenological changes as they were observed and experienced. The 'more' being demanded here is a detailed anatomisation of Arthur's personal and professional life. A stronger analysis of Arthur's decision to look to literature to record some of his accounts of living with epilepsy at the end of the nineteenth century can be understood as a gesture of resistance to the probing insatiability of the medical gaze and the concomitant reductive medical rhetoric proscribing epileptic identity.

Taylor and Marsh ponder the conditions that might have finally brought about Arthur's death. Could the cause be traced back to the experiential disturbances caused by his epilepsy, compounded by the combined social and professional factors that had come to severely constrict both his public and private life? Was the 'true hamartien' or 'tragic flaw' due to the tiny lesion supposedly generating erratic neuronal discharge in his brain? Or was his downfall due to a more potently problematic brew of bromism and long-term chloral intoxication? Perhaps it was the latter possibility that drove medical colleagues to labour so long over trying to resuscitate him. Taylor and Marsh include a report from *The Times* dated 15 January 1894 which indicates the efforts made by Arthur's medical friends to protect him from the social, legal and religious consequences associated with possible suicide. When 'Dr Frederick George Drewitt of Manchester Square' was called to attend Arthur at 2 Manchester Square – the home Myers had moved into in 1893 and shared with friend and colleague

Dr Dawtrey Drewitt – Frederick found Arthur lying 'insensible' on the bed: 'and although six doctors kept up artificial respiration for 32 hours he remained in a comatose condition until he died on Wednesday'.[23] This, then, may well explain the advanced state of decomposition of his brain noted in the autopsy report rather than the weather, as suggested by Colman. I wonder, though, whether at least some of the underlying causes of death lie buried somewhere in the circuit of culture which ascribed meaning to Arthur's epilepsy and configured his identity as an epileptic.

Many of the medical stories of epilepsy from Myers' time contain at least one anecdote or reference to the explosive and sudden danger represented by the epileptic in society. The French psychiatrist Étienne Esquirol, for instance, informed his colleagues that:

> The fury of epileptic patients ... is of a very dangerous kind, blind, and in some degree automatic. Nothing can tame it; neither the sight of powerful instruments of restraint, nor moral influences, which means generally succeed with ordinary maniacs. Their violence is so terrific, and so much dreaded, that I saw, in an asylum of the South of France, all the epileptic patients tied down to their bed every evening, so great was the apprehension they created.[24]

The image created of uncontrollable violence echoes the apocalyptic fury reified in the Herculean myth. This view remained an integral referent well into the twentieth century for the latent threat embodied by the epileptic. The belief that people with epilepsy not only were a danger to themselves but also presented an inherent and undeniable danger to the community in which they resided became a determining factor in both the social ostracism with which the condition was met and the vigour of the response with which medicine attempted to control the possibilities presented by this ungovernable fury.

In 1876, Henry Maudsley argued that any murder committed without seeming motive or explanation suggested that the perpetrator of the crime may be afflicted with epilepsy. His view of the epileptic affected by paroxysms of mania or furore was both oddly sentimental and dramatic in its rendering of the phenomenon:

> It is one of the saddest experiences of asylum life to witness the pitiful fate of those patients who have not sunk below the consciousness of their condition. Gentle, amiable, and industrious through their long intervals of lucidity, they hope against hope that each recurring paroxysm will be the last; they eagerly try all remedies, in the hope of curing the disease; they see others leave the asylum restored to health, and confidently anticipate that their turn will also come; but confidence wanes as the attacks recur, the mind is slowly weakened by the storms

> of fury through which it passes, and they sink finally into the apathy of dementia – a state of mere oblivion, in which they cease to hope or care more.[25]

Maudsley's juxtaposition of the gentle, amiable, industrious and lucid, with the apathetic, demented and oblivious, foregrounds a heightened sense that contestation between the normal and abnormal personae rages unabated in the epileptic until disorder prevails. This potted chronicle also constructs a figure helplessly unable to maintain agency in controlling murderous impulses.

By the late nineteenth century, many journal publications had developed a rhetoric of benevolence that intimately entwined compassion and prejudice to justify the necessity of epileptic colonies. Medical writing had already stereotyped the male epileptic body as dangerously volatile, vulnerable to vice and feminised by its tendency to disorder and lack of self-control. By the end of the nineteenth century the epileptic had become a troublesome marker at the limits of mainstream society; a cipher that held the borderlands between normality and abnormality.

It is difficult to see where Arthur could have located himself and his empirical understanding of epilepsy in this economy. The medical narratives of his day reason from the extreme to the particular, with no nuances in between. Epilepsy in this representational economy is all-encompassing and necessarily devastating to all aspects of the autonomous self. Myers' insistence on describing his condition as 'occasional epilepsy' again suggests his resistance to this rhetorical totalitarianism. The impossibility of his situation goes some way in explaining his attraction to his brother's work in psychical research, and also his appeal to the works of Coleridge, Tennyson and Dickens, in attempts to articulate a truer self beyond the boundaries of late nineteenth-century medical discourse, where 'epileptic' and 'physician' remained contradictions in terms. We know that he believed some writers of poetry and literature effectively captured his sensory experiences of dreamy state or double consciousness with their words, but whether his hopes were justified in looking to them for the seeds of a truer self remains to be seen.

V

Unlike Dr James Anderson's patient, Dostoevsky was certainly not reluctant 'to talk about the scene' when it came to the pleasurable visual and sensory changes associated with his own epilepsy. His claims about these aspects of his symptomatology tend to be far more celebratory than those recorded by Myers. One of Dostoevsky's friends wrote that the author often spoke of his prodromal, or pre-seizure, phase as a period of ecstasy. He claimed to have experienced:

> a contentedness which is unthinkable under normal conditions, and unimaginable for those who have not experienced it. At such times I am in perfect harmony with myself and with the entire universe. Perception is so clear and so agreeable that one would give ten years of his life, and perhaps all of it, for a few seconds of such bliss.[26]

Many of these pleasurable aspects of cerebral paroxysm, as well as the darker and more difficult sensory changes, are written into characterisations in Dostoevsky's fictional works. In *The Idiot,* Prince Myshkin's pre-seizure states sometimes elevate him to a 'lofty calm', where 'his mind and heart were flooded with extraordinary light';[27] however, his seizures also plummet him to the lowest mode of existence.

Dostoevsky's characterisations also demonstrate the author's familiarity with medical accounts of epileptic symptomatology. Myshkin's seizures, like those of Yelena in *The Insulted and Humiliated,* are preceded by a 'frightful, unimaginable scream':

> In that scream everything human seems obliterated and it is impossible, or very difficult, for an observer to realise and admit that it is the man himself screaming. It seems indeed as though it were someone else screaming from within the man. That is how many people at least have described their impression. The sight of a man in an epileptic fit fills many people with positive and unbearable horror, in which there is a certain element of the uncanny.[28]

In an indexical turn, Dostoevsky describes Myshkin as having 'that strange look from which some people can recognise at the first glance a victim of epilepsy'.[29] Dostoevsky's point of departure from received medical understandings of epilepsy is with the character of the prince.

In the early stages of development of the novel, Dostoevsky had moved from creating an epileptic character more akin to Smerdyakov and Monks than the idealised figure that later becomes Myshkin. He brought about the transformation of his protagonist by displacing his more negative traits onto other characters in the published text, most notably the character of Parfion Rogozhin. As with Stevenson's Jekyll and Hyde, and, to a lesser degree, Hardy's Lucetta and Elizabeth-Jane, the result brings about a splitting between the appropriate and the illicit, between order and disorder. Rogozhin is the dark to Myshkin's light, semiotically coded as Myshkin's other. Despite their differences, when they first encounter each other on a train to Petersburg, the dark, fiery Rogozhin and the fair Myshkin are mutually fascinated by their unexpected and new found connection. They both experience 'a desire to enter into conversation' with each other.[30]

This disjunctive doubling of the characters allows Myshkin to remain untainted, free of the passions and excesses usually associated, in literature and medicine, with epilepsy. Instead, the traits become the provenance of his counterpart and Myshkin and Rogozhin function symbiotically: two halves of a fragmented whole. Like the figure of the epileptic hovering at the threshold of a seizure, their disjunction evokes the fragility of the barrier between prevailing order and transgression and suggests the unstable juxtaposition between a repressed, improper carnality and the symbolically sanctioned body. The non-viability of the fragmented self is heralded by the novel's conclusion. While seeming to understand this, but at the same time trying to preserve individuation, Rogozhin attempts to keep Myshkin at a distance. As they make their last journey together to the scene where he has murdered Nastasya Filippovna, Rogozhin insists that he and Myshkin walk separately but parallel on the street. He tells Myshkin: 'you go straight along here to the house.... But I'll walk on the other side.'[31]

When they arrive at the flat, Nastasya's body is already in the early stages of decomposition. On seeing her corpse Myshkin begins to tremble so much Rogozhin observes that he appears as though he is about to have a fit. He insists that he, the Prince and Nastasya must not be separated: 'So let her lie here now beside us, beside you and me'.[32] The three are symbolically reunited in an epileptic tableau as Rogozhin and Myshkin lie together on their makeshift couch at the foot of Nastasya's death bed. Myshkin is trapped in an automatism of comforting gestures, repeatedly passing his 'trembling hand' softly across Rogozhin's hair and cheeks. Rogozhin is 'completely unconscious and raving', shaking convulsively, making incoherent sounds, and from time to time emitting short screams. Nastasya's leaking corpse suggests the death-like post-ictal sleep following a *grand mal* episode. Neither character survives the reunification. Rogozhin is exiled to Siberia for his crime, his sentence ameliorated because of his 'brain fever'. Myshkin hurtles into the abyss of madness and is sent back to Schneider's Swiss clinic.

N. M. Lary, Jacques Catteau, James Rice and other scholars have noted that Dostoevsky displays a propensity to 'leak' traits and behaviours associated with medical models of epilepsy and hystero-epilepsy onto non-epileptic characters in his texts. In a sense, the strategy constitutes a literary simulation of hereditary taint and cross-contamination. Vanya's health problems flagged at the beginning of *The Insulted and Humiliated* eventually come to manifest resonances of

Yelena's paroxysmal episodes. After a distressing conversation with Nikolai Sergeich, Vanya appeared pale and felt unwell: his 'head began to spin and [he] fell down in the middle of the room', remembering 'nothing but Yelena's shriek'.[33] A second retreat into a state of 'absence' is sparked by a disturbing encounter with Prince Valkovsky. The Prince's fully revealed awfulness plunges Vanya into such a state of emotional turmoil that he loses all sense of time and place. He has no memory of his journey home, but when he arrives he finds that Yelena is in a delirium, having suffered a seizure. Yelena suffers, in all, seven paroxysmal episodes identifiable as epilepsy or hystero-epilepsy. Vanya experiences two episodes, also brought on by powerfully conflicting emotions that resemble hysterical or hystero-epileptic episodes. The sensitivity of Yelena and Vanya to psychological turmoil presents as a mutual disease, linked through the signification of Yelena's scream immediately prior to Vanya's first episode and confirmed by his prodromal sensations of the seizure she has suffered in his 'absence' after the Prince Valkovsky encounter.

Parfion Rogozhin and Nastasya Filippovna in *The Idiot* are also fragmented characters, their emotional fragility manifesting from time to time as 'convulsive' and 'hysterical' behaviours. Nonetheless, the traits and behaviours projected onto Filippovna, Rogozhin and Vanya are not labelled 'epileptic'; therefore these and other characters exhibiting the characteristics are not pathologised as such. In Dostoevsky's novels, tendency to fragmentation, instances of double consciousness, episodes of ecstasy, loss of time and memory, and even the occasional convulsive moment, all function as part of a spectrum of signifiers potentially available at various times to all characters. While there are similarities between Dostoevsky's representations of the epileptic figure and the medically inflected constructions evident in Dickens' work, the impulse to disseminate epileptoid signifiers onto other characters subverts the notion that the epileptic is reliably and exclusively defined by these properties. Just as non-epileptic characters are subject to moments of paroxysm and social disorder, so too are those with epilepsy subject to sustained social agency, reflectiveness and intellectual focus. The strategy destabilises socio-medical links between the epileptic and social disorder. It also goes some way in freeing the syndrome from the model of degeneration – with its ties to class and criminality – found in Dickens' texts. In a sense, Dostoevsky's impulse to democratise those possibilities of human experience increasingly yoked to contemporary medical models as key signifiers of epilepsy disorder becomes a literary precursor of Michael Persinger's research efforts in twenty-first-century Canada (see Introduction).

Dostoevsky also reproduced and perpetuated medical stereotypes at certain critical moments in his fiction. In his fictional and autobiographical writing, however, he insisted that there is a redemptive component to epilepsy. This insistence, coupled with persuasive descriptions of the harmony he experienced while in the prodromal phase of his own paroxysmal episodes (harmony he extends to Myshkin), was seized upon by medical writers to augment their understanding of epileptic experience. Hennri Gastaut, one of the first to incorporate Dostoevsky's descriptions into the medical model, was later to lament that medical acceptance of the writer's claims 'incorrectly enriched the symptomatology of temporal lobe epilepsy with symptoms which never occurred except in the imagination of the author':[34] an observation that seems to miss the point. Surely those changes to mentation and psychological state characteristic of temporal lobe phenomena are experienced firstly through the interpretative framework of the affected individual – a framework that includes imagination? Gastaut's conclusion, that Dostoevsky's empirical account of his symptomatology had no equivalent in the privileged medical model, mimes Myers' failure to find a cogent rendering of his own subjective experience in medical discourse.

In 1983 P. H. A. Voskuil revisited the issue and offered new evidence to support claims for ecstatic aura. He argues:

> It is important to note that the personality of this patient was likely to have influenced the symptoms of the seizures. One can imagine that the color of the symptoms of a psychic aura or seizures indeed depends on the patient's emotional world, and in Dostoevsky's case on his desire for a world of bliss and harmony.[35]

Voskuil draws on recently published electroencephalographic evidence of ecstatic seizure to revisit Dostoevsky's claims for an ecstatic aura and although, to some extent, he shares Gastaut's reservations about the precise diagnostic parameters of Dostoevsky's paroxysmal condition, he argues that it is not possible to completely discount a particular manifestation of partial complex epilepsy. Whatever Dostoevsky's subjective experience of symptomatology might have been, it was clearly his own. Gastaut foregrounds the point that Dostoevsky was adept at exploiting his disease artistically, and – significantly – Voskuil notes that the writer refused to take medication for his condition. This latter observation is a persuasive indicator that Dostoevsky understood only too well the cost to his creativity of a regime of contemporary drugs and chemical anodynes.

This latter observation also implicitly gestures to an issue raised in various chapters of this book: that is, the unspecified links between personality traits associated with epilepsy conditions and some medication regimes. What degree of fragmentation is directly attributable to paroxysmal neuronal discharge, and what level of intellectual viscosity, lability, psychological instability, defective memory and so on can be sourced back to a pharmaceutical intervention? Could Dostoevsky have continued to exploit his disease quite so artistically if he had been on a long-term regime of bromide, for example, or the chloral hydrate taken by Myers? Gastaut notes that while Dostoevsky may have 'unconsciously' mythologised his symptomatology:

> The seizures neither dulled nor diminished his genius, and the genius in no way was based on his epilepsy. This lesson constitutes a very strong defense in favor of the innumerable epileptic persons who are inexcusably prejudged to have a reduced intellect due to their seizures, and in favor of the rare epileptic geniuses whose exceptional abilities should not be considered a by-product of their disease![36]

In accord with Gastaut, literary critic Jacques Catteau argues that Dostoevsky's creative energy and health obtained despite rather than because of his epilepsy. He further claims that, as his career progressed, Dostoevsky was able to transcend any delimiting effects his condition might have posed for his craft: 'the pathological as such was eradicated, dissolved in a psychology which goes beyond the distinction between healthy and unhealthy'.[37] Dostoevsky was able to move beyond the normal/abnormal binary 'not because [he] celebrated illness', writes Catteau, 'but because he accepted it'.[38] James Rice suggests that Dostoevsky's way out of the normal/abnormal binary not only was forged through an acceptance and mastery of his paroxysmal condition, but was further consolidated by 'the discovery (and invention, to be sure) of polymorphous and polyphonic values precisely within his pathological condition, which he consciously and ingeniously negotiated through art'.[39]

It is the fidelity to medical models of epilepsy that empowers Dostoevsky's more subversive impulses. As he endorses through repetition the medical language of epilepsy, he also constantly reviews and revalues the implications and meanings of the paroxysmal moment. Through the character of Myshkin, Dostoevsky reflects on the sensory states of epilepsy and the dialectical relation between the expanded awareness associated with his prodromal phase and the abjection of the fit:

> And yet he came at last to an extremely paradoxical conclusion. 'What if it is disease?' he decided at last. 'What does it matter if it is an abnormal

> intensity, if the result, if the minute of sensation, remembered and analysed afterwards in health, turns out to be the acme of harmony and beauty, and gives a feeling, unknown and undivined till then, of completeness, of proportion, or reconciliation, and of ecstatic devotional merging in the highest synthesis of life?'... He did not insist on the dialectical part of his argument, however. Stupefaction, spiritual darkness, idiocy stood before him conspicuously as the consequence of these 'higher moments'; seriously, of course, he could not have disputed it. There was undoubtedly a mistake in his conclusion – that is, in his estimate of that minute, but the reality of the sensation somehow perplexed him. What was he to make of that reality?[40]

The heightened apprehensions of the aura, Myshkin concludes, were not 'abnormal' or 'unreal' sensations like those 'from hashish, opium, or wine, destroying the reason and distorting the soul'.[41] He is able 'soberly' to review and analyse these 'moments' when the fit is over and mentation has recovered. While acknowledging the cost of illumination, he questions whether 'Stupefaction, spiritual darkness, [and] idiocy' are the inevitable consequence of those 'higher moments' and the subsequent fit.

I am not suggesting here that Dostoevsky can be drawn seamlessly into a heuristic exercise organised around Myers' quest to reclaim a subjectivity that was not merely defined by his epilepsy, although Dostoevsky's success in negotiating from the borderlands an enunciative position that compelled medical engagement and dialogue goes some way in addressing the unliveable oppositions confronting Myers. Nor am I suggesting that Dickens and Dostoevsky were the only two writers working in the latter decades of the nineteenth century to feature characters with the symptomatology of epilepsy. What I am arguing is that these two writers, between them, were instrumental in constructing an epileptic figure that became a stock device in twentieth-century cultural aesthetics and narrative traditions in English: a point I will return to. Furthermore, and despite Dostoevsky's innovations, there persisted a range of signifiers in the textual ethos that accreted to form an epileptic identity located at the extremes of the psychosocial spectrum. By the mid 1900s, it was the aesthetics and politics of the more extreme cultural representations that continued to validate the sharply divided subject positions organised around the pathological and normal. To paraphrase Myshkin, what was to be made of that reality? The answer would appear to be: more of the same.

VI

Stevenson was a fan of Dostoevsky, reading the Russian author's work in French translation. He took Myshkin's 'reality' and reconfigured it to resonate with Victorian sensibilities. In some ways, it is Stevenson's tale of the irreconcilably dislocated self that can be read as a metaphor for Arthur's predicament. Jekyll is representative of the middle-class intellectual and moral values of Victorian society. A physician, he has 'every guarantee of an honourable and distinguished future'.[42] He also embodies impulses that must be repressed or hidden in order to maintain his status in society and to preserve his own 'high views' of what that status entails. In a literalisation of double consciousness, Jekyll writes of his split identity: 'My two natures had memory in common, but all other faculties were most unequally shared between them'.[43] He argues in his final letter to Mr Utterson that human nature is intrinsically split: 'man is not truly one', he claims, 'but truly two'. He begins to experiment with ways to formalise the separation of what he sees as mutually exclusive states of being.

In the main, Jekyll wilfully represses his cruder impulses, until such time that he must spend himself in those unspecified pleasures otherwise forbidden his public self. In reflecting on these concealed pleasures, he is burdened with 'an almost morbid sense of shame', which drives him to seek redemption by labouring 'in the eye of day, at the furtherance of knowledge or the relief of sorrow and suffering'.[44] Until the cycle inevitably begins again. Rather than try to reconcile these conflicts in his character, he seeks to exorcise one from the other. Initially, it is an attractive solution that allows him to maintain the status and dignity accorded the one, while enjoying uncensored the licentious freedoms of the degenerate other. Reflecting the duality of its owner's nature, the shared space of Jekyll/Hyde is situated on the threshold between London respectability and disreputability. One aspect of the house is located on a street that stands in censorious comparison to the racier aspects of the neighbourhood. However, the solid respectability of this middle-class façade is radically compromised by the 'sordid negligence' of the rear door used by Hyde to gain entrance to the building. Although Hyde has his own abode in the seedier environs of Soho, his freedom of movement across the threshold of Jekyll's home suggests the vulnerability of Victorian social and class boundaries.

At the outset of Jekyll's experimentations in doubling, his sensory experiences are not wholly unpleasant. After the 'agonies' of transformation have subsided, he feels 'strange', but 'indescribably new' and 'incredibly sweet':

> I felt younger, lighter, happier in body; within I was conscious of a heady recklessness, a current of disordered sensual images running like a mill race in my fancy, a solution of the bonds of obligation, an unknown but not an innocent freedom of the soul.[45]

Hyde literally fleshes out Jekyll's socially and intellectually forbidden carnality, the transformation shaking 'the doors of the prison-house' of Victorian propriety. Eventually, Jekyll loses control of his wilful splitting and, after the murder of Sir Danvers Carew, becomes subject to episodes of 'horrid nausea' and 'the most deadly shuddering' whenever he contemplates the increasing dissonance between his intellectualised middle-class identity (mind) and those acts committed by Hyde (brute flesh).

Hyde gains pre-eminence as Jekyll sickens at the memory of the extent of his transgressions and the physician is increasingly 'seized' by the 'indescribable sensations' and 'premonitory shudder' that herald the 'change'. Tellingly, Jekyll is most vulnerable to these paroxysms when he sleeps or 'even dozed for a moment' in his chair.

> Under the strain of this continually impending doom and by the sleeplessness to which I now condemned myself, ay, even beyond what I had thought possible to man, I became, in my own person, a creature eaten up and emptied by fever, languidly weak both in body and mind, and solely occupied by one thought: the horror of my other self.[46]

The other self that so appals Jekyll is 'caged in his flesh' and 'struggles to be born'.[47] It is a birth that he is unable to prevent. In a triumph of matter over mind, Jekyll becomes trapped in the disorderly body of Hyde. Intellectual normality finally succumbs to fleshly deviance. Nevertheless, order does prevail. Victorian morality resurfaces long enough for Jekyll/Hyde to self-administer a fatal poison, thus eradicating the potential to transgression. The resolution posits the views that split identity (double consciousness) is somehow anathema to sustained life and that the status quo will ultimately prove resistant to corporeal contamination.

Stevenson's novella demonstrates a keen awareness of the wider concerns circulating in the last decades of the nineteenth century. The narrative's theme of duality taps into those issues of class, criminality and degeneration fermenting at the core of London society in the 1880s. Stevenson likens the relationship between Jekyll and Hyde to that of father and son: 'Jekyll had more than a father's interest; Hyde had more than a son's indifference'.[48] The comparison suggests the paternalistic authority claimed by the middle classes over the lower working classes and residuum. Jekyll's failure to bring this unruly 'son' to order reflects wider anxieties about the breakdowns in administration and control of the middle echelons of London society over their degenerate charges.

It has been noted that Stevenson's novella examines and implicitly comments on Victorian society's increased awareness of the deep and barely suppressed contradictions at its core.[49] Jekyll is coded in accord with that society's vulnerability to an unmediated return of all that lies beneath the threshold between what Frederic Myers would call the supra- and the subliminal self. Jekyll's departure from the protocols of scientific orthodoxy and his hubris in seeking to order and control his own human condition suggest the 'true hamartien' that marks him for corruption and an ultimate downfall. By liberating his carnal desires from the confines of intellectual and social restraint, he wilfully opens the way to chaos, thus embracing the irrational and disorderly.

Stevenson's account of repression and split social consciousness so applicable to the London of the 1880s rests on an older story of urban conflict and fragmenting identity. It has been argued, most extensively by John Gibson, that the progenitor of Stevenson's characterisation is a figure from Edinburgh's history: one William Brodie, 'Deacon of the Wrights, a powerful figure on the Town Council' and 'a big man in the town'.[50] By day, Deacon Brodie commanded the respect of his fellow citizens in eighteenth-century Edinburgh society, if only because of his professional status. By night, he commanded a gang of miscreants who were lining their pockets by breaking into and stealing from the homes of Edinburgh's wealthier classes. After his connection to the spate of burglaries had been detected, Brodie was almost successful in escaping legal retribution by fleeing to Europe; however, he was captured and returned from Holland to his home city. Brought to trial for his nocturnal transgressions, he was sentenced to death by hanging, the sentence to be carried out on 1 October 1788. Curtailment of the earlier flight to freedom, the trial and subsequent sentencing were not enough to entirely quench Brodie's hope of cheating the hangman's noose. He had, with the help of friends, been able to formulate a plan that would have him survive his death sentence. The plan, for all its ingenuity and application, did not work. Brodie failed to be revived after his friends had hastily retrieved his body from the scaffold and he was quietly buried in one of the city's churchyards. Or so the story goes.

The magnitude of Brodie's double life captured the city's imagination. Edinburgh, in the late eighteenth century, stood at the threshold of extensive social and cultural change: its cultural identity was being whittled away by the encroachments of the English language; its political, religious and philosophical distinctiveness subject to intense debate. Brodie came to personify the city's fragmenting identity, living on in folk tales of the subversive and illicit. A large mahogany cabinet built by the Deacon had come to rest in the Stevenson family's Edinburgh home and the young Stevenson became acquainted with the item's maker through stories told to him by his childhood nurse. The effects of this confluence of events on Stevenson's literary imagination have been well documented.[51] Furthermore, his own life, particularly as a young man in his father's house was marked, like Dostoevsky's, by the conflicts imposed by social demands for conformity and the pull of private desires. Like Dostoevsky, it was a theme he chose to explore in his guise as author.

If Brodie came to personify the schism in eighteenth-century Edinburgh's identity as a respectable centre of commerce and learning by day and a hot spot of sex, gaming and deeds dastardly by night, his fictive descendant has become emblematic of an ailing nineteenth-century London. In this city, in the final decades of the century, the disorder was epileptiform in nature: a spasmodic impulse to deviance that threatened the ordered surfaces of mainstream society with degeneration. The hidden nature of Hyde's deviation from Victorian normativity can be read as a metaphor for epilepsy as it was conceptualised and represented in many of the medical journal articles of the age.

Jekyll/Hyde's transformative spasms and increasingly uncontrollable bodily movements locate the character in the signifying borderlands of the condition. When Utterson and Poole break into Jekyll's laboratory, they find 'the body of a man sorely contorted and still twitching'.[52] Jekyll's vulnerability in sleep to the internal disordering effects of his other self is evocative of nocturnal seizures associated with epilepsy and further suggests the epileptiform nature of his deviance. Jekyll/Hyde represents, as Australian physician F. Norton Manning said of the epileptic, the extremes of human possibility, being at both the 'zenith and nadir of intellectual capacity'.[53] Furthermore, this transgression from corporeal, social and scientific orthodoxy is feminised in Stevenson's narrative: Poole tells Utterson that he has heard Jekyll/Hyde – or, in an act of linguistic emasculation, 'it' – weeping: 'Weeping like a woman or a lost soul'.[54] That other self 'caged' in Jekyll's flesh struggling 'to be born' is evocative of birth and serves to complete the dissolution of Jekyll's Victorian masculinity. This feminisation of corporeal disorder is put to use as a key image and recurring motif in the 1941 film version of Stevenson's novella directed by Victor Fleming. Throughout the film Spencer Tracy's transition from Jekyll to Hyde is figured through images of the good woman (Lana Turner as his fiancée, Beatrice) and the slut (Ingrid Bergman as the barmaid, Ivy). The film offers up a Freudian interpretation of conflicted sexuality to model Jekyll's split identity.

Richard Enfield informs Utterson of his first perceptions of Hyde when he encounters him on the dark streets of London: 'It wasn't like a man; it was like some damned Juggernaut'.[55] Hyde's progress in this instance connotes the irresistible momentum of automatic behaviour and, in a move reminiscent of contemporary medical discourse, Enfield's impulse is to displace this 'alienness' from the centre of English identity by associating it via the term 'Juggernaut' with the cultural practices of the racial other.[56]

Hyde is also subject to rage crises. His potential for explosive and catastrophic fury rhetorically links him to the mythic furores of Seneca's Hercules and Shakespeare's Othello. Jekyll claims that Hyde is a 'devil' that 'had been long caged, [and] came out roaring'. It is in one of these blind rages that he kills Danvers Carew. As Poole describes Hyde to Utterson: 'there was something queer about that gentleman – something that gave a man a turn – I don't know rightly how to say it, sir, beyond this: that you felt it in your marrow – kind of cold and thin'.[57]

Stevenson's rendering of split identity is a distillation of what, on the surface, does appear as a paradox in Deacon William Brodie's life. Yet whatever argument or theory we might apply to the conditions and circumstances that brought Brodie to such an ignominious end, he himself seemed more or less able to comfortably accommodate the breadth of experience yielded by his choices. Letters to family and friends written just before he embarked on his penultimate voyage convey a wry acceptance of his situation and put forward practical suggestions for containing the damage of his crimes for himself and loved ones.[58] Dramatically transformed by Stevenson's narrative of moral and urban conflict, Brodie's literary metamorphosis into Jekyll/Hyde reduces a range of complex yet integrated behaviours to radically polarised extremes: symbolically, the good and evil of human potential are dichotomised along neatly defined axes. Good and evil are also located with different kinds of bodies. Jekyll is 'a large, well-made, smooth-faced man of fifty, with something of a slyish cast perhaps, but every mark of capacity and kindness'.[59] Hyde epitomises degenerate corporeality: he is 'pale and dwarfish; he gave an impression of deformity without nameable malformation, he had a displeasing smile' and 'he spoke with a husky, whispering and somewhat broken voice'.[60]

Whether Arthur Myers ever read Stevenson's novella can only be a matter of conjecture. The text was certainly contemporary and his references to other writers of fiction and poetry suggest a more than casual acquaintance with the literary culture of his time. If he was cognisant of Stevenson's narrative, however, it was not to this that he looked for clues on how to reconcile his epileptic and professional/social identities. This is perfectly understandable, given the narrative's austere thesis on the implacable irreconcilability of a disordered body and intellectual integrity. Instead, Arthur quotes Dickens when attempting to give representational form for his 'occasional epilepsy'. Even here, however, he exercises a meticulous care in choosing his narrative devices. Clearly, the system of representation that gave cultural presence to Monks' epileptic character cannot have provided a viable alternative for Arthur. As I have already suggested, despite providing medically validated renderings of epilepsy symptomatology, Dickens constructed a narrow range of possibilities for his epileptic characters.

VII

Of all the possibilities available to Arthur, Bradley Headstone in *Our Mutual Friend* is perhaps the most developed of Dickens' epileptic characters, although, from his over-determined 'decent' entry into the narrative, he too is flagged as bearing the seeds of his own inevitable degeneration:

> Bradley Headstone, in his decent black coat and waistcoat, and decent white shirt, and decent formal black tie, and decent pantaloons of pepper and salt, with his decent silver watch in his pocket and its decent hair-guard round his neck, looked a thoroughly decent young man of six-and-twenty. He was never seen in any other dress, and yet there was a certain stiffness in his manner of wearing this, as if there were a want of adaptation between him and it, recalling some mechanics in their holiday clothes.[61]

The character's vulnerability to a barely suppressed disorder is indicated by the 'settled trouble' of his face, a face 'belonging to a naturally slow or inattentive intellect that had toiled hard to get what it had won, and that had to hold it now that it was gotten'.[62] Headstone is painfully self-conscious of his 'obscure' origins and in this passage the inauthenticity of his claims to middle-class respectability is suggested through the association of his 'want of adaptation' with that of 'mechanics in their holiday clothes'.

In the book, Eugene Wrayburn dismisses him as being a 'curious monomaniac'. Like Monks, Headstone is driven to paroxysmal fury by strong passion. His violent infatuation with Lizzie Hexam combines with his jealousy of Wrayburn to propel him explosively towards attempted murder. The split between Headstone's earnest decency and violent passion prefigures the wilful split sought by Jekyll in his attempt to retain an appropriate public masculinity free of carnal and emotional passions. In her reading of masculinity in English literature, Eve Sedgwick has argued that this split in Dickens' novel can be extended to the Headstone–Wrayburn relationship and figures repressed 'homosocial' desire. Sedgwick's analysis provides further insight into the demands of licit (patriarchal, Victorian) masculinity and the fragmenting consequences (opportunities) for male characterisation in the nineteenth-century English novel.[63] Headstone's decline from a hard-won respectable life and keen attention to the pastoral care of his students endows the characterisation with a pathos not associated with Monks. However, Headstone's impulse to decency and his aspiration to middle-class respectability are not enough to save him; for Dickens, his essentialised epileptic nature cannot be completely erased by the influences of culture and education.

In the novels *The Life and Adventures of Martin Chuzzlewit, The Old Curiosity Shop* and *David Copperfield,* Dickens deploys the 'fit' as a narrative device to achieve transition from one state to another in plot development. Old Anthony Chuzzlewit, after an evening by the fire, falls into seizure: 'It was frightful to see how the principle of life, shut up within his withered frame, fought like a strong devil, mad to be released, and rent its ancient prison-house'.[64] When he regains consciousness after the episode, his speech is garbled. Although he utters words, 'they were such as man had never heard' and he 'gabbles' to his son Jonas in an 'unearthly tongue'. Jonas had planned on poisoning his father, but Chuffy, the old man's faithful clerk, eventually reveals that Anthony had stumbled upon his son's plan and, in fact, dies from a combination of grief and a broken heart. Chuffy explains that 'his dear old master's' mind was fatally affected by his son's perfidy. Anthony's death frees Jonas from paternal restraint and he pursues his villainous ambitions to their logical conclusion. J. E. Cosnett has attributed Anthony's death to 'late-onset epilepsy … due to cerebral vascular disease', with accompanying paraphasia and aphasia.[65] The retrospective diagnosis indicates the fidelity of Dickens' descriptions of symptomatology to contemporaneous medical writing.

In *The Old Curiosity Shop,* Little Nell tells Kit: 'grandfather has been taken very ill, I found him in a fit upon the floor'.[66] Although her grandfather eventually recovers from this crisis, he remains mentally debilitated by the episode:

> the mind was weakened and its functions were impaired. He was patient, and quiet; often sat brooding, but not despondently, for a long space; was easily amused, even by a sunbeam on the wall or ceiling;

> made no complaint that the days were long or the nights tedious; and appeared indeed to have all lost all count of time and every sense of care or weariness.[67]

The seizure episode signals a transition for Nell and her grandfather from their relatively stable life in the Curiosity Shop, which the grandfather has managed to gamble away to Daniel Quilp, to a precarious life on the road, which will end first in Little Nell's death, and, eventually, her grandfather's.

The fit as a device of transition also occurs in *David Copperfield*. After being forbidden by Francis Spenlow to pursue his affections for Spenlow's daughter, Dora, David is freed from his master's prohibition when Spenlow suddenly dies. The lawyer is found lying by the roadside after having fallen from his phaeton. Mr Tiffey tells David:

> Whether he fell out in a fit, or got out, feeling ill before the fit came or – or even whether he was quite dead then, though there is no doubt he was quite insensible – no one appears to know. If he breathed, certainly he never spoke. Medical assistance was got as soon as possible, but it was quite useless.[68]

In these texts the fit heralds either sudden death, as in the case of Anthony Chuzzlewit and Francis Spenlow, or triggers a chain of events that leads to untimely death, as with Nell Trent.

None of these constructions of the epileptic can have proved comforting to Arthur. Dickens' faithfulness to medical discourses of epilepsy and 'epileptic' social behaviours reinforces the premise of an inevitable and predictable degradation of self associated with the condition. Nell Trent's grandfather adores her but is incapable of reining in personal behaviours that undermine her security. He is an inveterate (and unsuccessful) gambler, regularly leaving the child alone in the shop when he goes out for his nightly 'fix'. His seizure episode somatises an impulse to fecklessness, infantilises him and finally leaves him completely dependent on Nell. Despite Francis Spenlow's concerns that David's prospects make him an unsuitable match for his daughter, he himself dies, leaving his financial affairs in disarray and without leaving a will to secure Dora's financial security. Monks and Bradley Headstone are by turn completely impotent in managing their potential for disorder, and murderously destructive. Anthony Chuzzlewit's fit is symptomatic of betrayal.

The quotation Arthur takes from Dickens to illustrate his experience of symptomatology belongs to David Copperfield. On returning to Canterbury, David revisits Wickfield's house, where, in conversation with Mr Micawber, he is for a moment, through the pull of his attraction to Dora, privy to an awareness of the continuity and depth of his feelings for Agnes:

> We have all some experience of a feeling, that comes over us occasionally, of what we are saying and doing having been said and done before, in a remote time – of our having been surrounded, dim ages ago, by the same faces, objects, and circumstances – of our knowing perfectly what will be said next, as if we suddenly remembered it! I never had this mysterious impression more strongly in my life, than before he uttered those words.[69]

Micawber has told David that were it not for the fact that his young friend had declared his commitment to Dora, he, Micawber, would have thought the 'superior' and 'remarkable' Agnes the favoured one. There is nothing in David Copperfield's history to suggest that his experience of double consciousness in that moment is a result of epilepsy. In light of this, it makes Arthur's choice an interesting one, and perhaps an understandable one given the orthodoxy of Dickens' constructions of epilepsy and the epileptic. Significantly, this is not the only example of David's propensity to double consciousness. It is, however, the only instance that reflects a self-awareness of suppressed yearning.

David Copperfield is a hybrid figure in the novel, able to move easily across class boundaries. After Clara Copperfield dies, David's primary maternal figures, Clara Peggotty and Betsey Trotwood, become representative of this social mobility. He moves easily and with confidence between the middle-class society of Canterbury, Dover and London to the working-class robustness of the Peggotty family and their social circle near Yarmouth. He is able to sustain a professional profile with Spenlow and Jorkin's law firm while maintaining his long-term friendship with Mr Micawber, a character always in various stages of retreat from legal retribution because of debts.

His episodes of double consciousness are important to plot progression and repeatedly carry him to a level of awareness beyond the moment. When he and Uriah Heep are discussing the Wickfields, and specifically Agnes, in his London rooms, David is so moved by his 'delirious idea' of running Uriah through with 'a red-hot poker' that he is mentally transported:

> [Uriah] seemed to swell and grow before my eyes; the room seemed full of the echoes of his voice; and the strange feeling (to which, perhaps, no one is quite a stranger) that all this had occurred before, at some indefinite time, and that I knew what he was going to say next, took possession of me.[70]

This rendition of double consciousness, with its violent overtones, is perhaps more suggestive of medically scripted epilepsy symptomatology than the one drawn upon by Arthur. David experiences this sudden change in perceptual state 'with a shock, like a ball fired from a rifle'. In another instance of enhanced awareness, and portending Emily's defection from hearth and home, David is all but overcome at Barkis' funeral with a premonitory 'dread' of what is to come.

Although he has repeated experiences of variable intensity of double consciousness throughout the novel, David's memory of 'the strange feeling' from episode to episode is flawed. The provoking factor for both the delirious idea of skewering Uriah Heep with a red-hot poker and the forced reminiscence sparked by his conversation with Micawber is reference to Agnes. In a sense, she functions as the epileptogenic trigger for his mental diplopia. Yet despite errors in judgement, and a spasmodic tendency to *déjà vu*, David Copperfield goes on to win out over tragedy and trying professional circumstances. His value to Arthur's quest lies with the character's sustained autonomy in both his personal and professional lives. And of course he is able to retain a social and sexual viability unavailable to those 'others' prone to neuronal paroxysmal episodes in Dickens' medically oriented characterisations. Furthermore, and again unlike Arthur, the fictional David retains authorial power over his own self-written history.

The fragmented or hybrid figure is a complex trope in the nineteenth-century novel. In examining the function of the hybrid figure in Gothicism, Gerry Turcotte points out that it becomes representative of divided experience and the forbidden, instantiating on some level a dialogue between self and other.[71] The hybrid is a figure of liminality located on the threshold of the mundane and the normal. It is quite often a figure in transition, a figure of possibility, as with David Copperfield. It can also be a figure symbolising the tumult of category crisis, necessarily fragmented, necessarily other. Integrated identity is at once sought and deflected. The hybrid figure is either inculcated into the dominant regime and the category crisis resolved through reunification with the dominant order, or it is marginalised to the unliveable zones of the abject. According to Jan Gordon, in texts drawing on elements of the Gothic, the fragment represents the incomplete or unfinished. It can be interpreted, she argues, as a mediation between nature and culture, and 'from one perspective at least, [it] may be seen as culture being reclaimed by nature'.[72] The possibly fatal consequences of an attempted reunification – a resuturing of split identity to a socially acceptable cohesion – is signified by the death of Jekyll/Hyde; the death of Lucette Le Sueur and Yelena; and the death-in-life to which Rogozhin and Myshkin are consigned. Death is the final victory of nature over culture.

By 1900 the hybridised figure of the epileptic had been well established as a locus of disease and social paranoia. Two factors that saw both medical and cultural responses to the category crisis represented by the epileptic body gloss the fact of its ambiguity. Somehow this *particular* hybrid figure could be detected at a glance, the measure of its deviation from normativity clearly indexed on the body. With few notable variations, the epileptic figure in late nineteenth-century fiction bore a remarkable resemblance to its counterpart in medical narratives. The male epileptic body, medically stereotyped as violent, volatile and vulnerable to vice, finds representation in Monks, Smerdyakov and Headstone, who are all unable to control their more explosive passions. For all his beauty and kindness, Myshkin is oddly impotent. When asked by Ganya if he would marry a woman like Nastasya Filippovna, Myshkin replies: 'I can't marry anyone, I am an invalid'.[73] Ascribed social mobility and cultural capital notwithstanding, Dostoevsky does not allow the character to ultimately live beyond the identity category of the disabled other.

Dostoevsky's characterisation of Myshkin, and despite the medical debates generated by the author's descriptions of his own symptomatology, had only a limited effect on representations taken up by the cultural circuit producing late nineteenth- and early twentieth-century epilepsy narratives. Arthur Myers' attempts to recruit alternative possibilities for representing epileptic experience do not survive him. Rather, it is Stevenson's dual characterisation of Jekyll and Hyde that becomes the smuggled contraband crossing the temporal borders between centuries and the discursive borders between representational systems. Frederic's efforts to provide an alternative identity story for his brother are also subsumed when in 1919 Sigmund Freud publishes an essay on aesthetics and the uncanny that takes up the historically ratified associations between convulsiveness, automatism and epileptic danger.

VIII

In this essay, Freud suggests that the uncanny 'is undoubtedly related to what is frightening – to what arouses dread and horror; equally certainly, too, the word is not always used in a clearly definable sense, so it tends to coincide with what excites fear in general'.[74] He traces the meaning of the English 'uncanny' through its etymology in the German *unheimlich*, meaning 'unhomely', and points out that its meaning 'is obviously the opposite of "*heimlich*" ("homely"), "*heimisch*" ("native") –

the opposite of what is familiar'.[75] Through this etymological mapping, clear boundaries between meanings attributed to these oppositional terms begin to erode:

> among its different shades of meaning the word '*heimlich*' exhibits one which is identical with its opposite, '*unheimlich*'. What is *heimlich* thus comes to be *unheimlich*.... In general we are reminded that the word '*heimlich*' is not unambiguous, but belongs to two sets of ideas, which, without being contradictory, are yet very different: on the one hand it means what is familiar and agreeable, and on other, what is concealed and kept out of sight.[76]

Freud's discussion throughout the essay deals primarily with occurrences of the uncanny in literature. He suggests, however, that, beyond the aesthetics of literature, the uncanny can be located with a living person.

The effects of epilepsy and madness, he argues, are instances where the layman is confronted with 'the working of forces hitherto unsuspected in his fellow men, but at the same time he is dimly aware of them in remote corners of his own being'.[77] In differentiating between those instances of the uncanny produced through literature and those experienced as part of real-world existence Freud maintains:

> We can also speak of a living person as uncanny, and we do so when we ascribe evil intentions to him. But that is not all; in addition to this we must feel that his intentions to harm us are going to be carried out with the help of special powers.[78]

According to Freud the uncanny effects of epilepsy and madness are grounded in these origins of suspected harm and fear. In this extrapolation from literary artefact to corporeal signification, he follows not only Ernst Jentsch (whose claims he is undermining here) but also a fashion discernible in the medical writings of other late nineteenth-century physicians.

Freud's efforts to pin down a meaning of the uncanny are undermined somewhat by his over-determined and ambiguous claims for its definitive boundaries. In an attempt to capture and explain that which nevertheless remains radically inexplicable, the essay explores and enacts its own anxiety in problematic tracings and recuperations of the discontinuities, connections and envelopments that mark Freud's departure from, and ultimate return to, Jentsch's premise that somehow the uncanny hinges on intellectual uncertainty.

The French theorist Hélène Cixous argues that the very 'indefiniteness [of the *unheimlich*] is part and parcel of the "concept"' and necessarily erodes any possibility of Freud's knowledge claims about its enunciation. She insists that, at best, he has only sought 'the *basic* sense' of the idea: 'Thus the analysis is anchored, at once, in what is denoted. And it is a question of a concept whose entire denotation is a connotation.'[79] Cixous's detailed critique of what she deems to be a tendency to intellectual sleight of hand in Freud's essay has merit. Her observation that the indecisiveness of the *unheimlich* is part and parcel of the concept might also be said to apply to epilepsy. Freud's medical contemporaries claimed to know what it is, but when it came to concise definition, knowledge claims proved to be less than stable. Freud's work on the uncanny, and by extension the evocation of the uncanny in social responses to epilepsy and madness, remains a productive component in my examination of turn-of-the-century responses to the epileptic.

The body that suddenly falls in convulsion excites powerful and complex reactions in the bystander: shock, anxiety, fear, helplessness, confusion about what is taking place, embarrassment, superstition, revulsion. Some of these responses are due to the suddenness of transition from consciousness to unconsciousness, to frenetic, uncontrolled activity: as Freud puts it, the observer is confronted with 'feet which dance by themselves'.[80] Drawing on his idea that 'What is *experienced* as uncanny [fearful] ... can be traced back without exception to something familiar that has been repressed',[81] I suggest here that much of the anxiety and alienation generated by the convulsing body remains grounded in this confrontation between the socialised, ordered self and a vision of a repressed, uncontrolled other.

The notion that the familiar and symbolically proper remain vulnerable to a repressed and disordered other is also suggested by Freud's involved mapping of the etymological roots of the uncanny. He uncovers supposedly repressed associations between the *heimlich* and its conceptual opposites: mysticism, unconsciousness, the obscure, the inaccessible to knowledge. Notions of the *heimlich*, signifying that which is familiar, normal, orthodox, are further complicated as this linguistic unfolding continues: 'to behave *heimlich*, as though there was some thing to conceal; *heimlich* love-affair, love, sin; *heimlich* places (which good manners oblige us to conceal)'.[82]

His journey through this essay brings him very close indeed to the territory that Frederic Myers had tried to navigate and rationalise in his work, and Freud's attempts to clearly define the boundaries between psychoanalysis and the occult have been the subject of some debate. Pamela Thurschwell argues that these attempts were at times marked by a certain ambiguity: 'Freud's volatile relationship with telepathy, a systematic wavering between embracing it and refusing it, covers most of his career'.[83] She points out that in his biography of his old teacher, Ernest Jones discusses at length Freud's sustained interest in the occult. He writes of urging Freud to maintain a distance between the developing discipline of psychoanalysis and exploration into the occult. In a reply to Jones' concerns that at least linguistically invokes Frederic, Freud responds by telling his colleague: 'If someone should reproach you with my Fall into Sin, you are free to reply that my adherence to telepathy is my private affair like my Jewishness, my passion for smoking, and other things, and the theme of telepathy – inessential for psychoanalysis'.[84]

Medical literature from the turn of the century often becomes mired in a boggy conceptual terrain between medical denotation and cultural connotation. Freud's acts of discovery of the illicit at the heart of the decorous suggest the internal conflicts (discernible at the interstices of *langue/langage*) troubling medical aspirations to objectively define the neurological processes underlying the observable effects of epilepsy. In this regard, his engagement with the conceptual object of his work bears an uncanny resemblance to medical attempts to define and clarify the condition. In Cixous' words, nineteenth-century neurologists sought 'the *basic* sense' of epileptic disorder. Although their explanations struggled to capture precisely *what* denoted epilepsy in medical terms, through the late nineteenth century and beyond, the medical project was often side-tracked into a pursuit of a concept whose medical denotation was primarily constituted by its cultural connotations. It is worth noting Hughlings Jackson's claim that 'the [medical] student … imagines there is some entity of which epilepsy is the proper name'.[85] Like Freud's take on the uncanny, the term 'epilepsy', it seems, was also a word not always used in a clearly definable sense.

By the end of the nineteenth century and into the twentieth century, 'epilepsy' was still used to describe and define a range of social events and behaviours not attributable to the model of discharging cerebral lesions implicated by Jackson and others in medical accounts of the syndrome. Within these textual productions the uncanny, and its embodied representation, the epileptic, are codified to the point of near incomprehensibility. Nonetheless, late nineteenth-century neurology also anxiously insisted on the heterodoxy of the epileptic figure within regimes of biomedical and social normalcy, and rigorously policed the terms of its exclusion.

The flailing, leaking body of the epileptic generates a misrecognition of those aspects of the subject that become repressed with maturation and socialisation. Entry into a symbolic order which privileges the clean, controlled and obedient body is contingent on the continued suppression of the disordered body. The convulsing body, once so familiar, so akin to our own, so knowable, suddenly crashes through those psychical barriers revealing the *unheimlich* located at the core of the *heimlich*. The other part of ourselves that is concealed, and 'kept from sight, so that others do not get to know of or about it',[86] is exposed to the interpretative gaze. In emphasising the negative connotation embedded in the sign of repression, *'un'*, Freud introduces a definition attributed to Friedrich Schelling which imports ideas of lapsed modesty or failed social decorum into the realm of the uncanny. Schelling's version of the above quote invokes the possibility of choice in maintaining a veil over that which should be repressed or concealed from the public gaze: '"*Unheimlich*" is the name for everything that *ought* to have remained ... secret and hidden but has come to light'.[87]

Freud's conceptualisation of the *unheimlich* prefigures Judith Butler's observation that the abject and marginal are never completely exterior – they are folded in as the constitutive substance of the centre.[88] The excluded 'not-subject' remains, in fact, at the very heart of subjectivity. Julia Kristeva argues for a differentiation between the uncanny and the abject body. Abjectness is 'more violent', she writes; it is 'elaborated through a failure to recognise its kin; nothing is familiar, not even the shadow of a memory'.[89] The epileptic body in *grand mal* seizure complicates this concept, I think. It *is* unfamiliar, even alien, at the cataclysmic centre of a neuronal tempest. Yet it is still recognisable as a material body. And this is precisely what makes an encounter between this particular manifestation of abjectness and the non-affected observer so confronting. This violent loss of control is, as one commentator has noted in relation to theories of stigma, 'something which normal people fear in themselves'.[90] It is a fear specific to an initial sense of connection between bodies, a recognition of *potential* kinship.

The possibility that our bodies can be suddenly overtaken by hitherto undetected forces from within is, of course, a classic theme in science fiction films of the twentieth century and I will return to this idea in Chapter 5. But for now, recall the 1979 film *Alien*[91] and that shockingly memorable scene when Kane (John Hurt), apparently recovered from his encounter with the creature from the alien ship, sits down to enjoy a well deserved breakfast with his crew mates. His body suddenly and violently explodes in a flurry of non-volitional jerks and shudders, his face contorted by grotesque muscle spasms. He appears to be having a seizure. Then horror of horrors! The cause of his spasms erupts from *within* his body – a body that, up until this moment, appeared so familiar, so 'normal' – in the form of a neonatal alien. The power of the moment to shock lies with its juxtaposition of the homely breakfast scene and the *unheimlich* birth scene. As Kristeva notes of the abject, 'It is ... not lack of cleanliness or health that causes abjection but what disturbs identity, system, order. What does not respect borders, positions, rules. The in-between, the ambiguous, the composite.'[92]

Lennard Davis argues that the key to Freud's reading of certain kinds of bodies as uncanny is located with the intimate relation between the *unheimlich* and the *heimlich*:

> The disabled body is seen as *unheimlich* because it is the familiar gone wrong. Disability is seen as something that does not belong at home, not to be associated with the home. Freud notes that the terror or repulsion of the uncanny is ambivalent, is found precisely in its relation to and yet deviance from the familiar.[93]

The *heimlich* body – that body at once homelike, agreeable, intact, predictable – is founded on a series of repressions. Davis suggests that Freud appears to ignore this factor and its implications for 'the inherently fragmentary nature of the original body *imago*'. He notes that a reanalysis of this relationship between the familiar (normal) and unfamiliar (abnormal) via the French psychoanalyst Jacques Lacan revisions the *unheimlich* body as 'the originary, familiar body made unfamiliar by repression'.[94]

The subject with epilepsy, specifically epilepsy uncomplicated by other symptomatology, inhabits that liminal or interstitial space in the dyad between normality and abnormality, poised on the threshold of an always threatening transition between *heimlich* and *unheimlich*. Signifiers of this particular form of neurological difference are veiled by a seemingly normal exterior. This perceived homogeneity exacerbates the shock felt by the onlooker when that symbolic boundary between hitherto fixed identities proves vulnerable to rupture. There is a doubling between what was known and what was thought to be unknown, what was concealed and now appears confusingly before our eyes. Through the spectacle of the convulsing other, the normative subject is confronted with the spectre of a half-forgotten, pre-socialised self. The boundary between the known and the unknown, between the repressed and the public self fails. Carefully defined delineations between normality and abnormality, between ability and disability, are destabilised as erratically firing electrical impulses inscript the seizing body with signs of the neuronal chaos that compels its reconfiguration of spatiality. Of course, the irony here is that, post-seizure, the affected subject has no memory of just how disordering the disorder has been for the observer. The epileptic body in *grand mal* or generalised tonic/clonic seizure has come to represent the fragility of the hold that the symbolic order has over the material body. Consequently, it is a locus *and* a repository of both medical and cultural anxiety because of its category instability. The danger, stigma and value of the epileptic body are locatable in its ambiguity and power to disrupt scripted boundaries between order and chaos.

The threshold vulnerable to breach becomes an unstable and dangerous margin between tractable normality and unruly abnormality if it fails to bear the defining weight between dichotomous and otherwise mutually exclusive categorisations. It is the threshold, after all, that retains the boundaries between normality and abnormality, between abled and disabled. These boundaries sustain the crucial difference between conflicting cultural identity positions. Without that demarcating and containing threshold, separation of the *heimlich* (normal, orthodox, knowable) and *unheimlich* (the hidden, inaccessible to knowledge) disintegrates, drawing otherwise opposite concepts inexorably towards an uncanny border where clear distinction begins to break down and the powerfully symbolic currency of the dichotomy is placed in danger of collapsing in on itself. The epileptic body can conceivably locate itself on either side of this defining threshold, the fact of its hybridity further undermining the signifying integrity of both classifications. Faced with William Lennox's dictum that 'Man is built to convulse',[95] we are compelled to consider that convulsing just *may* be part of a spectrum of human experience rather than discrete aberration. Historically, the cultural and medical response to the seizure-prone body has been to deny this possibility and vigorously insist on the maintenance of that threshold at all costs, and so to locate the spectre of epileptic disorder unequivocally beyond the bounds of normality.

It is not just the sight of the convulsing body that generates disease in the general population. Freud reviews Jentsch's thesis that feelings of the uncanny can be evoked by 'doubts whether an apparently animate being is really alive'. The 'effects of epileptic fits and manifestations of insanity' are cited as instances that 'excite in the spectator the impression of automatic, mechanical processes at work behind the ordinary appearance of mental activity'.[96] While Freud claims not to be in complete accord with this theory of the uncanny, he nevertheless appropriates its basic tenets in the development his own thoughts on the subject. He extrapolates on Jentsch's location of the uncanny with the body of the epileptic and the madman, arguing that the origin of this effect is not only due to the glimpsing of unsuspected forces but also the recognition that those forces are part of our own darkest psychical recesses. Freud does not expand on what he means precisely by epileptic fits in his essay. I take it that both he and Jentsch are referring to instances of *grand mal* seizure rather than automatisms or episodes of epileptic furore. Automatisms and epileptic furore or mania certainly suggest the illusion of the mechanistic or non-human. Aretaeus described these aspects of the epileptic persona as 'inhuman'.[97] Referring to epilepsy as 'the uncanny disease with its incalculable, apparently unprovoked convulsive attacks' in his 1927/28 essay 'Dostoevsky and parricide',[98] Freud confirmed his earlier thesis on the *unheimlich* effects of the disorder on general sensibilities.

Suspicion that the epileptic is somehow culpable in her or his own disorder, that there is agency in the links between furore states and Freud's ascribed 'evil intentions', is ambiguously inscribed in nineteenth-century biomedical productions of epilepsy. The 'epileptic' is constructed as both wilful and mindless, simultaneously an agent in her or his own aberrance and the pitiful victim of a cruel neurological fate. Concomitant with this suspicion, that those with epilepsy somehow wilfully and immodestly exceed the boundaries of self-control, is the fear that non-insane epileptics controlled their potential for disorder too well, veiling from public and medical scrutiny the signifiers of hereditary taint. Their ability to pass undetected in normate society posed a threat to the boundaries between normal and abnormal, and by extension they undermined the processes of biological evolution by breeding with the normal population.

IX

The notion of an essentialised epileptic duality continued to grip the medical imagination well into the twentieth century and it was Stevenson's imagery of the radically divided self that came to the fore in medical representation. In attempting to organise a complex range of theories and information about epilepsy and its consequences for those subject to epilepsy, the twentieth-century neuropsychiatrist Leopold Szondi argued for an 'epileptiform drive factor', which he termed 'the ethical factor'. He claimed that this factor dictated those aspects of the human condition we call good and evil. Dietrich Blumer summarises the argument thus:

> The epileptiform or ethical factor thus determines the forces of 'good' and 'evil,' the paroxysmal nature of humans, which can be observed in three phases: the penting up of crude affects; the explosive discharge or attack; and the phase of making up – the ethical–religious phase. This process of general significance tends to be most dramatically expressed in certain epileptic disorders. Thus follows the paradoxic finding of the

> 'two-faced epileptic' or the 'Jekyll-and-Hyde' nature of many patients. Although many patients appear stabilized in the hyperethical phase, the paroxysmal force of the process tends to be episodically destabilizing and frequently results in marked emotional lability.[99]

Although this ethical factor constitutes part of the drives that fuel all human endeavour, it is most dramatically expressed, so the argument goes, in certain forms of epilepsy, typically those paroxysmal conditions located in the temporal lobe. In some cases of temporal lobe epilepsy, the spectrum of human behaviours attributable to Szondi's ethical factor become polarised to the point of caricature: law-abiding conscientiousness and fair-mindedness (good) apocalyptically replaced by anger and intolerance (evil).

Obviously this is an argument that requires some scrutiny. Certainly the medical literature offers up a plethora of anecdotal evidence on the extremes of behaviour triggered by cerebral paroxysm. However, as Blumer and others have argued, seizure behaviours do not occur in a vacuum. While there can be little doubt that cerebral events can and do have a catastrophic effect on certain behaviours at certain times, Blumer notes that 'the emotionality of certain epileptics merely represents extraordinary variants of the norm'.[100] In other words, these behaviours will usually occur at the extremes of a spectrum of possibilities specific to the individual.

Although Deacon Brodie lends historical countenance to the ethical factor, there is nothing to suggest that his fluctuations between diurnal good and nocturnal evil were either paroxysmal in nature or symptomatic of a split in personal identity as such. Profound polarisation in social behaviours is not necessarily an indicator of internal fragmentation. Certainly this was the view of Braxfield, the Lord Justice Clerk at Brodie's trial. In reviewing for the court and the defendant Brodie's deviation from what might be duly expected of a man with his background and social status, he frankly attributed the accused's 'melancholy situation' to a taste for high living and the pleasures of gambling:

> It's much tae be lamented that thae vices, which are called gentlemanly vices, are sae favourably looked upon in the present age. They hae been the source o' yer ruin; and, whatever may be thocht o' them, they are sic as assuredly lead tae ruin.[101]

Gibson argues that extracts from letters written by Brodie and contemporary documents of his behaviour during the trial and sentencing suggest an integrated self-awareness and acceptance, albeit rueful, of his own potential to transgress the limits demarcating social and legal propriety. Nevertheless, it is easy to see the value of Brodie in Stevenson's literary explorations of an irreconcilable split between conformity and disorder, just as we can see the attractiveness of Stevenson's imagery for medical systems of representation.

Enfield notes an indefinable 'something' about the character of Hyde that is enough to bring out a 'sweat' on him, to inspire 'loathing' on sight and to turn the physician tending the child Hyde has trampled 'sick and white with the desire to kill him'.[102] Like Monks, Hyde's 'wrongness' is indexed on the body, and yet is resistant to ready or accurate deciphering. His uncanny presence at the centre of Jekyll's life conforms to Freudian theories the *unheimlich*. Jekyll's alter-ego is frightening to Enfield, but not in any clearly definable sense. He embodies what has been hitherto repressed or concealed from Jekyll's public life, indeed, those traits, to recall Freud, that 'ought to have remained ... secret and hidden but [have] come to light'. This deviance from appropriate Victorian masculinity is figured in accordance with those characteristics and stigmata identified by Cesare Lombroso and others. Hyde's physical deformity transparently conveys his degenerative nature. Furthermore, the 'epileptic' episodes function as the defining coda of this characterisation. Lombroso argued, after all, that epilepsy 'united the criminal and the morally insane in one natural family'.

The Myers brothers can only have been discouraged by this style of representation. In reviewing and assessing his own behaviour after seizing while examining a young male patient, Arthur writes of coming back into conscious awareness of the situation to find that the patient was no longer in the consulting room. About an hour later, when tracing his movements during that lost time, he found that his patient had been put to bed (presumably by the child's mother or other hospital staff) and his examination notes inscribed with his diagnosis of 'pneumonia of the left base'. He writes:

> I re-examined him with some curiosity, and found that my conscious diagnosis was the same as my unconscious – or perhaps I should say, unremembered diagnosis had been. I was a good deal surprised, but not so unpleasantly as I should have thought probable.[103]

Frederic argues strongly for the probability of an essential continuity – albeit disrupted – between the supra- and subliminal self rather than a multiplicity of selves: an argument that seems to be supported by Arthur's observations of his own altered states.

Debates about the extent and significance of the links between epilepsy conditions, social behaviours, moral responsibility and intellectual capacity are wide ranging and complex. Sustained engagement with that field of literature is beyond the boundaries of this book. Most medical writers on the subject of the epilepsies have something to say about the effects of cerebral paroxysm on human behaviour. Arthur's account of his own seizure-inflected behaviour, however, suggests a continuity of the self that undermines the Jekyll-and-Hyde image drawn upon by Szondi and others to connote epileptic fragmentation.

Nevertheless, from the interpretative frame sketched here, it is possible to understand the attraction of Stevenson's text in Szondi's attempts to convey some of the more confounding traits associated with epilepsy conditions. Stevenson's novella is a rich resource for a range of powerful and dramatic imagery and characterisation that depict the extreme and nuanced conflicts in human behaviour. However, the function of the characterisation in the statement 'Thus follows the paradoxic finding of the "two-faced epileptic" or the "Jekyll-and-Hyde" nature of many patients' is worth further review. Could the phrase still function as a useful metaphor in a twentieth-century context? Did it enrich that century's medical discourse and facilitate clarification of epilepsy conditions? Or was it more akin to catachresis: an abuse of language that reduced temporal lobe experience to a dated literary dramatisation — a triumph of myth over matter, so to speak?

'Metaphor', as Donald Davidson suggests, 'is the dreamwork of language and, like all dreamwork, its interpretation reflects as much on the interpreter as on the originator'.[104] The construction and interpretation of metaphors are equally creative endeavours, Davidson argues, and the success of collaboration between 'dreamer' and 'interpreter' – even if they are the same person – will, to a degree, rely on a shared frame of reference. The metaphoric value of this strategy in Stevenson's examination of Victorian morals and social fragmentation is undoubted. Jekyll/Hyde is a figure for the times. However, the consequence of conveying the complexities of epileptic behaviours via this dramatic distillation in twentieth-century medical discourse would seem to invite obfuscation rather than illumination.

Tracing John Locke's contemplation on the place of figurative language in philosophical discourse, Paul de Man refers to Locke's claim that with catachresis 'of mixed modes … the word can be said to produce of and by itself the entity it signifies and that has no equivalence in nature'. Moreover, de Man claims that 'Something monstrous lurks in the most innocent of catachresis'.[105] Rather than enhancing understanding of a metaphorical link between properties, potentialities and ways of being, catachresis disrupts the text/ure of knowledge claims. This, I argue, is the legacy of the intertextual function of the Jekyll/Hyde allusion in twentieth-century medical discourse.

Stevenson's narrative of paradox and duality is, itself, a transformative and, on one level, reductive dramatisation of nature. It is encoded with nineteenth-century medical concepts of degeneration, as well as discourses of moral insanity and epileptic disorder. The novella, in turn, provides a powerful metaphor for medical explanations about the fragmentation and social deviance associated with epilepsy. While the vivid evocativeness of the Jekyll/Hyde figure is no doubt attractive, its value in twentieth-century endeavours to refine and clarify knowledge claims about the epilepsies is at best spurious. At worst, it perpetuates a textual violence on the complex historical, cultural and empirical realities of living with an epilepsy disorder. Whether the idea it conveys has a precise equivalent in the symptomatology of epilepsy syndromes is also highly questionable. That being the case, Szondi's intertextual deployment of Stevenson's characterisation, rather than functioning as a metaphor for the fragmentation associated with the epilepsies, smuggled the figurative monster of catachresis across temporal and generic borders.

If, like Szondi, however, we indulge for the moment in the pleasures of intertextual play and read fiction onto life, there are, of course, some uncanny comparisons to be made between the social conditions reproduced and explored in Stevenson's text and those confronting Arthur's attempts at self-definition, particularly in relation to issues of identity and the consequences of social and scientific unorthodoxy. A sample of the moral judgement visited upon Jekyll when he strays from the paths of 'proper' science can be glimpsed in the *Lancet*'s published response to Frederic's psychical research. Jekyll's textual emasculation generated by his split identity resonates with the professional impotence that overtook Arthur in the last year of his life and saw him having to resign from his work. The image of emasculation also suggests the hyposexuality so frequently associated with temporal lobe epilepsy. Furthermore, Arthur was largely exiled from social and professional positions that, if it had not been for his epilepsy condition (his disordered body), would surely have guaranteed him that fate Stevenson casts for Dr Jekyll: 'an honourable and distinguished future'. Despite his medical training, however, Jekyll loses control of his disorder. He finally kills what he cannot cure.

The intertextual play discussed in relation to Szondi, and indulged in by myself in the paragraph above, is deemed inappropriate by many illness narrators. Illness is not a game. The place of figurative language in medical discourse is the subject of some debate, the objection being that to metaphorise illness is to commit a textual violence on illness experience. In *Illness as Metaphor* Susan Sontag argues: 'My point is that illness is not a metaphor, and that the most truthful way of regarding illness – and the healthiest way of being ill – is one most purified of, most resistant to, metaphoric thinking'.[106] The project to diminish the power of language to mediate our experience of disease is current and ongoing. But is it possible, or indeed feasible, to think that we can ever work with a system of signs, a system of representation, completely 'purified' of intertextual play? To narrativise disease or illness experience seems immediately to place one back into the flow of language, in all its forms and possibilities.

As de Man has suggested, 'The use and abuse of language cannot be separated from each other'.[107] This is a conclusion reached by Sontag herself. Writing of AIDS, she decides: 'metaphors cannot be distanced just by abstaining from them, they have to be exposed, criticized, belabored, used up'.[108] Which, of course, is not to say that they can be eradicated. Arthur's search for a healthier way of living with temporal lobe epilepsy takes him beyond the metaphors available to him within a medical context, but not away from metaphor as such. Rather, his reference to poetry and fiction seems to be part of a quest to find a more meaningful metaphor to bridge the gap between epilepsy as medical object and epilepsy as lived experience.

X

In Chapter 1, I appropriated Hughlings Jackson's notion of double consciousness as a strategic device for the purpose of examining some of the more problematic strands in medical narratives about and clinical responses to 'the epileptic'. Jackson used ' double consciousness' to denote a state of ideational and cognitive splitting. The alteration in perception, he claimed, was not merely a function of pathology but could also occur in so-called healthy states for a variety of reasons. He expanded somewhat on this definition through reference to punning. In identifying links between visual and mental diplopia, he argued that with double consciousness mentation is subject to a process similar to that causing this phenomenon in vision.

> Vision is stereoscopic; in a sense it is slightly diplopic, for there are two dissimilar images, although there seems to be but one external object, as we call it. To borrow the ophthalmological term, we can say that mentation is 'stereoscopic;' always subject–object, although we often speak of it as single ('states of consciousness,' etc.).[109]

Double consciousness, he argues, entails in various parts a simultaneous manifestation of two otherwise mutually exclusive states of awareness; a sense of something quite specific, yet beyond precise definition; a sense of something familiar, yet strange. According to Frederic Myers it can also encompass the simultaneity between subliminal and supraliminal self. These definitions of double consciousness bear a remarkable resemblance to Freud's definition of the uncanny as belonging to 'two sets of ideas, which, without being contradictory, are yet very different'.[110]

Where did Arthur Myers founder in this dangerous terrain? Did he become fatally disoriented in the borderlands between 'complete resemblance' to medical–cultural stories of epilepsy and 'vast difference'? Did he glimpse distorted images of himself through rhetorical refractions of the violent, duplicitous, greedy, lazy, malicious, irresponsible, decadent, degenerate epileptic personae inscribed in the pages of the *Lancet* and *British Medical Journal* because of his tendency to seize? How was it possible for him to reconcile this pathologised identity with his professional persona as a medical practitioner and his social position as a member of London's intellectual aristocracy? Conversely, did he identify with that other axis of epileptic possibility and consider himself a genius, ingenious or unusually creative?

It is impossible to know. His letters to family and self-written case notes suggest an individual of average, or perhaps above average, intelligence. In letters to his mother and Frederic particularly, he comes across as an affectionate, insightful and loyal man striving to maintain professional and personal relationships despite periodic bouts of cerebral disorder. As Jackson noted of double consciousness, the medical texts defining Arthur's epileptic identity and the texts deriving from his personal and intellectual life suggest two dissimilar images, 'although there seems to be but one external object', 'the epileptic'. The impossibility of living the subject positions available to him as an epileptic – of locating himself in the subject–object borderlands so to speak – at least as these positions were scripted at the end of the nineteenth century, is underscored by the possibility of his suicide.

African-American writer William Edward Burghardt Du Bois has claimed in relation to racial identity that in the North American culture of the late nineteenth century African-Americans were permitted no 'true self-consciousness'. Rather, identity could be perceived only 'through the revelation of the other world'. He wrote: 'It is a peculiar sensation, this double-consciousness, this sense of always looking at one's self through the eyes of others, of measuring one's soul by the tape of a world that looks on in amused contempt and pity'.[111] Du Bois' observation *vis-à-vis* the identity politics of his day suggests wider application in the analysis of binary identity systems and more recent instances of 'othering'.

Without wishing to co-opt the cultural specificity of Du Bois' experience, I want to suggest here that his conceptual framework provides a productive critical space from which to examine Taylor and Marsh's summation of particular manifestations of Myers' symptomatology as 'amusing'. This categorisation of Myers' automatisms is prompted by his evident capacity 'to act apparently rationally and with intent whilst not fully subject to the monitoring process usually attributed to the self'.[112] It is again worth noting that it is only those seized episodes which effect Myers' *own* well-being that are thought amusing; those which impinge on the comfort zones of others – for example, the pin episode in Jackson's office – are deemed not so benign. As I have suggested above, it is a view that fails to consider the impact of this fracturing of self-awareness on Myers' own sense of identity. The tape by which Taylor and Marsh set about measuring Arthur's identity is calibrated only to the surfaces of his seized states. They examine his writing not for any first-hand insights he might have to offer to his profession about the lived realities of his condition, but for further signs of symptomatology.

The medico-social subject position to which Myers found himself consigned was constituted by a range of observable neuronally provoked changes: social transgressions, absences and uncontrolled bodily movements. This position was further ratified through the social relations and competing power structures specific to his time and culture. His essentialised epileptic nature, as described and reinforced by the bulk of medical writing discussed above, precluded the possibility of self-analyses, self-knowledge, assessments and change. As an epileptic, he might, by Maudsley's reckoning, at times be hopeful, but it is a futile hopefulness, inevitably swamped and washed away by the neuronal storms that periodically held sway over his sensibilities.

The compelling question that remains unasked of the abjected individual is, in Du Bois' words, 'How does it feel to be a problem?' How does one negotiate the schism between an identity exclusively written on the body, particularly a body that is devalued within the dominant order, and claims for a potentially evolving self-knowledge? Du Bois has argued that a doubling of self-awareness for African-Americans, the constant striving to reconcile two 'warring ideals', radically impeded efforts to merge the 'double self' into a 'truer self'. How was it possible, he mused, 'for a man to be both a Negro and an American, without being cursed and spit upon by his fellows, without having the doors of Opportunity closed roughly in his face'?[113] Du Bois' observations are geared to the politics of racial identity in a particular historical and cultural context. Nevertheless, his idea of split identity, of an unreconciled self-awareness, also gestures to the conflict faced by Arthur as a physician and an epileptic at the end of the nineteenth century. It may well have been a conflict that cost him his life.

Notes

1 Walter Colman, 1894, quoted in David C. Taylor and Susan M. Marsh. 'Hughlings Jackson's Dr. Z: the paradigm of temporal lobe epilepsy revealed'. *Journal of Neurology, Neurosurgery and Psychiatry*, vol. 43, 1980, pp. 764–65.

2 For more biographical detail of the brothers' lives see the following entries in the *Oxford Dictionary of National Biography*. Oxford: Oxford University Press, 2004: 'Myers, Arthur Thomas (1851–1894)' (by Alan Gauld); 'Myers, Ernest James (1844–1921)' (by A. C. Bell, revised Megan A. Stephan); 'Myers, Frederic William Henry (1843–1901)' (by Alan Gauld).

3 Frederic W. H. Myers. *Human Personality and Its Survival of Bodily Death*. Ed. Leopold Hamilton Myers. 1903. London: Longmans, Green, 1907, p. 14.

4 John Hughlings Jackson and Walter S. Colman. 'Case of epilepsy with tasting movements and "dreamy state" – very small patch of softening in the left uncinate gyrus', 1898, in James Taylor, ed. *Selected Writings of John Hughlings Jackson*. 2 vols. London: Hodder and Stoughton, 1932, vol. 1, pp. 458–63.

5 Quoted in John Hughlings Jackson. 'On a particular variety of epilepsy ("intellectual aura"), one case with symptoms of organic brain disease', 1888, in James Taylor, ed. *Selected Writings of John Hughlings Jackson*. 2 vols. London: Hodder and Stoughton, 1932, vol. 1, p. 389.

6 Jackson, 'On a particular variety of epilepsy', p. 388.

7 'Psychical research'. *Lancet*, 22 December 1881, p. 1104.

8 Taylor and Marsh, 'Hughlings Jackson's Dr. Z', p. 761.

9 William James. 'Frederic Myers's service to psychology'. 1901. *Antimatters*, vol. 1, no. 1, August 2007, pp. 193–200, page number of quote unavailable.

10 Taylor and Marsh, 'Hughlings Jackson's Dr. Z', p. 761.

11 Jackson quoted in Kenneth Dewhurst. *Hughlings Jackson on Psychiatry*. Oxford: Sandford, 1982, p. 101.

12 Taylor and Marsh, 'Hughlings Jackson's Dr. Z', p. 765.

13 See: B. Barraclough. 'Suicide and epilepsy', in E. H. Reynolds and M. R. Trimble, eds. *Epilepsy and Psychiatry*. Edinburgh: Churchill Livingstone, 1981, pp. 72–76; Christopher Ounsted, Janet Lindsay and Peronelle Richards. *Temporal Lobe Epilepsy 1948–1986: A Biographical Study*. London: MacKeith Press, 1987, pp. 15, 22, 57; Janusz J. Zielinski. 'Epidemiologic overview of epilepsy: morbidity, mortality, and clinical implications', in D. Blumer, ed. *Psychiatric Aspects of Epilepsy*. Washington, DC: American Psychiatric Press, 1984, pp. 90–91; Lena Nilsson, *et al.* 'Risk factors for suicide in epilepsy: a case control study'. *Epilepsia*, vol. 43, no. 6, 2002: 644–51; Samden D. Lhatoo and Josemir W. A. S. Sander. 'Cause-specific mortality in epilepsy'. *Epilepsia*, vol. 46, suppl. 11, 2005, pp. 36–39.

14 Jackson, 'On a particular variety of epilepsy', p. 386.

15 Taylor and Marsh, 'Hughlings Jackson's Dr. Z', p. 758.

16 William Gordon Lennox. *Epilepsy and Related Disorders*. 2 vols. London: Churchill, 1960, vol. 2, pp. 714, 787, 719.

17 Dietrich Blumer, 'The psychiatric dimensions of epilepsy', in Dietrich Blumer,

ed. *Psychiatric Aspects of Epilepsy*. Washington, DC: American Psychiatric Press, 1984, p. 23.

18 Taylor and Marsh, 'Hughlings Jackson's Dr. Z', p. 760 (italics added).

19 Taylor and Marsh, 'Hughlings Jackson's Dr. Z', p. 763. Unless otherwise indicated, all further quotes in this paragraph are from this page.

20 John Hughlings Jackson. 'Observations on the localisation of movements in the cerebral hemisphere, as revealed in cases of convulsion, chorea, and "aphasia"', 1873, in James Taylor, ed. *Selected Writings of John Hughlings Jackson*. 2 vols. London: Hodder and Stoughton, 1932, vol. 1, p. 79.

21 Quoted in Macdonald Critchley and Eileen A. Critchley. *John Hughlings Jackson: Father of English Neurology*. Oxford: Oxford University Press, 1998, p. 47.

22 Donald A. MacKenzie. *Statistics in Britain 1865 – 1930: The Social Construction of Scientific Knowledge*. Edinburgh: Edinburgh University Press, 1981, p. 33.

23 Taylor and Marsh, 'Hughlings Jackson's Dr. Z', appendix IV, p. 766.

24 Quoted in Dr Todd. 'Epileptic mania'. *Lancet*, vol. ii, 1851, p. 372.

25 Henry Maudsley. *Responsibility in Mental Disease*. London: C. Kegan Paul, 1876, pp. 228–29.

26 The quote is attributed to Strakhov, cited in Henri Gastaut. 'Fyodor Mikhailovitch Dostoevsky's involuntary contribution to the symptomatology and prognosis of epilepsy'. *Epilepsia*, vol. 19, 1978, p. 188.

27 Fyodor Dostoevsky. *The Idiot*. 1868. Trans. Constance Garnett. Melbourne: William Heinemann, 1961, p. 219.

28 Dostoevsky, *The Idiot*, pp. 228–29.

29 Dostoevsky, *The Idiot*, p. 2.

30 Dostoevsky, *The Idiot*, p. 1.

31 Dostoevsky, *The Idiot*, p. 593.

32 Dostoevsky, *The Idiot*, p. 598.

33 Fyodor Dostoyevsky. *The Insulted and Humiliated*. 1861. Trans. Olga Shartse. Foreword E. Starikova. Moscow: Progress Publishers, 1976, p. 191.

34 Gastaut. 'Fyodor Mikhailovitch Dostoevsky's involuntary contribution', p. 187.

35 P. H. A. Voskuil. 'The epilepsy of Fyodor Mikhailovitch Dostoevsky (1821–1881)'. *Epilepsia*, vol. 24, 1983, p. 663.

36 Gastaut, 'Fyodor Mikhailovitch Dostoevsky's involuntary contribution', p. 198.

37 Jacques Catteau. *Dostoevsky and the Process of Literary Creation*. Trans. Audrey Littlewood. Cambridge: Cambridge University Press, 1989, p. 118.

38 Catteau, *Dostoevsky*, p. 126.

39 James L. Rice. *Dostoevsky and the Healing Art: An Essay in Literary and Medical History*. Ann Arbor, MI: Ardis, 1985, p. 234.

40 Dostoevsky, *The Idiot*, pp. 219–20.

41 Dostoevsky, *The Idiot*, p. 220.

42 Robert Louis Stevenson. *Strange Case of Dr Jekyll and Mr Hyde*. 1886. *Dr Jekyll and Mr Hyde & The Merry Men and Other Tales and Fables*. Hertfordshire: Wordsworth Classics, 1999, pp. 41–2. Unless otherwise indicated, all quotes from this edition.

43 Stevenson, *Dr Jekyll and Mr Hyde*, p. 48

44 Stevenson, *Dr Jekyll and Mr Hyde*, p. 42.

45 Stevenson, *Dr Jekyll and Mr Hyde*, p. 44.

46 Stevenson, *Dr Jekyll and Mr Hyde*, p. 53.

47 Stevenson, *Dr Jekyll and Mr Hyde*, p. 53.

48 Stevenson, *Dr Jekyll and Mr Hyde*, p. 48.

49 See: Robbie B. H. Goh. 'Textual Hyde and seek: "gentility", narrative play and proscription in Stevenson's *Dr Jekyll and Mr Hyde*'. *Journal of Narrative Theory*, vol. 29, no. 2, spring 1999, pp. 158–83; Alan Sandison. *Robert Louis Stevenson and the Appearance of Modernism*. Basingstoke: Macmillan, 1996; William Veeder and Gordon Hirsch, eds. *Dr Jekyll and Mr Hyde: After One Hundred Years*. Chicago, IL: Chicago University Press, 1988; Daniel Wright. '"The prisonhouse of my disposition": a study of the psychology of addiction in Dr. Jekyll and Mr. Hyde'. *Studies in the Novel*, vol. 26, no. 3, autumn 1994, pp. 254–67.

50 John S. Gibson. *Deacon Brodie Father to Jekyll and Hyde*. Edinburgh: Paul Harris, 1977, p. 21. Unless otherwise indicated, all further quotes are from this edition.

51 See David Daiches. *Robert Louis Stevenson and His World*. London: Thames and Hudson, 1973; J. C. Furnas. *Voyage to Windward*. London: Faber, 1952.

52 Stevenson, *Dr Jekyll and Mr Hyde*, p. 33.

53 F. Norton Manning. 'The epileptic: his treatment and care'. *Australasian Medical Gazette*, 20 June 1900, p. 217.

54 Stevenson, *Dr Jekyll and Mr Hyde*, p. 32

55 Stevenson, *Dr Jekyll and Mr Hyde*, pp. 4–5.

56 Juggernaut is a title given to Krishna. The *Oxford English Dictionary* states: 'The image of the god at Puri in Orissa is annually carried in procession on an enormous cart, under the wheels of which many devotees are said to have formerly thrown themselves to be crushed'.

57 Stevenson, *Dr Jekyll and Mr Hyde*, p. 31.

58 Gibson, *Deacon Brodie*, pp. 54–55.

59 Stevenson, *Dr Jekyll and Mr Hyde*, p. 14.

60 Stevenson, *Dr Jekyll and Mr Hyde*, p. 14, pp. 11–12.

61 Charles Dickens. *Our Mutual Friend*. 1865. Ed. and Introduction Adrian Poole. London: Penguin Classics, 1997, p. 218. All quotes are from this edition.

62 Dickens, *Our Mutual Friend*, p. 218.

63 Eve Kosofsky Sedgwick. *Between Men: English Literature and Male Homosocial Desire*. 1985. New York: Columbia University Press, 1992, pp. 161–79.

64 Charles Dickens. *The Life and Adventures of Martin Chuzzlewit*. 1843–44. Ed. and Introduction Patricia Ingham. London: Penguin, 1999, p. 296. All quotes are from this edition.

65 J. E. Cosnett. 'Charles Dickens and epilepsy'. *Epilepsia*, vol. 35, no. 4, 1994, pp. 904–5.

66 Charles Dickens. *The Old Curiosity Shop*. 1841. Ed. Angus Easson. London: Penguin Classics, 1972, p. 134. All quotes are from this edition.

67 Dickens, *The Old Curiosity Shop*, pp. 144–45.

68 Charles Dickens. *The Personal History of David Copperfield*. 1849–50. Ed. Jeremy Tambling. London: Penguin Classics, 1996, p. 515. All quotes are from this edition.

69 Dickens, *David Copperfield*, p. 523.

70 Dickens, *David Copperfield*, pp. 355–56.

71 Gerry Turcotte. '"Speaking the formula of abjection": hybrids and Gothic discourses in Louis Nowra's novels'. *Westerly*, vol. 3, September 1991, p. 61.

72 Jan B. Gordon. 'Narrative enclosure as textual ruin: an archaeology of Gothic consciousness', in Michael Timko, Fred Kaplan and Edward Guiliano, eds. *Dickens Studies Annual: Essays on Victorian Fiction*, vol. 11. New York: AMS Press, 1983, p. 213.

73 Dostoevsky, *The Idiot*, p. 33.

74 Sigmund Freud. 'The "uncanny"'. *Standard Edition of the Complete Psychological*

Works of Sigmund Freud. Ed. and trans. James Strachey. Vol. 17 (1917–19). London: Hogarth Press, 1955, p. 219. All quotes are from this edition.

75 Freud, 'The "uncanny"', p. 220.
76 Freud, 'The "uncanny"', pp. 224–25.
77 Freud, 'The "uncanny"', p. 243.
78 Freud, 'The "uncanny"', p. 243.
79 Hélène Cixous. 'Fiction and its phantoms: a reading of Freud's *Das Unheimliche* (the 'uncanny')'. *New Literary History*, vol. 7, no. 1, 1975, p. 528.
80 Freud, 'The "uncanny"', p. 244.
81 Freud, 'The "uncanny"', p. 247.
82 Freud, 'The "uncanny"', p. 223.
83 Pamela Thurschwell. 'Ferenczi's dangerous proximities: telepathy, psychosis, and the real event'. *Differences: A Journal of Feminist Cultural Studies*, spring 1999, p. 150. Accessed via Expanded Academic Index online, 19 April 2001.
84 Quoted in Thurschwell, 'Ferenczi's dangerous proximities'.
85 John Hughlings Jackson. 'A digression on epilepsy', 1866, in James Taylor, ed. *Selected Writings of John Hughlings Jackson*. 2 vols. London: Hodder and Stoughton, 1932, vol. 1, p. 5.
86 Freud, 'The "uncanny"', p. 223.
87 Freud, 'The "uncanny"', p. 224 (italics added).
88 Judith Butler. *Bodies That Matter: On the Discursive Limits of 'Sex'*. New York: Routledge, 1993.
89 Julia Kristeva. *Powers of Horror: An Essay on Abjection.* Trans. Leon S. Roudiez. New York: Columbia University Press, 1982, p. 5.
90 Graham Scambler. *Epilepsy*. London: Tavistock/Routledge, 1989, p. 47.
91 *Alien*. Dir. Ridley Scott. Prod. Gordon Caroll, *et al.* Perf. Sigourney Weaver, Tom Skerritt, John Hurt. Screenplay Dan O'Bannon. Twentieth Century Fox, 1979.
92 Kristeva, *Powers of Horror*, p. 4.
93 Lennard J. Davis, *Enforcing Normalcy: Disability, Deafness and the Body*. New York: Verso, 1995, p. 141.
94 Davis, *Enforcing Normalcy*, p. 142.
95 Quoted in Christopher Ounsted, Janet Lindsay and Peronelle Richards. *Temporal Lobe Epilepsy 1948–1986: A Biographical Study*. London: MacKeith Press, 1987, p. 2.
96 Freud, 'The "uncanny"', p. 226.
97 Quoted in Owsei Temkin. *The Falling Sickness: A History of Epilepsy from the Greeks to the Beginnings of Modern Neurology*, 2nd edition, revised. Baltimore, MD: Johns Hopkins University Press, 1971, p. 44.
98 Sigmund Freud. 'Dostoevsky and parricide'. *Standard Edition of the Complete Psychological Works of Sigmund Freud*. Ed. and trans. James Strachey. Vol. 21 (1927–31). London: Hogarth Press, 1961, p. 179.
99 Blumer, 'The psychiatric dimensions of epilepsy', p. 56.
100 Blumer, 'The psychiatric dimensions of epilepsy', p. 56.
101 Quoted in Gibson, *Deacon Brodie*, p. 109.
102 Stevenson, *Dr Jekyll and Mr Hyde*, p. 5.
103 Quoted in Jackson, 'On a particular variety of epilepsy', pp. 404–5.
104 Donald Davidson. 1978. 'What metaphors mean', in Sheldon Sacks, ed. *On Metaphor*. Chicago, IL: University of Chicago Press, 1978, p. 29.
105 Paul de Man. 'The epistemology of metaphor', in Sheldon Sacks, ed. *On Metaphor*. Chicago, IL: University of Chicago Press, 1978, p. 19.
106 Susan Sontag. *'Illness as Metaphor' and 'AIDS and Its Metaphors'*. New York: Anchor, 1990, p. 3.

107 de Man, 'The epistemology of metaphor', p. 19.
108 Sontag, *'Illness as Metaphor'*, p. 182.
109 John Hughlings Jackson. 'An address on the psychology of joking', 1887, in James Taylor, ed. *Selected Writings of John Hughlings Jackson*. 2 vols. London: Hodder and Stoughton, 1932, vol. 2, p. 359.
110 Freud, 'The "uncanny"', pp. 224–25.
111 W. E. Burghardt Du Bois. *The Souls of Black Folk: Essays and Sketches*. 1903. New York: Johnson Reprint Company, 1968, p. 3.
112 Taylor and Marsh, 'Hughlings Jackson's Dr. Z', p. 760.
113 Du Bois, *The Souls of Black Folk*, p. 4.

CHAPTER 4

The colonies

> Oh give me land, lots of land, with the starry skies above –
> Don't fence me in.
> (Cole Porter, 'Don't fence me in', 1942)

I

At the close of the nineteenth century, 'epileptic danger' proved to be as much about economic viability as about hereditary contamination. In the industrialised spaces of a waning century, the epileptic figure acquired different meanings and connotations than had been evident in earlier systems of representation. Prognostications about epileptics meshed with capitalist narratives of maximum production, output and profit. Ideas of epileptic taint and epileptic disability became infused with those theories of temporal efficiency and scientific management that had become the organising principles of the factory floor. Defined by its unpredictability within this new social and representational matrix, the epileptic body could only be found wanting. Medical practitioners, social reformers and philanthropists in Britain and the United States argued that the only way to save mainstream society from the danger of its epileptic populations – and, indeed, the only way to save epileptics from the danger they presented to themselves – was through judicious and humanitarian confinement.

Confinement was to take the form of 'labour colonies', 'farm colonies' or 'epileptic colonies', as they were variously known. These were to be places where the epileptic could be isolated from social conditions such as an undisciplined lifestyle, the temptations of big-city living –

specifically, alcohol and vice – and the economic penury thought to exacerbate the disorder. Rhetorical associations that had located the epileptic on the negative axis in the culture/nature dichotomy were about to be geographically realised. Furthermore, it was claimed that isolation of the disorder from the healthy social body would yield the added benefit of halting hereditary contagion. As well as confining epileptic 'danger' to a controlled environment, colonies would also secure for the medical observer a consistent opportunity for surveillance and, by extension, the opportunity to learn more about the syndromes at close quarters. However, the colonies were not merely products of medical concerns about the physiological, psychological and social difficulties associated with epilepsy conditions. Rather, they developed from a complex range of social and political issues extant in the closing decades of the century.

The final years of the century saw the medical story of epilepsy overtaken by stories of nation building and urgent calls to protect national borders from 'the dangers within'. Industrialisation and increased urbanisation had created unprecedented strains on cities. Crime, poverty and homelessness were rife. At the same time, theories of evolution and social progressiveness had seized the public imagination and provided a new language to talk about escalating social problems. Legal, social and medical reformers alike were caught up in identifying and addressing the pathogenic causes of society's ills. Increasingly, these putative social pathogens were located with the 'underclasses': the impoverished; the criminal; the insane. A central figure in this plethora of pathogenic bodies was 'the epileptic'. It was still a figure not readily amenable to identification and control; nor was it contained by class parameters.

As I have suggested in previous chapters, medical stories of 'the epileptic' at the turn of the nineteenth century became allegories for these wider social anxieties. This was particularly the case in Britain. So it was that epilepsy narratives came to register wider scientific and social concerns about increasing urban chaos, racial degeneration, poverty and disease. To understand the attitudes and events that cast 'the epileptic' as a central figure in narratives of an ailing commonwealth and common health, it is necessary to examine the radical restructuring of urban and productive space that had been taking place from about 1850 onwards.

In examining the conditions that give the epileptic colony movement its momentum, the first sections of this chapter take account of key debates circulating around this period and examine the ways they shape medical narratives of epileptic disorder and epileptic danger.

The latter sections of the chapter examine the comparisons and differences between the way the colony movement evolved in England, North America and Australia through the early decades of the twentieth century.

II

Donald MacKenzie argues that by the late nineteenth century urbanisation had given rise to an increasingly centralised and politically articulate professional middle class in Britain and that there was also a discernible belief that elements of the working class were becoming reassuringly inculcated to their place in the scheme of things.[1] Deploring the negative effects of Bohemianism on the English race, Francis Galton insisted that 'No man who only works by fits and starts is able to obtain his living nowadays'.[2] By 1869 Galton was claiming that the 'steady workman' had become the bulwark of the English economy, as the 'artisan part of our population is slowly becoming bred to its duties'. Coexisting with and disturbing this social mood of hierarchical complacency, however, were concerns that a growing class of physically and mentally degenerate poor threatened the social and economic security of bourgeois communities.

By the early 1890s there was a growing conviction that the English race was in imminent danger of degradation because of the risks posed by hereditary taint from disorders such as epilepsy and because of the effects of overcrowded and unhealthy living conditions in the large industrial centres. Gareth Jones has observed:

> If the theory of hereditary urban degeneration had been confined to one or two eccentric doctors, there would be little point in examining it, except perhaps as a quaint by-way of medical history. But this was not the case. In the 1880s and 1890s the theory received widespread middle-class support and was given authoritative backing by Booth, Marshall, Longstaff, and Llewellyn Smith.[3]

In turn-of-the-century medical journals, worries about epilepsy and its possible links to class degeneration and moral disorder rode in on a wave of social unease that had been gathering for at least fifty years. From the late 1840s multiple political and social forces had begun to coalesce around the management of the epileptic body.

Throughout the latter decades of the nineteenth century, politicians, social reformers and the medical profession were calling for solutions to a growing bank of socio-economic problems affecting the lower classes in Britain. Social Darwinism and determinist or evolutionary psychiatry had become decisive categorical factors by the 1870s. In 1883 Galton coined the term 'eugenics', a word he developed from the Greek for 'noble in hereditary' or 'good in birth'. Galton's ideas for a science of breeding stronger, more intelligent human 'stock' were to gain in popularity not only in England, but also, by the early twentieth century, in North America and Australia, where they were taken up to reinforce a rhetoric of nation building. It was not surprising, then, that by the 1880s members of the medical profession were debating in the correspondence section of the *Lancet* the implications of hereditary degeneration for future generations, via topics such as epilepsy and marriage.

Strenuous efforts to apprehend social decline were to be mounted simultaneously from several different directions. In England, some of the earlier sites tabled for legal and administrative overhaul were the interlinked statutes and institutions comprising the management of the poor and pauper classes under the Poor Law system. After decades of social upheaval, as well as economic and political conflict, the Poor Law Amendment Act, or the New Poor Law, was adopted in 1834. Poor Law ideology at this time was geared not only around notions of paternalistic obligation and beneficence by the gentry towards the lower working classes, but also around the geographical and social control of these classes. Through the first half of the nineteenth century the working class began to move into the cities in ever greater numbers, in accordance with an expanding industrial economy. This presented specific problems for Poor Law administrators, who found themselves having to cater to an exploding population of poor and pauper classes in the cities.

Poor Law ideology was structured around notions of systematic deterrence. By keeping its services to the poor down to, and sometimes below, the bare minimum of need, Poor Law guardians hoped to actively discourage dependence on its charity. Some nineteenth-century reformers went so far as to argue that, in fact, charity and relief funds for the poor and pauper classes only encouraged their dependence. Writing in 1868, J. R. Green suggested that assistance such as the Mansion Relief Fund ultimately inhibited any impulse for self-help in the dependent classes: 'The very clergy who were foremost in the work of relief last year stand aghast at the Pauper Frankenstein they have created'.[4] This ideology, along with increased need for relief, merged to create an unlovely and parsimonious environment for workhouses and infirmaries.

Poor Law criteria for what constituted genuine need were quite specific and finely drawn. The 'poor' were those who, all things being equal, were able to survive on their own resources but needed to turn to the Poor Law guardians for help when sickness, unemployment or old age forced them below viable levels of subsistence. While in receipt of assistance they were redefined as 'paupers'. The threshold between being classified as poor or pauper became slippery ground for the working-class individual with epilepsy and some of the reasons for this economic vulnerability are examined more closely below. Suffice to say for the moment, however, that late nineteenth-century medical responses to those afflicted by epilepsy were to organise as much around these economic factors as they were to be driven by the health care needs of the individual.

By 1840 many physicians and social reformers working with the poor had begun to speak up for a radical rethinking about the type and quality of medical services available through Poor Law facilities. The General Medical Order of 1842 was introduced in an effort to redress the omissions and inconsistencies of the 1834 Act *vis-à-vis* the provision of medical services. Through the next fifty years or so the struggle between Poor Law administrators and the medical profession continued over standards of health care for the poor and pauper classes, over control of the infirmaries, and over who should control the administration of statutory services provided to the sick. The *Lancet* placed itself at the forefront of this movement, forming its own commission of inquiry into Poor Law medical services. The pressure brought to bear on the Poor Law commissioners began to yield results and by 1867 implementation of the Act variously known as the Metropolitan Poor Law Amendment Act, the Metropolitan Poor Act or the Metropolitan Asylums Act began the process of giving doctors more say over the administration of both infirmaries and sick poor and pauper patients.[5]

Restructuring of the Poor Law statutes and services was to have a direct bearing on the course of medical and social responses to epilepsy over the next five decades or so. For a start, implementation of the 1867 Act placed the medical and social management of the lower-class, non-insane epileptic patient more squarely within the field of the medical profession. This boundary shift would eventually expand the medical gaze from the exigencies of neurological investigation and care to an intense scrutiny of the socio-economic management of these patients. However, changes to the Poor Law Act and boundary shifts in disciplinary authority were only part of the story. Concomitant with changes to the Poor Law Act, the epileptic body was to be subjected to other techniques of scrutiny and analysis. It became the cynosure of various mechanisms of power which, since the eighteenth century, had sought to standardise the corporeal body through regimes of surveillance and control.

III

Industrialisation had radically refigured the workplace in the major cities of western countries. By the mid nineteenth century the commercial demands of a capitalist economy required an increasingly efficient worker able to cope with the complex machinery used in factories and to comply with the rigorous time frames ordering the work space of the factory floor. The English working man, by 1869, was being epitomised by Galton and others as having 'great bodily strength, applied under the command of a steady, persevering will, mental self-contentedness, impassibility to external irrelevant impressions, which carries them through the continued repetition of toilsome labour, "steady as time"'.[6] As a consequence of changing social and industrial conditions, in the latter half of the nineteenth century the body was being almost exclusively described, represented and understood according to those mechanisms of power Michel Foucault identified as developing in the eighteenth century. The body that mattered in this new age of mass production, as Foucault argues and Galton's comments confirm, was the body that could be trained or managed to maximum efficiency.

For Foucault, the disciplinary methods created to produce and police this ideal(ised) body permeated not only the military but also the school system and the hospital:

> The human body was entering a machinery of power that explores it, breaks it down and rearranges it. A 'political anatomy', which was also a 'mechanics of power', was being born; it defined how one may have a hold over others' bodies, not only so that they may do what one wishes, but so that they may operate as one wishes, with the techniques, the speed and the efficiency that one determines. Thus discipline produces subjected and practised bodies, 'docile' bodies.[7]

It was through the systematic dissemination of these modes of 'discipline' that the body was inculcated with those positive forces – utility in economic terms and obedience in political terms – that were the salient links between labour and production in a capitalist economy. This paradigm obviously excluded, among others, any who were prone to episodic bouts of disability: those who were unable to produce and sustain a continued repetition of toilsome labour, 'steady as time'.

Further undermining this working-class ideal, particularly in London, was a floating and largely immeasurable population of those who have been called 'the casual poor'. This group constituted 'a disquieting alien presence [the *unheimlich*] in the midst of mid-Victorian plenty' and to contemporary Londoners they were indistinguishable from criminals and other degenerate classes.[8] The 'dangerous class' or 'residuum' of London society became an important subject of debate in the last twenty-five years of the nineteenth century. Jones writes that this 'residuum' was characterised by late nineteenth-century social theorists as consisting of:

> those who have a poor physique and a weak character – those who are limp in body and mind. The problem was not structural but moral. The evil to be combated was not poverty but pauperism: pauperism with its attendant vices, drunkenness, improvidence, mendicancy, bad language, filthy habits, gambling, low amusement, and ignorance.[9]

As politicians, social reformers and pamphleteers were turning their attention to the unemployment problems besetting the industrial cities of the north, it was becoming apparent in the last quarter of the century that London was experiencing these problems at crisis levels. By the 1880s, as London grew in national importance, so too did the conviction that while the metropolis was apparently impregnable from outside invasion, it might well be vulnerable to the growing disorder within its borders.

David Armstrong points out that through the late eighteenth and early nineteenth century, medicine began to turn its gaze to a body which had a new anatomy. He argues that this seemingly discrete body began to be recorded in separate case notes. It is a body, he suggests, that:

> was accessible because ... medicine began to use methods of physical examination; it was analysable because pathology became localisable to a distinct point within the body; it was passive because the patient's personal history was relegated from its primary position as the key to the diagnosis to a preliminary; and it was subjected to evaluation because patients were moved from the natural locus of the home to the neutral domain of the hospital. Thus, every time medicine had cause to deploy its new techniques and treat an illness, it drew an outline of a particular anatomy, a docile body.[10]

Although Armstrong is primarily examining relations between medicine and the social body during the twentieth century, it is possible to discern those relational impulses between the institution and society examined in Armstrong's text as already identifiable by the late nineteenth century.

The medical gaze defining this new anatomy in the late nineteenth century also began to identify disease over and above the corporeal body; it began to locate and identify disease more broadly in the social body. 'The new gaze', writes Armstrong of the twentieth century, 'identified disease in the spaces between people, in the interstices of relationships'.[11] However, by the late nineteenth century, the problem for the medical profession had already become one of trying to locate and map the wider boundaries of disease: one of trying to construct and maintain a social equivalent of the anatomical atlas identified by Foucault in relationship to the corporeal body. The 1890s saw the dispensary drawn into the disciplinary apparatus ministering the body. Armstrong asserts that, as a site of power and regulation, the dispensary became an extension of the panoptic vision. It required the social body to be monitored and so widened the gaze to detect, diagnose and prescribe the defining boundaries between normal (therefore appropriate) and abnormal (or deviant) interpersonal relationships and occupational pursuits. By early decades of the twentieth century, epileptic colonies had become an important arm of this apparatus of detection, surveillance and control.

The new medical gaze had already begun to focus on the lower classes by the mid nineteenth century. As part of the Poor Law revisions, commissioners gathered data on the moral, social and productive health of the labouring classes to better pinpoint and interpret areas of social degeneration and potential disorder. In the age of capitalist expansionism, industrial society demanded a docile, legible and therefore manageable body rendered knowable by the truth of medical science. Responding to this socio-economic climate, mid nineteenth-century English medical journals began to publish with increasing regularity papers and news items about the rise in physical and social disorders identified in relation to the proliferation of factories in the cities and towns.

This trend is exemplified in a paper published in the *Lancet* in 1859 by Dr William McTurk.[12] Physician at the Bradford Infirmary and Dispensary, McTurk turned to the issue of medical response to the demands of an industrial economy in an address to the National Association for the Promotion of Social Science. He argued that in industrial centres such as the city of Bradford, with its rapidly expanding wool trade, busy mills and fast-moving machinery, the epileptic was not only a danger to him- or herself but also a threat to the safety of fellow workers. As the century moved to its close McTurk's theme was amplified elsewhere. By the late nineteenth century it was being argued that the mechanisation and inflexible temporal organisation of the workplace, coupled with the complexity of industrial machinery, had generated a class of 'industrial rejects', for whom special provision would have to be made.

The title of McTurk's paper, 'The *apparent* increase of epilepsy among the working classes of the town of Bradford' (italics added), is also worth noting. It reinforces class boundaries through its focus on the problem posed by the defective worker in a capitalist economy, and use of the word 'apparent' is suggestive. McTurk's deployment of this term seems to gesture to an awareness that the 'apparent' proliferation of defective bodies may indeed be a consequence of those social and industrial forces reshaping the welfare and health care systems, on the one hand, and, on the other, the space of the factory and mill. It also suggests a proliferation of surveillance mechanisms. As Foucault has argued, the invention of the new political anatomy was neither sudden nor all of a piece. It was the product of a multiplicity of processes and methods that were, in almost every instance, a 'response to particular needs: an industrial innovation, a renewed outbreak of certain epidemic diseases'.[13] This idea of a manufactured deviance or disability was also to be voiced by Henry Maudsley, albeit with implicit emphasis on the idea of hereditary taint, but his chosen analogy evokes images of an industrialised deficit. 'Lunatics and criminals', he argued, 'are as much manufactured articles as are steam-engines and calico-printing machines.... They are neither accidents nor anomalies in the universe, but come by law and testify to causality; and it is the business of science to find out what the causes are and by what laws they work.'[14]

IV

Reflecting wider social concerns about increasing urban unemployment, from about the mid 1880s medical journals, in editorial comments and articles, began to exhibit an ongoing preoccupation with the socio-economic significance of epilepsy syndromes. Examination of the epileptic body from the perspective of economic efficiency had historical precedence. In antiquity, for example, the impulse to locate the presence of epilepsy was not merely driven by medical desire to understand and heal but was also informed by the commercial demands of a slave economy, where the body periodically affected by seizure represented significant disruption to service and material production. In ancient Babylonian law, Egyptian law and Greek law, detection of epilepsy in a newly purchased slave legally cancelled the transaction. In some cases it was legal for the buyer of this particular type of damaged goods to claim restitution for up to twelve months after purchase. In an ancient version of provocative diagnosis, prospective purchasers attempted to uncover epileptic potential by artificially triggering an attack: 'The rotation of a potter's wheel before his eyes would make the epileptic feel giddy and might be the cause of a seizure. Fumigation with kindled jet was [also] one of the recorded experiments by which the physicians tested the health of "slaves exposed for sale".'[15] Owsei Temkin argues that some of the more drastic methods for detecting or exposing epilepsy were the result of the economic import of hidden disorder.

As it surfaced in the British journals, the preoccupation with detection and socio-economic placement was accompanied by an insistence on the homogeneity of those with epilepsy conditions. All other systems of social stratification were subsumed by ascription of an epileptic identity. Decrying a lack of facilities catering to the needs of non-insane epileptics, the *British Medical Journal* records the observation that although those with epilepsy and insanity, or epilepsy and imbecility, were accommodated by the asylum system, 'for the patient suffering from epilepsy alone there is no public place for treatment'.[16] An editorial comment in the *Lancet*, while lamenting the crowding together of 'these poor people' in asylums, at the same time suggests: 'The very fact of their being together is a measure of safety. It is interesting to see how they help each other.'[17] Use of the word 'interesting' indicates the writer's preconceptions of an epileptic capacity for compassion.

It was being claimed with growing confidence by the 1880s that if only the epileptic body could be somehow more effectively managed, its destabilising influence on society might be checked. Consistent surveillance under ordered conditions was thought to provide the most attractive option for management and discipline. At a special meeting of the Council of the Charity Organisation Society in London, May 1886, Dr Rayner argued that 'any trade could be utilised for epileptics, provided that they were carefully watched for a time before being entrusted with employment, and that there was [ongoing] close supervision'.[18]

J. S. Risien Russell, one-time resident medical officer at the National Hospital, Queen Square, pondered at some length in 1891 the question of *how* to render 'useful' the lives of 'idiots and chronic epileptics' through disciplinary regimes. He deemed it such an important issue that he 'made no apology' for 'drawing attention to the excellent system' devised and practised by a Dr Bourneville in Paris. The system recounted by Russell, aimed primarily at children, entailed a strictly supervised regime of task-oriented education, exercise and various bodily hygiene therapies (hot and cold baths, frequent bowel evacuations, and so forth). Further behaviour modification was achieved by using a range of rewards for compliance and solitary confinement in bare, prison-like cells for recalcitrance. 'In cases where it is deemed necessary', Russell wrote, the non-compliant child is 'confined in a padded cell, and, if, necessary, it is darkened. An attendant is constantly present, and can observe the offender through a small aperture without his being observed.'[19] Unwelcome in the school system because of the disruptive potential of their seizure condition, it was extremely difficult for the young person with an epilepsy syndrome to achieve even the most basic skills that would facilitate earning a livelihood in later life.

In their survey of the state of epileptic colonies in Britain in the mid twentieth century, Kathleen Jones and Aileen Tillotson point out that changes to administrative boundaries and the education system in the latter part of the nineteenth century gradually led to separation of defectives and epileptics from the mentally ill.[20] The reshaping of these administrative groupings led to a special interest in children with epilepsy and their management into adulthood. In 1886 the Idiots Act paved the way for the establishment of 'idiot asylums' or 'mental deficiency colonies'; however, within the purview of the Act and the facilities it engendered, there was no comparable provision for children with epilepsy. This omission was addressed in 1899 with the implementation of the Elementary Education (Defective and Epileptic Children) Act, which empowered local authorities to spend funds on the groups of children specified and which in turn was to pave the way for epileptic colony schools.

In fact, far gentler versions of Russell's preferred philosophy for managing juvenile epileptic disorder had been part of an English therapeutic repertoire for some time. Hughlings Jackson had suggested the importance of diet in health regimes for those with an epilepsy syndrome. Hygiene management, along with moral management and 'wholesome mental exercise', had become important adjuncts to the chemical management of epileptic disorder through the last quarter of the nineteenth century. In an editorial item published in the *British Medical Journal*, John Kent Spender lauded the positive effects of 'more harmonious action' on epileptic sensibilities: 'But even when the faculties are acute and femininely sensitive, the stultifying effects of the long continued epileptic convulsion may be appropriately met by gymnastic exercises and systematic shampooing of the whole body'.[21] Yet the times seemed to demand far more stringent interventions into epileptic disorder than those advised by Jackson and Spender.

Employment for adults with epilepsy became another central theme in late nineteenth-century narratives about the condition. An advertised meeting of the newly formed National Society for the Employment of Epileptics was held at the Mansion House in London on 25 January

1893 to engage this issue. In preparation for the meeting an editorial in the *British Medical Journal* covered in some detail the economic restrictions faced by adults with an epilepsy condition in the current inhospitable employment climate:

> Every medical man is well aware of the unfortunate position of an epileptic, who is a burden and a care at home, and who might be usefully employed, in favourable surroundings, to his infinitely increased happiness and contentment, but is quite unfitted to gain a living in the open labour market.[22]

A National Society survey of seventy adult patients at the National Hospital in Queen Square had recently confirmed general medical opinion on the unemployability of those with epilepsy. Evidently, of the seventy surveyed, thirty-eight had lost positions because of their vulnerability to seizure; twenty-seven could get no work at all; one had to accept a much lower-paying and unskilled position; two were able to obtain occasional work but were always eventually discharged because of the fits; and two had managed to work in some capacity from their own homes.

Addressing the escalating economic problem presented by the adult epileptic, William Turner noted in 1897:

> An epileptic artisan is absolutely debarred from many trades and occupations, such as building, engineering, &c., while in other cases the services of an epileptic workman are not desired by an employer of labour unless he be of an exceptionally indulgent and charitable nature.[23]

Turner's observations capture the economic and social realities facing working-class folk with epilepsy because of the propensity to seize. Of course, they also rather neatly gloss the problematic and complex issues of why a tendency to fit from time to time *should* debar the person periodically disabled by the syndrome from working at all. The fact that it should is taken for granted. It is important to point out here that Turner was writing about manifestations of the syndrome constituted merely by the tendency to convulse, without any inter-seizure (non-chemical) impairment to intellect or general health. His contemporary William Broadbent suggested: 'In true epilepsy ... The patient in the intervals [between paroxysmal episodes] enjoys such health as is natural to his constitution, and there are no symptoms suggestive of any affection of the nervous system.'[24]

Nevertheless, earning a living was an enormous problem for those who were from the lower classes and affected by epilepsy conditions. By the early 1890s the question repeatedly asked in the medical journals was 'What is to be done with epileptics?' The epileptic body was neither docile nor passive. It neither lent itself unproblematically to regimes of discipline nor remained compliantly within the bounds of newly established diagnostic protocols. Neither was epileptic disorder localisable to a distinct point within the body; it had the potential to permeate the very fabric of society. Moreover, it threatened spasmodic destabilisation for the labour/production relations of capitalist spatiality. Given these combined factors, there indeed seemed to be no place for 'the epileptic' in the current labour market and the question being asked with increasing urgency by medical writers was eventually taken up as indication of the pressing need for epileptic colonies in the editorial section of the *Lancet*. 'The great problem is one which must be faced', the writer of one piece claimed; 'it is obtruding itself more and more every day…'.[25]

While those with epilepsy might be able to maintain their status as being merely poor by eking out a living in between seizure episodes, once their potential for cerebral paroxysm became known, more often than not they found themselves eventually recategorised as pauper. This entailed a double stigmatisation. Already marked as 'social lepers' (a phrase used repeatedly in the *Lancet*, the *British Medical Journal* and the *Australasian Medical Gazette* to emphasise the displacement of 'epileptics' in normative social hierarchies and to argue for the efficacy of developing epileptic colonies) because of their neurological condition, the working-class epileptics' spasmodic descent into pauperism brought its own disabling consequences.

Because of the late nineteenth-century administrative conflation of defectiveness and epilepsy, public attitude inextricably linked the two conditions, a factor that served to further exacerbate the economic vulnerability of those with an epilepsy syndrome. In advancing the call for farm colonies for epileptics, the editorial section of the *British Medical Journal* carried the following observation:

> The lot of an epileptic is always a sad one, but few people recognise how additionally sad is that of the person who becomes a pauper because he is an epileptic. The ratio of epileptics among pauper and non-pauper children is not materially different, but among adults the ratio of paupers who are epileptic far exceeds that in the non-pauper classes; showing that a large number of epileptics are paupers only because they suffer from epilepsy.[26]

It was estimated that the number of epileptics in England by 1895 'amounted to between 30,000 and 40,000, a number double as large as that of the blind, and four times as large as that of the deaf and dumb'.[27] However, even as turn-of-the-century physicians quoted statistics on the numbers of epileptics at large in society, they also evinced the suspicion that somehow these numbers under-estimated the reality.

William Turner, in citing epileptic population statistics from various European countries, North America and Australia, displayed a repeated and somewhat paranoid urge to adjust estimates upwards, arguing that difficulties in being able to detect the presence of epilepsy probably made for significant under-estimation of numbers in most, if not all, calculations.[28] In 1900, Australian physician F. Norton Manning was to worry his colleagues with the spectre of a 'large army' of so-called 'sane epileptics' threatening the stability of the Australasian colonies.[29] The perception was that there were more epileptics out there than contemporary estimates indicated – and the numbers were growing.

V

In 1895, opening Passmore Edwards House at the recently built Chalfont St Peter's Epileptic Colony in Buckinghamshire, the Duke of Devonshire notes the 'distressing' frequency with which those with 'the lamentable condition' find themselves in such impoverished circumstances that they have no choice but to seek refuge in workhouses or union infirmaries.[30] Two years later Turner argues that 'in all classes of society the epileptic whose fits debar him from occupation becomes a burden to his relatives; whilst among the poorer classes he swells the ranks of the unemployed, and eventually ends in the workhouse'.[31] Turner goes on to suggest that although epileptics may well be able to work productively in those intervals between seizure episodes, because of their propensity to fit, and the doubts this raises about the state of their inter-ictal mental capacities, by and large they are absolutely prohibited from all but the most menial and low-paying casual work. Given these conditions, he concludes it is not surprising that 'this makes one in every five of the total epileptic population of London an inmate of a workhouse'; furthermore, 'of the pauper inmates of the workhouse one in every sixty is an epileptic'.

Deprivation was a necessary condition of pauperism under the auspices of the Poor Law administrators. Pauperism also carried with it a shameful loss of status in the eyes of the community, reducing the adult subject to a state of abject dependence. Michael Flinn points out that the stigma of pauperism was 'signified in the brutal sixteenth century sometimes by actual branding, in the marginally more humane eighteenth century by badges, and in the nineteenth century by loss of pride'.[32] Although the pauper with epilepsy might not bear those physical markings of economic shame identified by Flinn, by the late nineteenth century the epileptic body, regardless of class status, was likely to be marked by the stigma of disorder through the extensive use of bromides to treat the syndromes. Thus, with their disorder chemically inscribed on their body, the working-class epileptic found it virtually impossible to 'pass' in the normative labour market.

Bromides are a class of binary salts consisting of bromine and another element or radical. Bromine – from the Greek *bromos* meaning 'stink' – is a reddish-brown, volatile liquid and is a chemical element of the halogen group. At ordinary temperatures it gives off a heavy, foul, suffocating vapour and, when taken internally, acts as a violent poison. Potassium bromide seemed to be the most commonly recommended form of the compound in the journals but ammonium, sodium and strontium bromides, either singly or in various combinations, were also used to treat epilepsy. The compound was administered orally. Dosages varied widely, sometimes beginning at one drachm (sixty grains) daily. However, M. de Saulle recommended a more cautious therapeutic approach:

> for the first fortnight [of treatment], the dose of Potas. Bromide should not exceed thirty grains daily. After that the dose may be increased by eight grains, so that at the end of three months a dose of from 60 to 120 grains is taken in the 24 hours.[33]

Temkin has pointed out that, by the turn of the century, huge amounts of the substance were being dispensed through hospital pharmacy departments. One nineteenth-century physician writes of a patient who over a five-year period consumed eighty pounds of the drug, seemingly with no ill-effects.[34] As I have indicated in Chapter 2, however, along with other side-effects, bromides can cause florid eruptions of acne on the patient's skin. At the turn of the century, arsenic was one of the preferred treatments for bromide acne. Unfortunately, a side-effect of arsenic ingestion is often significant pigmentation loss. This, though, was deemed by most physicians to be preferable to the acne rash.

The bromides came to medical attention during the 1850s. Sir Charles Locock, obstetrician to Queen Victoria, had evidently read that bromide had been effective in curbing sexual desires in a German physician. M. Huette, in reporting on the effects of bromide on the body, had written in the *Medical Gazette of Paris* in 1850 that 'the bromides possessed also remarkable power in inducing torpidity of the genital organs'.[35] At a meeting of physicians held in London in 1857 where Edward Sieveking presented an account of fifty-two cases of epilepsy, Locock commented that he had been treating some of his female patients who were prone to hysterical epilepsy associated with menstruation with potassium bromide with some success.

Reasoning from this chance observation seems to have developed along the lines that if bromide compounds calmed the sexually oriented disorders of Locock's female patients and if, as had been reported, they could cause a self-induced impotence in the German physician, then there just might be therapeutic potential for the treatment of epilepsy. Because masturbation, or onanism, had long been thought one of the causes of epilepsy, it was argued that by suppressing the libido it might be possible to suppress the disorder. Given the causative links proposed by western medicine between sexual deviance, epilepsy and insanity, it is not difficult to imagine the associative leap that brought the bromides into the fold of the 'anti-epileptic' pharmacopoeia.

The mid nineteenth century had ushered in a developing medical impulse to identify the specifics of epilepsy. The age of blood-letting, purging and blistering was finally being re-evaluated and the time became ripe for innovation. Medical practice embraced this latest addition to its therapeutic armoury with some enthusiasm. By 1861 Charles Radcliffe had written that 'the name of Sir Charles Locock ought to be remembered with gratitude by every epileptic'.[36] Radcliffe's glowing accolade notwithstanding, within just over a decade some physicians were beginning to question the overall efficacy of extensive bromide use for patients. By 1870, for example, Hughlings Jackson was warning that withdrawal from the substance could generate seizures of even greater severity than those warranting medical intervention in the first place.[37]

A therapeutic inquiry into the effects of bromide on the healthy body was published in the *Lancet* in May 1884. Dr Hughes Bennett set out to test the growing general belief that prolonged use of bromides could cause a physical and mental depression worse than the malady for which they were prescribed. Bennett engages in what he claimed to be an unbiased analysis of the effects of bromides on the epileptic body. 'In attempting to throw light on this subject', he argues, 'two preliminary considerations must be recognised – 1st, the physiological actions of the drug on the healthy subject; and 2nd, the inter paroxysmal symptoms of the epileptic constitution'.[38] His findings were that in the healthy individual medicinal doses of bromide lowered intellectual functions, impaired memory, caused confused thinking, made the test subject dull, stupid and apathetic, generated a tendency to somnolence, slowed and impeded speech, enfeebled limbs (causing a staggering and uncoordinated gait), impaired or abolished sexual function and, in advanced cases, could generate imbecility or paralysis.

In other words, bromides inscribed the healthy body with the symptomatic signifiers attributed to epilepsy.

Bennett concludes that the bromides certainly have a toxic effect on the healthy body. In his considerations of the effects of bromides on the epileptic body, however, he begins from the premise of a body already 'naturally' subject to those symptoms identified as the toxic consequences of bromides for the healthy body:

> Admitting, then, that the prolonged and excessive administration of the bromides causes a series of abnormal symptoms in the healthy individual, affecting mainly the general nutrition, the mental faculties, and the sensory and motor functions, and also that the epileptic state is itself frequently accompanied by impairment of innervation [*sic*] of a somewhat analogous nature, it follows that when the drug is given for the relief of the disease care must be taken not to confound the two series of phenomena with one another.[39]

Despite admitting that prolonged use of bromides causes adverse symptoms in the healthy body, Bennett argues that physicians should not necessarily rethink therapeutic strategies in relationship to the patient with epilepsy. The epileptic body was, after all, already diseased:

> The general health [of the epileptic] is frequently unsatisfactory, the functions of the body being impaired in vigour, the digestion is weak, and the circulation feeble. The entire nervous system is in an unstable condition, the patient being at one time irritable and excitable, and at another, depressed and despondent. There is a very common condition of so-called 'nervousness' which is accompanied by headache, pains, tremors, and a variety of other subjective phenomena. The mental powers are enfeebled, the memory defective, and these intellectual alterations may exist in any degree, even to permanent and intractable forms of insanity. The physical conditions may also be changed, the nutrition of the tissues is often imperfect, the skin is pale, the muscles flabby, and the motor powers generally enfeebled, all of which may also present different degrees of severity so as to culminate in actual paralysis.[40]

Bennett sees what he expects to see when regarding the epileptic. He assumes that the state of disorder already in existence somehow immunises the epileptic against the toxic effects of the bromides. His description of the 'natural' state of the epileptic body bears an uncanny resemblance to the state of Mr P— *after* his encounter with those therapeutic regimes critically described by Joseph Williams in 1852 (see Chapter 1). Although Mr P—'s treatments preceded the bromide era, his physicians before Williams failed to diagnose the debilitating consequences of their therapeutic interventions precisely because the dominant medical gaze was encoded to see a body already, *and essentially,* in-toxic-ated by epilepsy.

To support the claims he makes for bromide therapy, Bennett offers as proof four case histories of patients who, although on long-term bromide therapy (for a mean of six years), exhibit no adverse side-effects. Of the four patients (three female, one male), he notes that three have impaired memory with some 'irritability' and two of the females display a tendency to 'great nervousness'. Nevertheless, Bennett registers no signs of bromism. The fourth patient (a twenty-two-year-old female) is deemed 'robust and active, and takes her full share in domestic work'.[41] There is no comment on her intellectual function. Medicinal dosages for three of the patients (two female and the male) were calculated at one and a half drachms daily of either potassium bromide or a combination of potassium and ammonium bromide, while the fourth patient was prescribed one drachm daily. In Bennett's study, all cases being observed were purported to be on a minimum dose of 'one drachm and a half daily, which, if necessary, was further increased in quantity'. By M. de Saulle's reckoning, three of the patients specifically cited in Bennett's study were on a middle to low range maintenance dosage (ninety grains per day), and the fourth on a minimum (sixty grains per day) maintenance dosage. The results of the analyses were calculated on an aggregate of 141 cases.

In the short and medium term, Bennett's argument for the unproblematic use of bromides failed to convince a few of the more sceptical medical practitioners. Jackson's observations were already a matter of record and some fifteen years later, in North America, William Spratling was flagging the questionable efficacy of bromide therapy, arguing that the compounds offered no hope of cure; all they did was suppress the disease. While in some cases the bromides may have limited value, he claimed, 'indiscriminately used, as they so often are, they do more harm than good'. He wrote: 'We speak of this drug in particular because of the evil effects we have seen from its widespread and irrational use'.[42]

In England, Sir William Broadbent also questioned the soundness of medicine's chemical response to the syndrome and wondered if 'the relief of symptoms, the diminished frequency and mitigated violence of the fits, may not in many instances be too dearly purchased'. He went on to conclude:

> That such is the case is distinctly my opinion.... I have seen patients reduced to a condition of practical dementia by long-continued dosing with bromides, and when the attacks have ceased it has seemed to be because the nerve centres had no longer energy for an attack.[43]

His comments acknowledge that on a regime of bromide medication even the healthiest individuals being treated for epilepsy would have trouble applying themselves to obtaining and sustaining a livelihood between seizures. Complicating this state of affairs further, the corporeal brand signifying epileptic identity (florid acne-form rash, secondary arsenic-induced loss of pigmentation) brought with it the probability of pauperism for working-class individuals, a double stigmatisation that proved virtually impossible to surmount.

For the majority of Bennett's contemporaries, however, the compounds remained the drug of choice and they were to stay at the forefront of therapeutic intervention for some time to come. Australian physician Norton Manning was arguing in 1900 that 'The bromides are, of course, the great stand-by in the treatment of the malady, and they must be given as regularly and steadily as you give food'.[44] Manning claimed that he was not among those 'who had any dread of their use'. All physicians had to do was to remain attentive to dosage regulation according to increases and reductions in the patient's weight, for 'in some cases the patient seems to feed and fatten on the bromides'. Underscoring the complacency exhibited by Bennett and Manning about the efficacy of the prolonged use of large doses of bromide is the example cited by Temkin of a patient (a fourteen-year-old boy) presented before a North American medical meeting at the turn of the century. The attending physician tells his colleagues: 'As you see he is broken down in appearance, has large abscesses in his neck, and is all together in a bad condition. But this is better than to have epilepsy.'[45]

Broadbent is one of the few physicians to have argued against this pharmaceutical trend. Other doctors noted adverse side-effects from the compounds but were unwilling to consider the possibility that the epileptic patient could be harmed by a heavy-handed or prolonged bromide regime. Or they argued, like the physician in Temkin's example, that as debilitating as some of these side-effects might be in some patients, some of the time, nothing was as bad as suffering the effects of epilepsy.

Writing somewhat against the grain, Broadbent suggests that even more important than the tell-tale rash, the unacceptable loss of energy, spirit and ableness must bring doctors around to rethinking the therapy. Even more surprisingly, he posits the view that adults with epilepsy who experience seizures over intervals of six weeks or more should be encouraged to take responsibility for their own convulsive cycles, to learn to recognise the patterns and self-medicate with small to moderate doses of bromide as needed. To recommend this level of agency for a patient was innovative; to endorse it for a patient with epilepsy was to speak heresy – and not only in the nineteenth century. As a normalising strategy, bromide sedated the troublesome epileptic personality. It certainly suppressed any libidinous impulses to moral contagion. It may have even consoled some in mainstream medical and non-medical communities that the threat of epileptic disorder might be ultimately constrained. According to the *Oxford English Dictionary*, bromide can also mean 'Something or someone boring, commonplace, or conventional; esp. a soothing platitude or trite remark'. Yet for all its promise, neither the chemical substance nor its social equivalent worked to decisively disinfect normate society of epileptic dis-ease.

VI

Despite advances made in mapping the human brain and increased medical knowledge of brain function, aspirations to understand and control epilepsy still remained largely unrealised. In the United States, Spratling worried about the resistance of the epilepsies to medical knowledge. His frustrations echo those being voiced by his British counterparts. Broadbent began a lecture on the subject in 1902 by observing:

> Epilepsy is a disease of which we know extremely little definitely, and with certainty nothing at all. We are up to a certain point agreed as to what cases are to be included under the term; we have much real and trustworthy knowledge as to the etiology of the disease; but its pathology is largely conjectural, and its treatment mainly empirical.[46]

Cure was as far beyond the reach of late nineteenth-century medical men as it had been for their predecessors. Efforts to prevent epilepsy from tainting the gene pool of future generations became fuelled by its intractability to medical resolution once detected. By the turn of the nineteenth century, these efforts were to be articulated and circulated as discourses of physical containment: if the syndrome could not be cured, its carriers would be isolated from the healthy social body. The medical gaze had adjusted its focus somewhat. If current therapeutic practices could not control the propensity of the epileptic body to seize, physicians, in a panoptic turn, could at least extend the gaze to prevent epileptic disorder from seizing the social body. Practically and ideologically, responses to epilepsy again looked to past dictums for their solutions: 'For it is easier to prevent what is threatening', the Greek physician Soranus had argued in the the second century CE, 'than to expel what is present'.[47]

Over the last five years of the nineteenth century, concerns about hereditary taint and escalating unemployment lent new urgency to the question of what was to be done with chronic epileptics. It was a question that had begun to assume mantric qualities and hinged specifically around sane epileptics. Those epileptics who were deemed consistently deranged in some way were covered by lunacy laws and as such were the responsibility of the asylum. On the other hand, sane epileptics, while not judged wholly capable and representing economic dependence on society, remained beyond the parameters of official containment. Furthermore, it was now being argued that not only were sane epileptics being economically disadvantaged because of ostracism in the workplace, not being able to work actually exacerbated the tendency to convulse. Both the *British Medical Journal* and the *Lancet* began to publish articles, news items and letters that emphasised such claims as: 'Epileptics are distinctly benefited by employment'.[48] The problem remained: *where* were they to work, and at *what*?

The question was thought serious enough to warrant the formation of the National Society for the Employment of Epileptics, a board of medical, legal and political reformers who regularly published the results of their meetings in both the *Lancet* and the *British Medical Journal*. Although this board was ostensibly set up to alleviate problems of unemployment for folk with epilepsy, they also adhered to the philosophy that 'the epileptic' was quite 'unfitted' to earn a living in the open labour market. Given this basic tenet, solutions to the issues facing the board were not immediately evident. It was now well accepted that the workhouse system and the asylum had both proved hopelessly inadequate in meeting the problems located with the sane epileptic. There was a residential home at Maghull in Lancashire and the Meath Home of Comfort and Rest for the Reception of Epileptic Women and Girls at Godalming in Surrey (set up in 1888 and 1892, respectively), but they were relatively small and relied on charity and philanthropic gifts for financial survival.

Concerns framing the question of where to place epileptics in relation to mainstream society were summed up by this item published in the *Lancet*:

> The need for a home or refuge of some kind to which epileptics could be sent has long been felt by those who have been brought much into contact with such patients. Every convalescent home is closed against them, they are frequently incapacitated by their unfortunate malady from occupying positions for which in other respects they are well fitted, and they cannot be regarded, except temporarily, as suitable for treatment in hospital, even in those institutions which more particularly deal with such cases.[49]

In England, the colony movement gained momentum from increased industrialisation in the cities, escalating unemployment among the casual poor, boundary shifts in community care services, and conceptual developments in thinking about the socio-political and economic import of the deviant body in mainstream society. These factors had merged to bring those with epilepsy to public attention as never before. Although the homes at Maghull and Godalming marked a beginning in accommodating epileptics away from the travails of mainstream society, they were not really equipped to address the problems highlighted by reformers. The National Society for the Employment of Epileptics turned outwards for inspiration and it soon became the mobilising force behind the epileptic colony movement in Britain. One of its founders – Miss Burden-Sanderson – had notes on the Bielefeld epileptic colony in Germany.[50]

Notions of labour farms or colonies as an answer to the threat posed by the residuum to the respectable working class were already being circulated by 1886. As Gareth Jones has argued, efforts to allay some of the more volatile fears troubling reformers such as Galton and Maudsley about protecting the working classes from the pathogenic effects of the degenerate classes were thought to require far more proactive policies than had been implemented to date. Furthermore, the problems represented by these 'dangerous' classes had, by the mid 1880s, far exceeded the wherewithal of Poor Law authorities. It was being argued that slum conditions significantly exacerbated or even, in some cases, caused degeneration. To continue to hope for some sort of natural abatement to the problem (that is, the eventual failure of the degenerate class to reproduce itself) constituted dangerous negligence.

Samuel Barnett, Alfred Marshall and Charles Booth were also among those advocating a more strenuous and systematic response to the issues personified by the demoralised residuum. They developed plans that would not only resolve the unemployment problem bedevilling London but also address an acute housing shortage for the respectable working class. The solution, they argued, was the establishment of farm colonies beyond the boundaries of the great industrial cities. The unemployed could then be removed from mainstream society and drafted into a more productive and ordered lifestyle.

> The object of these colonies would not be to provide employment but to provide training in habits of industry and to inculcate rudimentary agricultural skills. The farm colony would thus be a solution not only to the problem of unemployment and urban degeneration, but also to rural depopulation. For once rehabilitation had taken place, the chronically unemployed would be resettled on the land as agricultural labourers.[51]

Into an environment already seeded with this social model, and armed with notes on the Bielefeld epileptic colony, the National Society for the Employment of Epileptics launched an appeal to support a British epileptic colony system that was so successful that the Lord Mayor of London became involved in the work as President of the Society.

VII

There was early uncertainty about what, precisely, these institutional sites signified for administrators and soon-to-be residents, an uncertainty that was reflected in equivocation over appropriate nomenclature. An editorial item published in the *Lancet* at the end of 1892 used the phrase 'labour colony' in its heading. Two years later, in a similar vein, the *British Medical Journal* favoured the phrase 'farm colony' in its reportage of the soon-to-be realised facility at Chalfont St Peters. In announcing the laying of the foundation stone for the facility to be built at Chalfont, the *Lancet* referred to it as an 'Industrial colony', although the phrase 'epileptic colony' formed part of the header for the item on the subject. Asylums they were not, although the proposed residents of the facilities were considered not to be wholly or consistently sane. Nor were they hospitals, although they were to manage medicalised disorder. By 1895 the journals had settled on 'epileptic colonies' as the uniform descriptor.

Contributors to the British medical journals dubbed this latest response to epilepsy 'the great experiment'. This phrase was used in a variety ways in both the *Lancet* and the *British Medical Journal* from 1890 until the turn of the century. At a meeting of the Council of the Charity Organisation Society held in London on 10 May 1886 the need for special facilities to 'train' sane epileptics in such trades that would render them useful to themselves and society was addressed by Queen Square physician Dr Buzzard, who 'strongly advocated the proposal that some experiment should be made'.[52] Physicians, politicians and other interested parties were at various times exhorted to lend their support to consolidating and expanding the experimental facilities. William Turner alerted his colleagues to the shortfall of the British programme. Germany and America, he wrote, were not only more organised in their responses to this most pressing of socio-medical problems but also responding in a far more satisfactory way by establishing much larger colonies than were currently available in England. Delegates attending the North-Western Poor Law Conference in 1898 at Bangor, Wales, were told by Dr J. M. Rhodes that 'the public institutions of a country were the standard of its civilisation, and that England must not lag behind America and Germany in its provision for the epileptic and feeble-minded class'.[53]

Bielefeld became the prototype for the British epileptic colonies and by the turn of the century most of the British colony founders had visited the German institution. The Bielefeld colony was located in Westphalia and had been in official operation since around 1867 (although actually founded in 1841). References to the Bielefeld colony appear in nearly every item addressing the need for an epileptic colony system in Britain published between 1892 and 1900 in both the *Lancet* and the *British Medical Journal*. One proponent, in a rush of colonialist fervour, referred to the facility as the 'colony of mercy'. Throughout much of the western world, Bielefeld was held up as a curative model for society's disaffection with the epileptic and by 1899 the establishment was said to accommodate over 3,000 epileptics in a mixed farming community. The colony was located on the edge of the Teutoburgian forest and the 'cheap and willing labour supplied by the male inmates after a time reduced to a state of comparative cultivation what was formerly mere waste land'.[54] The colony was eventually to supplement this male population of colonists with similarly affected females and children culled from normate communities.

The primary aims of the colony concept were: to remove people diagnosed with epilepsy from the mainstream community; to place them in an ordered environment where all aspects of their lives could be placed under the surveillance of responsible carers; to monitor and control all possible exciting causes of their disorder; and systematically to administer medication (inevitably bromides). Theories on colony management also emphasised the importance of diet in regimes of therapeutic control.

Colony advocates took up the mantle of geographic and social control of the epileptic population shed by an overburdened Poor Law system. The colony idea yielded the extra attraction of presenting the wherewithal for those with epilepsy to finally be able to earn their keep, or at least contribute to the cost of their confinement. The colonies were to provide a designated 'epileptic' space beyond the boundaries of normative society, but not beyond the purview of normalising regimes. In a news item about a proposed 'labour colony', the *Lancet* noted some concern that the potential flaw in 'working such an experiment as this consists in the moral contagion almost inevitably associated with nervous disease'[55] but this was not felt to be an insurmountable problem. Certainly the sedative effects of bromides were a way of inhibiting possible outbreaks of moral contagion. Women were seen as a blemish in the productivity scenario and finding suitable commercial employment for them proved difficult.

Despite some reservations, the possibilities presented by the 'great experiment' proved too tempting for other normative societies to resist and colonies for sane epileptics soon began to spring up in France, Switzerland, Belgium, North America and Australia, as well as Britain. For the main part, the rhetoric used to justify such places was geared around a mixture of urgent socio-economic need and a sentimentalised humanitarianism. Both factors were already well established tropes in colonialist discourse, where a rhetoric of benevolence had long been drawn upon to reinforce colonialist power over the colonised. In England it was also argued that the colonies would provide a place where epileptics might build self-esteem through productive employment: a function that would help them control the tendency to seize. They were to be places of refuge rather than places of enforced confinement, where epileptics might find peace and purpose.

It was argued that epilepsy was becoming more prevalent and that the numbers of non-insane epileptics in society presented an increasing drain on public coffers. It was claimed that this 'poor, unfortunate class' had become not only 'family lepers' but outcasts in the wider community, whereas 'in a colony each epileptic is readily brought to see that he is as useful a person as his more highly favoured brother if placed under proper conditions'.[56] The view was put forward that 'the very fact of their being together is a measure of safety'. This last comment conveyed the idea that folk affected by epilepsy generally displayed a greater gentleness and consideration for each other than they were usually shown by the wider community, although the claim also contains embedded traces of the perceived threat posed by epileptics for a normative society. The belief that those with epilepsy would be somehow better off if they were put together in specially constructed and contained communities was to be reiterated often and with some passion in pro-colony rhetoric.

In accord with Risien Russell's approval of the programme developed by Dr Bourneville at the Bicêtre Hospital (see above), William Turner argued that colonies would be particularly beneficial to children; they could be educated and trained to ordered living. He worried, though, that the tendency of parents to hide their child's disease would prevent a significant number of children from taking advantage of the system.

After the National Society opened its colony at Chalfont St Peters in Buckinghamshire in 1894, others soon followed. What had, up until this time, been the work of philanthropic individuals who were responding to a felt need in society became more organised along established institutionalised lines. If unable to cure the corporeal body of epileptic disorder, the new medical gaze could now at least extend its diagnostic scope to address the potential for paroxysmal disorder in the social body. Epileptic danger had been redefined and processes were now in place to excise it from the healthy social body. Foucault has pointed out that, in their institution of public health standards, members of the medical fraternity were among the first managers of collective space.[57] With the advent of the colony movement it seemed that, at least in the short term, medicine and mainstream communities had finally hit upon a social bromide to quell the threat of epileptic taint. Rather ironically, a side benefit extended to colony epileptics was often a reduction in their bromide dosage so that they could function more effectively and productively.

Because of the relative cheapness of rural land, and in keeping with nineteenth-century beliefs about moral management and the containment of contagion, the colonies were geographically remote from cities and major towns. Reporting on his visit to the Chalfont colony, a correspondent for the *British Medical Journal* recorded the following impressions:

> The geography of the district is ... decidedly ambiguous, and were it not for the assistance of the ordnance survey the site of the colony would be difficult to find. This freedom from publicity is a great point in favour of the spot selected for this important undertaking, and the wisdom of it is shown in the quiet simplicity of the daily life of the place.... It is a happy reflection to consider that here a helping hand is being held out to rescue those sufferers from epilepsy whose lives under ordinary circumstances would be one of blank inertia, useless to themselves and to others, till mind and memory became lost in madness, and they had qualified for the lunatic asylum.[58]

The colonies were usually purpose built or located in converted farms and manor houses that had been adapted to facilitate isolation of the disorder and comprehensive surveillance of the colonists. They were invariably developed as rural spaces, emphasising simplicity, discipline and a flexible temporality necessarily absent from industrialised society. The geographic isolation of these institutions also reflected the disinclination of nineteenth-century mainstream society to live with or near epileptic communities.

The epileptic body had been deemed anathema in a capitalist economy: the colonies instantiated the epileptic's expulsion from the modernist dream of order and technical efficiency. In an inversion of the Eden narrative, at least some of the industrial rejects thrown up by the nineteenth century were being returned to a perverse version of the Garden, to dwell under a paternalistic regime of benevolent order.

In a prescriptive article on the care and management of residents in epileptic colonies, William Turner outlined the principles of colony ideology as it was to be practised in Britain. He argued that colonies should be guided by the following aims:

> (*a*) removal of the epileptic from the towns to the country; (*b*) the regular employment in the garden, fields, orchard, workshops, &c, of the colonists under the supervision of capable persons; (*c*) the maintenance of a well-ordered and regular mode of life, with the avoidance of excitement and abstinence from alcoholic liquors; and (*d*) abundance of good nourishment of a simple nature. Living under such conditions it has been found that the epileptic requires only a minimal amount of medicinal treatment, and it is the custom to give each colonist thirty grains of bromide of potassium at bedtime.[59]

These principles became standard operating procedure, with the added proviso that if they were to bear fruit they should also incorporate a special laboratory with a skilled pathologist in residence so that epilepsy could be observed and studied *in situ*.

The initial stages of colony development in Britain were crucial to their ongoing acceptance and success. These early colonies were being sponsored by private citizens. For the idea to receive the backing of the Poor Law unions, with the possibility of subsequent development of public establishments, they had to be seen to be working. With this in mind, the first colonists were selected with great care. This strategy of maximising success in any medical enterprise faithfully echoed the Galenic maxim that 'the physician ought to accept only such patients as would promise obedience to his dietetic regulations'.[60]

By 1906, including the expanded facilities at Maghull and Godalming, there were eight colonies in Britain. Three more colonies had been established by 1935.

VIII

The colony movement in North America began on a much more ambitious scale than was the case in England. Ellen Dwyer has argued that an impulse to 'grandeur', both in size and in décor, of the more public buildings, was very much a part of the philosophy driving the flurry of asylum construction that took place in North America from 1843. This impulse, she suggests, not only signified the importance and gravity of the therapeutic mission to be conducted within the walls of these edifices but was also intended as an antidote to any feelings of degradation that patients might experience.[61] The North

American colony project also differed from the English endeavour in its central concerns. Rampant unemployment and social reforms had formed the impetus behind the colony movement in England and although issues of employment for those with epilepsy formed part of the concerns of North American physicians, by the turn of the century the emphasis was very much on eugenic matters.

Opened informally in 1896, the flagship of the American colony system was the Craig colony, located at Sonyea in the Genesee Valley, Livingstone County, New York. The colony was 1,900 acres in size and located on the site of a defunct Shaker community. The site already had well developed fields, orchards, pastures and market gardens, extensive work having been done by the Shakers, who had worked the area for fifty years prior to its purchase by the state. A substantial number of good buildings, workshops and quarries made the site even more attractive to its new owners. The Shakers were celibates and as their numbers diminished they were unable to sustain the farm, hence its sale to the state.[62]

If we are to accept the evidence of retrospective diagnosis, the site had already enjoyed a long association with epilepsy; both Cesare Lombroso and William Lennox suggested that Ann Lee, founder of the Shakers, suffered from epilepsy. The associative possibilities between both the founding group of this community and their successors are obvious and tempting to make if only through the sect's appellation. However, William Spratling, the superintendent of Craig colony, resisted this temptation and instead chose to focus on other possible links between the settlement's successive inhabitants. In 1901, he argued that 'the time will come, and should come, when every state will enact laws to prohibit, if possible, the marriage and intermarriage of epileptics. I think such prohibition would be best for the epileptic, best for society at large, best for posterity, and best for the State for economic reasons.'[63] Spratling was in no doubt that epileptics should go the way of the Shakers who preceded them at Sonyea.

As in England, the Bielefeld colony had been the inspiration behind the North American colony movement, Dr Frederick Peterson reporting in the *New York Medical Record* in April 1887 on the 'marvellous success' of the German venture.[64] In the 1902 *Bulletin of General Information* on the New York facility, Spratling paints a vivid word picture of the geographical beauty of the site, in which he draws heavily on its historical associations with the 'proud Iroquois', who had named the area the 'Beautiful Valley'. Rather poetically, he writes:

> The term Sonyea, the name of the old Indian village on the site of which the Colony is founded, signifies in the Indian language 'a warm and sunny place'. This fair domain for the helpless, homeless beings

> to whom the State has extended a gentle, ministering hand, lies on the west side of the valley, the surface in the southern region portion rolling gently to the east, and in the northern part extending into alluvial bottomlands. The situation seems admirably adapted by nature for the humane purpose to which it is devoted by the wise benevolence of a great commonwealth. Through the centre of the tract, dividing it into two about equal portions, flows Kishaqua Creek, the name of which in Indian significance is 'loving stream'.

He proceeds to inform his readers that the 'loving stream' also 'serves an admirable purpose in providing a natural barrier for the separation of the two sexes'.[65]

As with the colony sites in England, the New York colony was touted as a rural idyll, albeit on a far grander scale than the British establishments. Spratling evokes the Edenic trope notable in the rhetoric of his English colleagues and amplifies it by gesturing to the site's ennobled past. Why the proud Iroquois no longer inhabited such a salubrious space is left unremarked and Sonyea's Indigenous caretakers are reduced to a signifier of (evacuated) pre-industrial perfection. Nevertheless, association of the Craig colony site with Native American tradition is evocative, particularly when one considers late nineteenth-century medical views on the links between industrialisation, city living and degeneration. Like the asylums built earlier in the century, the epileptic colonies were represented as places of refuge from the stresses of American industrialisation and big-city living.

The Craig colony was designed to house primarily those epileptics in poor or indigent circumstances and the board of directors were keenly interested in maximising the economic efficiency of the enterprise. For a patient to be in residence for less than two or three years was thought to be counterproductive to the business of ordering the disorderly and also impeded the facility's chance to reap any economic benefit from a newly disciplined productiveness. Spratling urged that 'many ought to feel that the Colony is the best home for them so long as they need one'.[66] The Craig colony, despite the large scale of its land holdings and the impressive size of its executive buildings, ultimately aimed to accommodate residents in a series of 'cottages' housing from fifteen to thirty patients each. Other American colonies later reproduced this pattern, developing ground plans and street layouts that mimed the 'normal' space of small-town America. The Abilene colony in Texas, for example, organised its administrative, utility and residential buildings in grid patterns demarcated by '1st Street, 2nd Street' and so forth, 'Maple Street' and 'Lakeside Drive'. Spratling went so far as to suggest that a patient entering the Craig colony in the near future might well choose to 'build a cottage for himself on the premises, subject to conditions to be prescribed by the Board of Managers'.

Although in the *Bulletin of General Information* Spratling briefly acknowledges the site's association with the Shaker community – his brevity perhaps an attempt to deflect the image of the religious, prophesying epileptic much in circulation in medical texts at this time – the emphasis of his 'sales pitch' is very much geared towards images of a latter-day Eden. His description of the facility's geographical beauty suggests a place of grace and gentle confinement with the potential for rebirth into mainstream society as an ordered, organically sound citizen. This is a suggestion strengthened by his account of 'V.S.'

V.S. arrived at the colony in February 1896, a hopelessly disordered young man, and emerged cured two and a half years later to take up his place in society as an industrious, self-supporting citizen. When he came to the colony aged twenty-eight he had been prescribed large doses of bromide for some time and on admission was taking forty grains of potassium bromide three times a day. Spratling acknowledged the adverse effects of this prolonged high dosage on the patient's mental and physical state and radically revised the treatment. On discharge V.S. was taking a maintenance dose of five grains of bromide three times a day, was seizure free, alert and able to pursue a career in printing while supporting his mother. His ongoing well-being depended, so Spratling argued, on his continued adherence to those principles of living learned as a colony resident:

> There was for this man a lesson of the most definite and vital importance to be learned under the good influences of Colony life, and he was ambitious enough to learn it well, and having done that to remember it. Should he fail in his knowledge and practice of how to live, he may again have convulsions; but he shows no sign of failure at this time.[67]

There can be no doubt that reduction of this young man's bromide dosage was central to his recovery from what seems to have been a medically exacerbated epilepsy. It is again worth recalling that the British physician Joseph Williams achieved similarly stellar results for his patient Mr P— some four decades earlier, beyond the confines of a colony (see Chapter 1).

If Spratling saw the Craig colony as paving the way to an ever-more efficient medical and social response to epilepsy, he also saw it as a line of last defence against society's further contagion from the disorder. He argued that the colonies could not only become economically self-sufficient given time and good management, but also that rigorous surveillance and analysis of pathology would ultimately yield up the secrets of the epileptic body.

Spratling notes with some pride in the 1902 *Bulletin* that the on-site Peterson Hospital is a well equipped, fully staffed facility:

> There are competent surgeons on the resident staff who do a great deal of abdominal and brain surgery, in addition to the surgical work required in a village of 1,000 persons unusually liable to accidents.[68]

When this seemingly innocuous claim for the first-rate medical care available to the 'unusually' accident-prone epileptic is measured against the 'great deal of abdominal and brain surgery' also carried out by the resident surgeons, a more sinister picture begins to emerge. Lisa Cartwright has noted that Spratling was more than a little proud of the institution's 'excellent results' from the high rate of abdominal surgery performed on twelve- to fifteen-year-old females.[69] Supposedly the surgery was performed to manage their epilepsy; however, it is worth recalling that Spratling also had a committed belief in prohibiting the reproductive potential of those with cerebral paroxysmal conditions.

In his analysis of the development of the eugenics movement in both Britain and North America, Daniel Kevles argues that the positive eugenics advocated by the likes of Galton (that is, breeding to the strengths rather than the weaknesses of human stock) was to be eventually augmented by an impulse to negative eugenics. Galton's protégé, Karl Pearson, insisted on the futility of improving schools for the lower classes on the grounds that 'No training or education can *create* intelligence. You must breed it.' Although Pearson privately acknowledged that the 'children of incapables' were a blight on human evolution, he stopped short of arguing for legislation to allow eugenic sterilisation.[70] Debates about what kind of ethical intervention might be taken to ensure that negative blood lines did not proliferate took place on both sides of the Atlantic and intensified as the new century dawned.

Segregation and sexual prohibition in institutions housing those deemed unfit, defective or degenerate were viewed as being only partially effective. Education programmes to develop eugenic sensibilities in the wider community were advocated by the Eugenics Education Society. William Whetham, an English physicist and eugenics proponent, and his wife, fellow eugenicist Catherine Whetham, argued that eugenic policies were necessary to the future of the human race and to the future of national security.[71] As a last resort, sterilisation of those who posed a threat to the ongoing evolution of the human species was also being considered, even by otherwise cautious eugenicists.

America's leading eugenicist at the turn of the century, Charles Davenport, like Galton and Pearson, argued for identifying and breeding good human stock: middle-class, white, intellectual. According to Kevles, Davenport 'looked forward to the day when a woman would no more accept a man "without knowing his biologico-genealogical history" than a stockbreeder would take "a sire for his colts or calves ... without pedigree"'.[72] To hasten this evolutionary dream, however, Davenport argued for the necessity of detecting 'defective germ plasm' – that is, plasm from the 'imbecile, epileptic, insane, criminalistic, alcoholic, and sexually immoral'. It was time, so the more radical eugenicists in both England and North America urged, to actively protect prime human stock from what the Whethams generally referred to as the 'contaminating strains of worthless blood'. Although systematic sterilisation of the defective had been debated by both British and American eugenicists, few British eugenicists became convinced of either the necessity or the wisdom of legislating for such a procedure.

In the United States, however, the concept of eugenic sterilisation was greeted with what Kevles calls 'a strong consensus'. As early as 1889 some officials in American institutions had begun to argue for eugenic sterilisation of their charges. Over the next two decades sterilisation of those deemed defective gradually began to creep into policy for a growing number of institutions housing the criminal, those with mental health problems and those with epilepsy: 'If the state could take a person's life', so Davenport claimed, the state could also 'deny the lesser right of reproduction'.[73] William J. Robinson, a New York urologist, argued that eugenic sterilisation could in no way be seen as an infringement of personal liberty or rights. He insisted: 'Such individuals have no rights. They have no right in the first instance to be born, but having been born, they have no right to propagate their kind.'[74] Davenport's anxieties about an ongoing proliferation of defective germ plasm and the Whethams' claim for an urgent need to staunch the worthless blood contaminating future generations paralleled a growing medical disaffection with the epileptic.

Compounding frustration at an inability to curb seizures (beyond the very limited effects of treatments such as bromides) was the conviction that the epileptic was by turn prone to childish dependency on the physician, unrealistic euphoria, religious arrogance, chronic ill-humour, deceitfulness and antisocial sentiment/behaviour. Following William Gowers' lead, by 1900 physicians on both sides of the Atlantic and in Australia were beginning to discuss the 'epileptic personality' as a discrete and necessary component of cerebral paroxysmal conditions. L. Pierce Clark, a physician at the Craig colony from 1900 to 1917, wrote extensively on epileptic personality and assembled a collection of tell-tale traits – all undesirable – attributed as general characteristics of epilepsy syndromes. Frequent reiteration of these characteristics by medical authors in time endowed them with a law-like inevitability and they became figured as a constitutive aspect of epilepsy conditions, as is evident in discussion in the *Australasian Medical Gazette* (see below).

Lennox points out that these early twentieth-century models of the epileptic personality, at least in North America, were formulated and popularised by physicians who, by and large, worked and resided in colonies and thus were the consequence of a vision limited by context. Nevertheless, the models resonate with the images set into play by Gowers in his thoughts on an essentialised defective moral control exhibited by epileptics. He argued, after all, that for those with epilepsy: 'Mischievous restlessness and irritability in childhood may develop into vicious and even criminal tendencies in adult life'.[75] Closely following this mode of representation, Pierce Clark observed in 1917:

> The child who is to be epileptic is vicious, already irritable and impulsive. His motives are futile, he isolates himself or runs away, and has sombre ideas. At the slightest reprimand he speaks of suicide, or absents himself for days after a chiding. He is sexually precocious, an onanist, has night terrors and somnambulism, etc.[76]

Given the irredeemably negative picture projected by the dominant psycho-physiological model of epileptic disorder, one that circulated well into the new century, it is little wonder that radical excision from the healthy social body was thought to be the optimal response. And that after excision, the embodied site of potential contamination should be sterilised.

Spratling's approach to an expansive and multifaceted surveillance of the epileptic body was to see him initiate a film project in 1905 that recorded the seizures of his patients. He was also a primary petitioner to the State of New York for changes to the laws governing autopsy. As a result of his petitions, the Craig colony was granted the right to perform autopsies on patients who had died while resident at the institution even in the absence of the patient's prior consent. These changes to the autopsy law in New York State were particular to the perceived needs of the Craig colony: no other facility had quite the same degree of power over the patient. Spratling argued that 'Such a law as this will aid in the elucidation of the problems underlying the etiology of *the strangest disease in human history*, and every public institution in the State should have a similar one'.[77] Cartwright notes that the law 'guaranteed

Spratling a supply of fresh bodies for neurological research'. Spratling's authority over his largely destitute charges was considerable. They also provided free labour for the colony which, under his stewardship, fairly quickly ran at a profit. These factors, Cartwright suggests, may go some way to explaining why Spratling seemed to consider his 'living charges as a stock of potential cadavers'.[78]

Spratling's concerns about the economic health of the colony echoed wider interests in the productive body. Theories of time and motion management were being developed in the United States to further serve capitalist demands for maximum worker efficiency. These theories are rather famously ratified in Frederick Winslow Taylor's principles of scientific management. Taylor's ideas on the scientific management of the body and productive space began gaining public attention towards the end of the 1880s. Taylor had trained as an engineer and his interests in production techniques and the power relations of the workplace led him to develop his theories of 'the managed life'. Regardless of what forms his stories of managed efficiency took, Martha Banta has argued that, inevitably, they all moved towards the same point: 'the need to apply the guiding hand that is simultaneously visible and invisible (now you see it, now you feel it)'.[79] It is a principle that brings to mind the management programme for epileptic children developed by Bourneville and advocated by Risien Russell.

'In the past', Taylor claimed, 'the man has been first; in the future the system must be first'.[80] Banta argues that Taylor aspired 'to contain human needs within a grand design possessing the capacity to envisage the whole significance of industrial management, from the art of cutting metals to all its results in human lives'.[81] It is not immediately obvious how the epileptic body can be manipulated or trained according to this vision. It is a wild card in the schema of managed (disciplined) bodies: seemingly hard wired to, at any time, and unpredictably, disorder – seize – those well greased links between man and machine. This potential to disrupt an ordered temporal and spatialised regime would seem to place it beyond the aspiration of the Taylorist man/machine. Nevertheless, both the Taylored body and the body of the colony epileptic were subject to similar regimes of surveillance and discipline by 1910: both bodies were the product of what Banta identifies in relation to Taylorism as 'managed lives'.

The care programme developed for the Craig colony displays a nascent awareness of Taylor-like principles of scientific management, if only as applied to agricultural and artisan production. In a letter to the *British Medical Journal* in 1899 Spratling thanks G. E. Shuttleworth for his kind remarks with regard to the Craig colony published in the journal earlier that same year. He goes on to expand on some of the points made in that discussion. The Craig colony, he writes, would gradually expand to house an epileptic population of 1,800 or more, in 'true and simple homes in every sense of the word'.[82] He is also at pains to inform his British colleagues that at the Craig colony steps were already being implemented to streamline the costs of running the establishment for the state. This economic rationalisation was being realised through a programme where least affected epileptics were trained to agricultural and domestic skills, thus offsetting the cost of their own upkeep as well as contributing to the cost of care for those more severely affected by the syndrome. Spratling's industry in managing the seemingly minimal economic potential of the epileptic body using those disciplines of surveillance and motivation that were to be valorised by later management theories paid off. Not only did the Craig colony gain economic self-sufficiency, but by 1905 the state actually made a profit from its agricultural and industrial production.

If Bielefeld had been the exemplar of colony structure and management throughout the latter decades of the nineteenth century, Spratling very quickly established the Craig colony as the North American paradigm in the first decade of the new century. With the Craig colony as his reference, Dr T. B. Bass, then superintendent of the Terrell asylum in Texas, recommended the construction of 'an eleemosynary hospital' for epileptics near Abilene, Texas. The task of overseeing the building of the Abilene colony fell to Dr John Preston, who then went on to occupy the position of medical superintendent for the first six years of the facility's development. In 1909 Bass, the conceptual architect of the project, took over the position of superintendent and functioned in that capacity for the next thirty-four years.

Under Bass's supervision the facility continued to grow in both size and population from those early years and to all intents and purposes he ran it with the same autocratic authority exhibited by his northern colleague. It is said that he experimented on his charges with various combinations of alcohol (usually whisky) in the early years of his stewardship. In the years just prior to 1913 he also experimented with dosages of rattlesnake vaccine as part of the hospital's therapeutic regime. If he recorded his findings from these experiments, the records seem to be no longer in existence. Furthermore, no official reports exist of the actual experiments.[83] Others, however, did report on their use of the substance and crotalin, or rattlesnake venom, enjoyed some popularity in the North American pharmacopoeia through the early years of the new century. Its potential value in the treatment of epilepsy was first reported in 1908, by L. Self, another Texan physician.

Evidently a patient had been bitten by a rattlesnake and one of the consequences of the bite was two years without seizures. Although initially greeted with interest and some enthusiasm by other American physicians at the time, Walter Friedlander points out that by 1914 the interest had just as quickly abated. Some deaths from the treatment were being recorded and eventually the medical fraternity was to conclude that crotalin had no substantial therapeutic value.[84]

Although residents of the Abilene colony were technically admitted on a voluntary basis, they were strongly urged (as were the Craig colony patients) to remain in the colony for extended periods, if not permanently.[85] If colonists fled the hospital, Bass was able to authorise state troopers to bring them back. By 1912, sixty per cent of the colonists were under twenty-one years of age and seventy-five per cent of the colony's epileptic population were capable of full-time work on the colony's farm and in its various production facilities as part of their therapy. Evidently there was a significant labour loss just after the outbreak of World War I, when many of the young male patients ran away 'to get rich picking cotton in East Texas'.[86]

The Abilene colonists were also subject to intense scrutiny in their day-to-day routines. As with those resident in the Craig colony, this surveillance extended to exploratory surgery and by the 1920s to 'X-Ray pictures'. Bass's quest for the definitive causal factors in epilepsy was to prove unsuccessful, however. Although he argued that head trauma and some acute infections such as meningitis and encephalitis could have a part to play in the aetiology of the disorder, in a 1930 paper published in the *Texas State Journal of Medicine* he also declared:

> It is, I think, a fairly well established fact that a child begotten while parents are drunk may be abnormal and possibly may develop epilepsy. In this way the prohibition law is striking at an evil. The propagation of the unfit should be discouraged as much as possible. Sterilization under proper control should be legalized in every state.[87]

Like the Craig colony on which it was patterned, the Abilene colony was structured to function like a village and, as far as possible, it was geared towards self-sufficiency. Indeed, as late as 1944 Hamilton Wright was to observe that 'Abilene citizens know little of the hospital and still less what it means in a financial way to the city'.[88] The observation suggests the liminal place that the colony and its inhabitants occupied in the socio-cultural psyche (and identity) of the town. Wright's flagging of the contribution the colony represented to the town's economic prosperity refers to trade links, in the form of perishable and emergency goods bought by the colony to supplement its own production, and a sizeable net payroll for those employed as ancillary staff. The colony's absence from the larger, collective town consciousness, however, suggests its place as an exclusionary zone beyond the borders of normative society. It was a place of abject beings; a place for those who had been cast off from mainstream congress, but who remained nevertheless constitutive of the town's identity.

IX

Australian medical professionals also looked to the colony system as a solution to the threat of epileptic disorder in society and like their North American colleagues chose to focus on the eugenic implications of such an enterprise. The rhetoric making it on to the pages of the *Australasian Medical Gazette* resisted the urge to humanitarian sentimentalism. Rather, writers for the journal pushed the point that the benefits of the colony system lay in facilitating the removal of the epileptic from the temptation of degenerate town living. Moreover, they claimed, this removal would isolate the disruptive potential posed by the epileptic for the general community. Most useful of all, it would expedite the implementation of moral treatment so necessary to curb the epileptic propensity for vice and general moral decadence.

Following the North American lead, it was argued that Australia needed to pay prompt attention to legislation aimed at controlling the epileptic population: 'For the large army of epileptics classed as sane no special provision has as yet been made in Australia, and the time is approaching when this will be felt to be a public want'.[89] In citing statistics on epileptic populations in countries other than England, William Turner concluded that the figures available to him suggested that Australia's numbers in 1897 were considerably below the estimate of European countries and America. However, as he did with European and American estimates, he queried the accuracy of the figures and suggested that 'it is not improbable that the ... numbers really under-estimate the total proportion of epileptics in the Australasian colonies'.[90]

In an article exploring the paradox of epileptic identity, Manning, who had once been the Inspector-General of the Insane for New South Wales, managed to give voice to a powerful medical antipathy towards the epileptic patient. He began his thesis by reminding his audience at the Australian Medical Association that the great curiosity about epileptics is that they occupy the extremes of human possibility, being at both the 'zenith and nadir of intellectual capacity'. On the one hand, the syndrome made for the genius associated with the likes of Paul the Apostle, Mahomet, Julius Caesar and Napoleon, yet, on the other, 'there is no being more degraded, more mindless, or more vegetative than the confirmed epileptic imbecile'.[91] Manning constructed for his audience a figure of both transformative potential and abject dissolution. With regard to the transformative possibilities offered by the genius aspect of this dyad, Broadbent makes the point barely two years later that after long-term treatment with bromides neither Julius Caesar nor Napoleon Bonaparte would have been capable of any sort of consistent day-to-day intellectual function, let alone the strategic planning and winning of battles.[92]

Manning's view of the epileptic is both bigoted and unforgiving and there are obvious parallels to be drawn between his rhetoric and that of Max Nordau in relation to the degenerate (see Chapter 2). Nevertheless, there is a sense in which the Australian physician captures a widely held, if superficially suppressed, belief and, as such, his views are worth quoting at some length:

> The epileptic ... is often a very interesting personality. He has sometimes a large intellectual capacity; he is sometimes thoughtful and well-read; he is occasionally of an artistic temperament; and he is always hopeful, and, except a little before the onset of the attacks, a cheery and companionable being. But the confirmed epileptic, especially where he has passed the bounds of sanity altogether, is very seldom a lovable creature. He has usually a Bible in one pocket, a prayer-book in another, a lie in his mouth, and a more or less plentiful supply of malicious accusations tucked away among his cerebral convolutions to be levelled, as occasion may seem to him to require, at all and sundry, but chiefly against those in immediate charge of, or thrown into immediate contact with him. Sometimes the religious and the malicious are curiously intermingled; the epileptic praying aloud, rails at his neighbours in good set terms, or sings hymns in what has been well described as a *noli me tangere* tone of voice. The mental and moral decadence are both curious, and are, no doubt, both largely pathological in origin.[93]

In confirming Manning's observations, Dr Angel Money noted that the *noli me tangere* behaviour highlighted in his colleague's address was especially evident at those times when the epileptic was feeling 'very well'. At those times, Money claimed, 'An epileptic is often exceedingly irritable'.[94] Money's comments about the insufferability of epileptic wellness might suggest secondary reasons for aggressive therapeutic bromide sedation.

Manning argued that although it was historically acceptable to divide epileptics into insane and sane categories, in fact this was a somewhat spurious division. The dividing line between the categories was so narrow and uncertain, and the borderland cases between the two so numerous, he claimed, that differentiating, except in the most extreme instances and for the purpose of institutional administration, was close to pointless. He proposed that although there were epileptics who might not be technically insane, this group could never be classed as totally sane either; the fact of their tendency to convulse precluded the possibility of sustained reason. Like his British counterparts, Manning also justified the efficacy of confining groups of epileptics together in one place as a way of increasing the possibility of their access to human kindness. He points out that 'a fellow-feeling makes even epileptics wondrous kind, [they] are very tolerant of the failings, compassionate of the weaknesses, and helpful in regard to the paroxysms of their fellow inmates'.[95] This is to say that 'epileptics' are as responsive to fellow feeling and community belonging as their normate 'others'.

By the time first decade of the twentieth century had come to a close, the altruistic tones that marked the early colony rhetoric of the British medical journals had all but disappeared. The movement was now overtly and unequivocally driven by socio-economic rationalisation and systematic attempts to curtail the disorder represented by the epileptic. The London correspondent for the *Australasian Medical Gazette* wrote that it was now up to the state to 'care for and train the cases of inherited epilepsy ... as surely as it confined in private or public asylums certifiable cases of insanity'.[96] To do otherwise for the non-insane epileptic was to merely bypass social responsibility in the guise of offering 'false freedom'; it was a 'cruel kindness, to allow them to be at large', the writer argued. Although the author of this text stops short of sanctioning official round-ups and 'Draconian' confinement of the offending group, he does propose that if the colonies are administered well enough, public opinion will be such that the 'average parent would be thankful to send his afflicted child into them'. The editors of the *Gazette* argue in an item published eighteen months later that although it was recognised that there was a great need to admit sane epileptics to colonies at the earliest possible time after diagnosis, too often patients did not enter these facilities 'until they [had] become intolerable to those belonging to them'.[97] In the same piece, reporting on the development of the Talbot colony in rural Victoria, the journal informed its readers that the inaccessibility of the site, near Clayton, although inconvenient for visitors, was a distinct advantage as far as the patients were concerned.

X

Despite its geographical isolation, Australia was not immune to the concerns plaguing the medical professions in England and America. Antipodean physicians were also considering the implications of links between disease, degeneration and social instability. Like their northern hemisphere counterparts, they were to turn their attention to eugenic issues and falling birth rates in the middle classes. In 1903 the New South Wales government appointed a Royal Commission to report on the serious decline in the birth rate over the past decade. The Commission concluded that Australian women were deliberately checking procreation by artificial methods, thus 'degrading the married state from one of honour to that of "monogynous [*sic*] prostitution"'.[98] Guy L'Estrange, writing for the *Australasian Medical Gazette* in 1910, argued that the feminist movement of the past thirty years had brought about this sorry state of affairs in Britain and Australia by encouraging middle- and upper-class women to abjure 'the duties and privileges of motherhood' and seek occupations in the public sphere.[99] Quoting statistics gathered over the past twenty years or so in Britain, he commented: 'To-day all at home and abroad lament the decreasing birth rate as a proof of a moral and physical degeneration which menaces the future of the Anglo-Saxon race'. L'Estrange hypothesised that if middle- and upper-class women were allowed to continue with this course of action then, too soon, the upper classes would be displaced by a lower order.

L'Estrange declares that the declining birth rate can be divided into two types: 'wilful and non-preventable'. Both types are seen as class related. The lower classes bred but bred true to levels of degeneration and L'Estrange argues that 'Nature, if slow in her methods, is sure, and is ruthlessly exacting her penalties in the form of mental and physical changes, while even the children which come at intervals, suffer from previous interference with physical laws'.[100] The preferred breeders, that is, the middle and upper classes, were, on the other hand, too 'immured' to luxury, travel and amusement to subject themselves heedlessly to the procreative process. The feminist movement, he insists, is a primary factor in this unwanted phenomenon: 'The duties and privileges of motherhood and family life are incompatible with a busy career, and no wage or distinction can compensate a nation for the loss of its increase or the healthy upbringing of children which are born'.[101]

Concerns about birth rates and which strata of the population were breeding were being fed by the eugenics movement, which had gained such prominence in Britain in the early years of the twentieth century that by 1912 there was a dedicated chair and special laboratories housed within the academic precincts of University College, London. University College received a grant of £45,000 on Francis Galton's death in 1911, which it used to establish the Galton Eugenics Professorship. In accordance with Galton's instructions, the position was given to Karl Pearson, Galton's long-time colleague and an early student. Galton and Pearson, along with Walter F. R. Weldon, had also co-founded the eugenics journal *Biometrika* in 1902.

A writer for the *Australasian Medical Gazette* reports enthusiastically on the work being done in Britain in this new field. Readers are informed that researchers William and Catherine Whetham, those pro-active prohibitionists of 'worthless blood strains', claim in their latest published work that improvement in environment is not enough to strengthen a people: 'some process of selection is also necessary'.[102] As the new century moved into the 1910s, the right and natural guiding lights for checking indiscriminate procreation became God and patriotism. It was argued that to adhere to the 'horrible morality' of allowing the current system to continue was to ensure the creation of an inferior race: 'the nation which grasps, and acts on, the essentials of the theory of Eugenics, will assume the position of the leading State in the modern world, and consequently obtain a prepondering influence in the affairs of the Nation'.[103] Germany had evidently already been paying close attention to the business of nation building. In the four decades since the Franco-Prussian War, when population numbers were thought to be about equal, Germany had raced ahead and by 1910 it was argued that the Germans now outnumbered the French by two to one. L'Estrange underscored his concerns about the situation by arguing that, in this instance, 'The empty cradle has accomplished what it took millions of money and thousands of lives to effect 39 years ago'.[104]

At a meeting of the Medical Association of Victoria, Australia, in September 1912, a Professor Doncaster from Cambridge insisted that legislative restriction needed to be put in place to curtail the reproduction of defective individuals.[105] In October of that same year a Dr Springthorpe's report on the findings of the Eugenics Congress held in London were conveyed to the readers of the *Australasian Medical Gazette*. In quoting the Congress's statistics, Dr Springthorpe claimed that findings supported the theory that 'epileptic taints in successive generations would form a very large part of the [defective] population'.[106]

By 1907, states in North America had already begun the processes necessary to legislate for a programme of negative eugenics and it became legal to perform eugenic sterilisation in Indiana. Positive eugenics was also being enthusiastically fostered. In a precursor to reality television, it was reported in 1913 that a 'jury of doctors' in New York were compiling a fund to support the carefully selected marital union and 'mating' of two 'examples of robust humanity' to test the veracity of eugenic science. One hundred pounds each was to be given to the bride and groom 'after the eugenics marriage is performed, and the other one hundred pounds will be theirs when the first child is born.'[107] Between 1895 and 1939, nineteen of America's United States passed laws prohibiting marriage for an epileptic. According to Lennox, as of 1960, in America eugenics sterilisation laws for epilepsy existed in only nineteen states out of a possible twenty-eight carrying sterilisation laws. In relation to epilepsy, Lennox also suggested that 'intelligently applied eugenics' would immeasurably enhance a medically fantasised utopia he dubbed the 'Land of Could Be a hundred years hence'.[108]

XI

By 1910, representations of epileptic colonies as imagined, utopian (Edenic) spaces invested with dreams of firmly and benevolently controlling epileptic disorder crash head on into the reality of these facilities as lived spaces for those with seizure conditions. The medical project to develop an enlightened physiological understanding of the epilepsies, begun so promisingly by the likes of Hughlings Jackson, had, by the first half of the twentieth century, devolved into a punitive castigation of the epileptic. To invoke Judith Butler's words: the colonies were places for 'those who [were] not yet "subjects", but who [formed] the constitutive outside to the domain of the subject'.[109] And with regard to the colonies, abjection designates precisely 'those "unliveable" and "uninhabitable" zones of social life'.[110]

It becomes clear from the texts analysed above that 'the epileptic' was viewed with a mixture of anger, revulsion, fear, rejection, interest, fascination and, too rarely, compassion. The imagined utopian spaces of the colonies peopled by (theoretically) docile epileptics function as an acerbic counterpoint to Lennox's eugenically idealised 'Land of Could Be a hundred years hence' and Galton's unpublished novel *Kantsaywhere*. Both writers hypothesise eugenic utopias blessedly free of epileptic disorder. That discourses of objective knowledge about epilepsy continued to evolve with parallel narratives of superstition and loathing is also evident from the readings discussed above. The presence of the epileptic in nineteenth- and early twentieth-century western society elicited intense and systematic responses. Circulating representations of those folk who experienced epilepsy invoked prolonged and sustained campaigns from mainstream populations to create, impose and police regimes of rigorous marginalisation. What still remains unclear is precisely *why* this figure evoked such complex and powerful reactions. As I have argued above, the body of the epileptic, with its multiple and often conflicting inscriptions, had come to occupy a volatile and disruptive place in the discursive formations that constructed it as 'other'. Historical and culturally powerful images informed and resonated with these discursive constructions in ways that had disappeared back into a forgotten past.

By 1914, the epileptic remained a figure of uncertain capacities and deficits. Elusive yet compellingly and stubbornly present at the heart of cultural fears about a chaos that threatened to overwhelm ordered civilisation, this figure came to stand for the menace from within. Ironically, when the catastrophe finally struck for those nations so intent on containing the *unheimlich* presence of their degenerate and epileptic populations, it came from beyond, in the form of World War I.

Into the later decades of the twentieth century the sheer diversity of signs and symptoms ascribed to those with epilepsy conditions continued to sustain a rich field of inquiry and theorisation for biomedical research. This diversity of symptomatology appropriated all aspects of the epileptic body into the domain of pathology and medical surveillance. Once interpellated into this economy, any negotiation of an enunciative subject position is delimited by the defining discursive regime. For 'epileptics' even to attempt an alternative narrative of who they are and what they are capable of remained fraught with danger. Questioning the efficacy of certain treatment regimes only reinforced medical assumptions about the epileptic personality. The more interrogative the neurological subject, the more pathological the persona.

Of all the voices articulating epilepsy through the course of the late nineteenth century and well into the twentieth century, the one that remained systematically silenced is the voice of the subject with epilepsy. Within the discursive systems and institutional sites surveyed in this chapter, in place of the enunciative subject with epilepsy, we have the mute and irrational figure of the 'epileptic'. So it is that in the patient census carried out in the British epileptic colonies by Jones and Tillotson in 1962, 'At the expressed wish of the colonies, no patient was approached directly'.[111]

Notes

1 Donald A. MacKenzie. *Statistics in Britain 1865–1930: The Social Construction of Scientific Knowledge*. Edinburgh: Edinburgh University Press, 1981, pp. 33–34.
2 Francis Galton. *Hereditary Genius: An Inquiry into Its Laws and Consequences*. London: Macmillan, 1869, p. 347.
3 Gareth Stedman Jones. *Outcast London: A Study in the Relationship Between Classes in Victorian Society*. Oxford: Clarendon, 1971, p. 128.
4 Quoted in Jones, *Outcast London*, p. 246.
5 For more extensive discussion of these changes and the underlying conditions see: Michael W. Flinn. 'Medical services under the New Poor Law', in Derek Fraser, ed. *The New Poor Law in the Nineteenth Century*. London: Macmillan, 1976, pp. 45–66; Kathleen Jones and Aileen Tillotson. *The Adult Population of Epileptic Colonies*. London: British Epilepsy Association and International Bureau for Epilepsy, 1963; Jones, *Outcast London*.
6 Mr Chadwick quoted in Galton, *Hereditary Genius*, pp. 347–48.
7 Michel Foucault. *Discipline and Punish: The Birth of the Prison*. 1975. Trans. Alan Sheridan. London: Penguin, 1977, p. 138.
8 Jones, *Outcast London*, pp. 14–15.
9 Jones, *Outcast London*, p. 11.
10 David Armstrong. *Political Anatomy of the Body: Medical Knowledge in Britain in the Twentieth Century*. Cambridge: Cambridge University Press, 1983, p. 6.
11 Armstrong, *Political Anatomy of the Body*, p. 8.
12 William McTurk. 'The apparent increase of epilepsy among the working classes of the town of Bradford'. *Lancet*, 10 April 1859, pp. 831–37.
13 Foucault, *Discipline and Punish*, pp. 138–39.
14 Henry Maudsley. *Responsibility in Mental Disease*. London: C. Kegan Paul, 1876, p. 28.
15 Owsei Temkin. *The Falling Sickness: A History of Epilepsy from the Greeks to the Beginnings of Modern Neurology*, 2nd edition, revised. Baltimore, MD: Johns Hopkins University Press, 1971, p. 49.
16 'Hospital-workshops for the epileptic'. *British Medical Journal*, 6 February 1886, p. 262.
17 'Care of epileptics', *Lancet*, 22 December 1881, p. 1104.
18 'Employment of epileptics'. *British Medical Journal*, 22 May 1886, p. 996.
19 J. S. Risien Russell. 'The management and education of idiots and epileptics at the Bicêtre Hospital in Paris'. *British Medical Journal*, 6 June 1891, pp. 1247–48.
20 Jones and Tillotson, *The Adult Population of Epileptic Colonies*.
21 Quoted in 'Importance of shampooing and gymnastic exercises in the treatment of epilepsy'. *British Medical Journal*, 2 May 1885, p. 890.
22 'National Society for the Employment of Epileptics'. *British Medical Journal*, 7 January 1893, pp. 31–32.
23 Aldren William Turner. 'The care and management of epileptics in colonies'. *Lancet*, 26 June 1897, p. 1734.
24 Sir William H. Broadbent. 'A lecture on epilepsy'. *British Medical Journal*, 4 January 1902, p. 1.
25 'Epileptic colonies'. *Lancet*, 16 April 1892, p. 82.
26 'Farm colonies for epileptics'. *British Medical Journal*, 3 November 1894, p. 1000.
27 'Care of epileptics'. *British Medical Journal*, 30 November 1895, p. 1386.
28 Turner, 'The care and management of epileptics in colonies', p. 1734.
29 F. Norton Manning. 'The epileptic: his treatment and care'. *Australasian Medical Gazette*, 20 June 1900, p. 219.

30 'Care of epileptics'. *British Medical Journal*, p. 1386.
31 Turner, 'The care and management of epileptics in colonies', p. 1734.
32 Flinn, 'Medical services under the New Poor Law', p. 46.
33 'Gleanings from the journals'. *Australasian Medical Gazette*, March 1882, p. 85.
34 A. Hughes Bennett. 'An inquiry into the effects of the prolonged administration of the bromides in epilepsy'. *Lancet*, 17 May 1884, pp. 883–84; 24 May 1884, pp. 928–30. See p. 929.
35 Quoted in D. F. Scott. *The History of Epileptic Therapy: An Account of How Medication Was Developed*. Nashville, TN: Parthenon, 1993, p. 43.
36 Quoted in Scott, *The History of Epileptic Therapy*, p. 44.
37 Quoted in Scott, *The History of Epileptic Therapy*, p. 45.
38 Bennett, 'An inquiry', p. 884.
39 Bennett, 'An inquiry', p. 884.
40 Bennett, 'An inquiry', p. 884.
41 Bennett, 'An inquiry', p. 929.
42 William P. Spratling. *The Craig Colony for Epileptics: Bulletin of General Information*. Buffalo, NY: Matthews-Northrup, 1 October 1902, p. 19.
43 Broadbent, 'A lecture on epilepsy', p. 4.
44 Manning, 'The epileptic', p. 222.
45 Quoted in Temkin, *The Falling Sickness*, p. 299.
46 Broadbent, 'A lecture on epilepsy', p. 1.
47 Quoted in Temkin, *The Falling Sickness*, p. 65.
48 'Hospital-workshops for the epileptic', p. 262.
49 'Home for epileptics'. *Lancet*, 6 August 1892, p. 319.
50 'National Society for the Employment of Epileptics'. *Lancet*, 1 October 1892, p. 787.
51 Jones, *Outcast London*, pp. 304–5.
52 'Employment of epileptics', p. 996.
53 'Treatment of pauper imbeciles and epileptics'. *British Medical Journal*, 1 October 1898, p. 996.
54 'Labour colony for epileptics'. *Lancet*, 12 November 1892, p. 1112.
55 'Labour colony for epileptics', p. 1112.
56 Turner, 'The care and management of epileptics in colonies', p. 1735.
57 Michel Foucault. 'Body/power', 1975, in Colin Gordon, ed. *Power/Knowledge: Selected Interviews and Other Writings 1972–1977*. Trans. Colin Gordon, Leo Marshall, John Mepham and Kate Soper. New York: Harvester Wheatsheaf, 1980, pp. 61–62.
58 'Visit to the new colony for epileptics'. *British Medical Journal*, 29 December 1894, p. 1502.
59 Turner, 'The care and management of epileptics in colonies', p. 1734.
60 Quoted in Temkin, *The Falling Sickness*, p. 71.
61 Ellen Dwyer. *Homes for the Mad: Life Inside Two Nineteenth-Century Asylums*. New Brunswick, NJ: Rutgers University Press, 1987, pp. 8–9.
62 Spratling, *The Craig Colony*.
63 Quoted in William Gordon Lennox. *Epilepsy and Related Disorders*. 2 vols. London: Churchill, 1960, vol. 2, p. 981.
64 Quoted in Spratling, *The Craig Colony*, p. 11.
65 Spratling, *The Craig Colony*, pp. 11–12.
66 Unless otherwise indicated, all quotes about the Craig Colony are from Spratling, *The Craig Colony*.
67 Spratling, *The Craig Colony*, pp. 37–39.
68 Spratling, *The Craig Colony*, p. 19.

69 Lisa Cartwright. *Screening the Body: Tracing Medicine's Visual Culture.* 1995. Minneapolis, MN: University of Minnesota Press, 1997, p. 66.
70 Quoted in Daniel J. Kevles. *In the Name of Eugenics: Genetics and the Uses of Human Hereditary.* New York: Alfred A. Knopf, 1985, pp. 34–35.
71 W. C. D. Whetham and Catherine D. Whetham. *The Family and Nation.* London: Longmans, Green, 1909; W. C. D. Whetham and Catherine D. Whetham. *Hereditary and Society.* London: Longmans, Green, 1911.
72 Kevles, *In the Name of Eugenics*, p. 47.
73 Quoted in Kevles, *In the Name of Eugenics*, p. 47.
74 Quoted in Kevles, *In the Name of Eugenics*, p. 94.
75 W. R. Gowers, *A Manual of Diseases of the Nervous System.* 2nd edition. 2 vols. London: Churchill, 1893, vol. 2, p. 748.
76 Quoted in Lennox, *Epilepsy and Related Disorders*, vol. 1, p. 696.
77 Quoted in Cartwright, *Screening the Body*, p. 57 (original italics).
78 Cartwright, *Screening the Body*, p. 57.
79 Martha Banta. *Taylored Lives: Narrative Productions in the Age of Taylor, Veblen, and Ford.* Chicago, IL: University of Chicago Press, 1993, p. 3.
80 Frederick Winslow Taylor. *Scientific Management.* 1910. Westport, CT: Greenwood Press, 1972.
81 Banta, *Taylored Lives*, p. 17.
82 William P. Spratling. 'The treatment of epileptics and imbeciles'. *British Medical Journal*, 28 October 1899, p. 1228.
83 W. B. Aston. 'Abilene State School 1901–1976'. Unpublished document. Abilene, TX: Special Library, Abilene State School, 1976, no page numbers.
84 Walter J. Friedlander. *The History of Modern Epilepsy: The Beginning, 1865–1914.* London: Greenwood Press, 2001, pp. 165–66.
85 T. B. Bass. 'Epilepsy'. *Texas State Journal of Medicine*, May 1930, p. 4.
86 Aston, 'Abilene State School 1901–1976'.
87 Bass, 'Epilepsy', p. 3.
88 Hamilton Wright. 'Abilene State Hospital in top rank of its type'. *Abilene Reporter News*, 14 May 1944, no page number.
89 Manning, 'The epileptic', p. 219.
90 Turner, 'The care and management of epileptics in colonies', p. 1734.
91 Manning, 'The epileptic', p. 217.
92 Broadbent, 'A lecture on epilepsy', p. 4
93 Manning, 'The epileptic', p. 217.
94 Angel Money. 'A few remarks on epilepsy'. *Australasian Medical Gazette*, 20 July 1900, p. 287.
95 Manning, 'The epileptic', p. 219.
96 'Correspondence: London'. *Australasian Medical Gazette*, 20 June 1911, p. 350.
97 'Talbot colony for epileptics, Victoria'. *Australasian Medical Gazette*, 7 December 1912, p. 590.
98 'Declining birth-rate'. *Australasian Medical Gazette*, 21 March 1904, p. 120.
99 Guy L'Estrange. 'Eugenics in the light of higher civilisation'. *Australasian Medical Gazette*, 20 January 1910, p. 5.
100 L'Estrange, 'Eugenics in the light of higher civilisation', p. 5.
101 L'Estrange, 'Eugenics in the light of higher civilisation', p. 5.
102 Quoted in 'Eugenics'. *Australasian Medical Gazette*, 20 April 1912, p. 414.
103 'Eugenics', p. 414.
104 L'Estrange, 'Eugenics in the light of higher civilisation', p. 6.
105 'Medical Association of Victoria'. *Australasian Medical Gazette*, 14 September 1912, p. 283.

106 'Physical conditions and conduct'. *Australasian Medical Gazette*, 19 October 1912, p. 407.
107 'Medical miscellany'. *Australasian Medical Gazette*, 13 December 1913, p. 548.
108 Lennox, *Epilepsy and Related Disorders*, vol. 1, p. 36.
109 Judith Butler. *Bodies That Matter: On the Discursive Limits of 'Sex'*. New York: Routledge, 1993, p. 3.
110 Butler, *Bodies That Matter*, p. 2.
111 Jones and Tillotson, *The Adult Population of Epileptic Colonies*, p. 10.

CHAPTER 5

Because you're 'you know. That way'

I am an electrical impulse. I discharge at random across a synapse, at the threshold of a seizure. Grand mal. Idiopathic. Without warning. She cries out. *I dance*. She waves her arms about, falls. Her pupils dilate, teeth bite into the tongue. *I am dancing*. Her face is the blue of cyanide. *I rampage*. Her muscles contract. She convulses. Saliva mixed with blood dribbles from her mouth. She has lost consciousness.
(Susan Hawthorne, *The Falling Woman*, 1992, original italics)

Getting to know you,
Getting to know all about you.
Getting to know you,
Getting to know what to say....
(Richard Rodgers and Oscar Hammerstein, 'Getting to know you', 1951)

I

Another century; other cities; other mediums; new technologies. Well into the twentieth century the convulsive figure given literary presence by Charles Dickens, Fyodor Dostoevsky, Thomas Hardy and Robert Louis Stevenson continued to thrive in literature. Visual representations of the seizure-prone body migrate from medical photographic and film projects to mainstream cinema. Films as diverse as *The Big Sleep*, *The Andromeda Strain*, *Romper Stomper* and *Deceiver*, as well as television shows such as *American Gothic* and *The X Files*, all draw upon the metaphorical capital of the epileptic or convulsing body to evoke the threat of chaos lurking beneath a patina of late twentieth-century order.

Twentieth-century representations of the female 'epileptic' owed more to Lucette Le Sueur than to Guster. Carmen Sternwood, the 'nymphomaniac' younger sister of Vivien in Raymond Chandler's novel *The Big Sleep*, is volatile and seductive.[1] Unlike her nineteenth-century predecessor, however, she is also figured lethal. The representation of Carmen Sternwood's seizure condition in both Chandler's text and Howard Hawks' 1946 film is used as the barely speakable explanation for her socially transgressive behaviour and a metaphor for her sexual promiscuity: she is a fallen woman who falls. For the most part, representations of males with epilepsy or seizure conditions are drawn from the palette that produced Monks and Smerdyakov. Myshkin has no direct descendant as such in the twentieth-century circuit of culture, but this style of representation nonetheless spawns some interesting possibilities. More often than not, though, epilepsy in mainstream literature, cinema and television is represented as no more than spectacle: background to the main action or a cinematic version of the textual catalyses discussed in Chapter 3 in relation to Dickens' deployment of the fit in *Chuzzlewit*, *Curiosity Shop* and *David Copperfield*.

By the latter decades of the nineteenth century, medical photography had become an increasingly popular medium for recording bodily difference. Cesare Lombroso was busily photographing epileptic and criminal 'types'. In 1889 Jean-Martin Charcot, in collaboration with Paul Richer, Gilles de la Tourette and Albert Londe, published *Nouvelle iconographie de la Salpêtrière* in a four-volume set. Photographic images and detailed drawings of convulsing bodies collected from his clinical practice at La Salpêtrière and his famous Tuesday lectures were reproduced in all four volumes. However, and despite best efforts to capture the essence of epileptic disorder visually, the images produced by Lombroso and Charcot *et al.* were unsatisfyingly flat and devoid of the energy associated with seizure.

In 1905 William Spratling gave permission for Walter Chase, a Boston neurologist, to make a series of cinematic films – the 'Epilepsy Biographs' – of his charges at the Craig epileptic colony. Capturing moving images of the defining signifier of epilepsy, the seizure, was by no means simple: the colony residents tended to seize out of camera range, either as they went about their daily tasks or at night, when asleep. It was fairly quickly understood by Spratling and Chase that more control was required if the project was to succeed. Chase noted:

> Realizing that it was impossible to set up the camera after the seizure had commenced, we had some one hundred and twenty-five male patients from the infirmary assembled in a convenient spot out of doors on a warm summer day. The clothes were removed and the patients covered

> with blankets, so that, a seizure occurring, the blanket could be readily dropped and the subject, within a very few seconds, placed in the range of the camera.[2]

Although Chase's method lacked any concern for the dignity of the seizing individual (who was presumably also being observed by 124 of his fellow colonists as he writhed naked on the ground), Lisa Cartwright reveals deeper causes of concern about some of these early visual projects. In discussing the connections between Chase's work and that of Francis X. Dercum, another neurologist filming seizures around the same time, she notes that Dercum artificially stimulated or triggered seizures in his test subjects. In a meeting where Chase showed his Craig colony films, Dercum observed: 'The convulsions introduced artificially were as genuine as any form of convulsive movement and there was no simulation on the part of the subject'.[3] This visual fascination with the seizure, whether medically induced or spontaneous, remains germane to medical imaging technologies and will be discussed in detail below.

By the middle of the twentieth century, however, beliefs that a hidden tendency to epileptic disorder could be somehow deciphered from the external surfaces of the body had been all but abandoned. The project to identify what epilepsy looked like in the absence of seizures had taken a new direction and another system of representation entered into the circuit of culture. With the advent of electroencephalographic (EEG) technology, neurologists had gained access to the electrical activity of the living brain. EEG readout tapes inscribed with the characteristic spike/wave patterns denoting paroxysmal brain activity became the most recent index by which physicians were trying to detect epilepsy disorder 'at a glance'. Researchers could now see and record what John Hughlings Jackson and William Gowers had only been able to hypothesise about. Nevertheless, a precise and reproducible measurement that would demarcate healthy brain function from the neuronal incontinence associated with the epilepsies had yet to be obtained.

Rather than metaphors of exoticism, class, deviance and degeneration, twentieth-century medical textual productions of epilepsy began to draw on metaphors of battle and militaristic imagery. In this representational economy, physicians – like Christ's apostles – are pitted against an evil adversary. So it is that the journal *Epilepsia* is published by the International League *Against* Epilepsy (italics added). American neurologist William Lennox, a past president of this association, is credited with the title of 'The Father of the Fight Against Epilepsy' by one of his obituarists. Frederic A. Gibbs points out that Lennox had remained confident that 'in the end all organisations working against epilepsy would co-ordinate their attack on the common enemy'.[4] In a medical culture where the historical tendency has been to conflate epilepsy with those affected by the condition, it is a problematic turn of phrase. Lennox argued that, eventually, in any affluent society, 'a way should be found to finance the war against man's ancient enemy, "the falling sickness"'.[5] Medications developed to treat the disorder in the late twentieth century are referred to as 'anti-epileptic'.

Only words and images, I know, but in the cultural circuit being explored here in order to better understand twenty-first-century medical stories of epilepsy and 'the epileptic', words and images are crucially important: they have material consequences.

II

As part of the 'war against man's ancient enemy', activating techniques to establish an epileptic threshold in the human brain became part of modern neurology's arsenal. Activation of epilepsy potential (also called provocative diagnosis) was intended to arouse those 'dormant abnormalities' not usually detectable with already-available diagnostic methods.[6] The premise underlying the practice is that in order to diagnose epilepsy, researchers and diagnosticians have to sometimes chemically induce or otherwise activate visible evidence: that is, the seizure. It was argued that effective treatment required decisive diagnosis, a view that was further reinforced by invoking the legal and social implications generated by the condition. Nevertheless, some researchers disputed the overall usefulness of this diagnostic methodology, arguing that it was an imprecise way of fixing an epileptic threshold and could, in fact, induce clinical seizures not of the type of the patient's habitual symptomatology.[7] These reservations notwithstanding, by the late twentieth century, activation methods had become an accepted diagnostic tool.[8]

In twentieth-century medical culture, so-called mild methods of activation entailed uncovering or detecting signs of neurological abnormality usually masked by conscious brain activity. It was argued that 'For epileptics, the hidden abnormal rhythms tend to expose themselves during sleep, and seizure discharges may be observed that are not present when the person is awake'.[9] Consequently, patients' brain waves were sometimes recorded after they had been given a short-acting barbiturate. Stimulating the brain to a condition of mild stress by getting patients to hyperventilate or by exposing them to an intermittent flashing light (photic stimulation) was also part of this mild method and had actually been standard diagnostic procedure since ancient times: versions of these methods were deployed by the ancients to detect epilepsy in newly purchased slaves.

From around 1935, physicians and researchers had begun to incorporate more drastic activation methods into this diagnostic regime. Researchers had found that intravenous injection of certain chemicals such as Metrazol could actually precipitate convulsive seizures. By 1956 Megimide was introduced into neurological diagnostic practice. The 1970s saw procaine and Megimide–pentothal also being used. While the procedures based on what Lennox termed the gentle stimulants (sleep, hyperventilation, light) induced dysrhythmia and excited neuronal activity, these latter means incurred significant discomfort and sometimes generalised seizures for the patient. By 1960 activation techniques usually comprised a combination of mild methods and the infinitely more problematic chemical provocations. Crudely put: while medical technology still could not provide a cure for epilepsy, 'spiking' the brain now yielded the means for a medically controlled production of signs and symptoms.

Focus on the effectiveness of activating methods to provoke or stimulate the signs and symptoms of the epilepsies wrought some complex changes in the medical gaze. Increasingly, its attention was held by the effectiveness of the diagnostic tools to stimulate electronically recordable changes to brain wave patterns and provoke observable pathological behaviours, rather than by the consequences that these methods might have for the immediate and long-term health of the individual. The technologies of epilepsy had begun to supersede patients' experiences of their symptomatology.

We can see some of the consequences of this radical change to the medical gaze in Henri Gastaut's 1978 recantation of his theory of ecstatic aura developed from Dostoevsky's writings, because he had seen no clinical evidence (subjective or otherwise) to support the author's account of what epilepsy felt like. The privileged place that technological proof of subjective experience has in the medical model is also evident in wider debates about Dostoevsky's accounts of his pleasurable pre-seizure states. In 1980 F. Cirignotta *et al.* published a case history which cited polygraphic proof of ecstatic aura.[10] In 1983 P. H. A. Voskuil[11] used Cirignotta's evidence to revisit Dostoevsky's case and in 1984, as a result of these publications, Gastaut published his acceptance that Dostoevsky's account of his ecstatic states indeed had veracity.[12] As David Armstrong has argued, 'In this sense the reality of the body is only established by the observing eye that reads it'.[13] The debate raises important questions about the relation between medical and personal interpretations of subjective experience: Reen Carter's recantation of her spirituality in favour of a medical story about diagnosis and treatment (see Introduction) is a case in point.

This redirection of medical focus is evident in a case report written up by M. Fischer-Williams, R. G. Bickford and J. P. Whisnant, and published in the journal *Epilepsia* in 1964. The case report is of an EEG series conducted on a forty-one-year-old woman undergoing epilepsy activation. At various times during the course of the testing, which was also recorded on film, the woman repeatedly expresses apprehension about the procedure and feelings of physical discomfort. When the frequency of the photic stimulation is increased to fifteen flashes per second, causing a 'generalized shaking', she asks her physicians to 'stop it' and tries to shield her eyes from the flashing light. Indeed, her physicians note that she 'repeatedly shouted "Stop it"'.[14] Testing persists until finally a seizure discharge is activated. The activated seizure discharge lasts sixteen minutes and leaves the woman feeling 'confused, disoriented, and amnesic for several hours'.[15] The physicians observe that 'a prolonged seizure was induced by photic stimulation. Rhythmic activity began in the right occipital region and spread to the right parietal and Sylvian areas and, after 2 to 3 minutes, to the left occipital and parietal regions'.[16] The EEG series was resumed the next day.

Soon after testing resumes in the following session, Fischer-Williams *et al.* note that 'a focal seizure began in the left occipital region that was in many ways the mirror image of the first one'.[17] They include at this point in the case study a series of EEG readouts recorded as the woman was asked such questions as 'What are you wearing?' They also include EEG readouts annotated with the woman's comments: '"Oh boy!" Looks scared. "I'm sorry I can't talk to you"' and '"I see all kinds of peculiar things"'. They comment:

> The patient turned her head away and was distressed by the light. In her own words, 'It bothers me', and, in the film that was made simultaneously, her behaviour appeared neurotic in that she laughed irrelevantly, tried to avoid photic stimulation, and appeared to be seeking undue attention.[18]

As a caption on Figure 3 in their paper, which depicts segments of the EEG records for this session, the physicians note that 'After initial photic stimulation, the seizure was self-perpetuating'.

In subsequent sessions the patient again expresses her discomfort and distress with phrases such as 'I don't like this'[19] (interpreted as 'petulance' by the doctors) and 'Oh, dear God',[20] as electrical seizure activity becomes generalised. The film of the fifth session shows that the woman draws the doctors' attention to a predicament with her eyes: they have deviated uncontrollably to the right. 'She said in a tone of exasperation "Oh, I hate this thing"'.[21] Continued activation of electrical discharge prevents her from elaborating on the situation but this does not deter her physicians from speaking for her: 'we may think that her phrase if completed would likely have been "I can't alter the direction of my gaze"'.[22] The woman's reluctance to subject herself to those conditions which precipitated the seizure episodes in previous sessions is glossed in the Fischer-Williams report as mere corollary to the EEG recording. At one stage a readout of the woman's EEG, recorded while she was making one of these statements, is inscribed with the comment 'Behaviour may seem neurotic'.

The privileged relationship in this case study is between the tools of diagnosis and the diagnosticians, while the woman's subjective responses to the events are treated as extraneous to the job at hand. The woman has become erased from the physician–patient–symptom equation: the patient *is* her symptomatology. No more. No less. The medical gaze remains fixated on the ways that various technologies stimulate electrical discharge in the brain. There is also a fascination with the seizure and the range of sensory and perceptual disturbances that can be produced via these technologies. Because the woman's expressions of distress, fear and discomfort are consistently interpreted as further evidence for diagnosis, they are evacuated of any compelling valency: a condition of research practice that allows the observing doctors to ignore any relationship between her agitation and their testing procedures. This, despite the fact that she repeatedly voices concern that the activation methods are making her feel nauseated, acutely ill and as though she is about to lose control of her bowels. There is a somewhat cursory acknowledgement by her physicians that they should 'probably' accept the explanation of fear for her resistant behaviour, 'since in the seizure of the day before ... she described the things she saw as "horrible"'.[23] They do not act on this acknowledgement.

Like Mr P— prior to Joseph Williams' intervention (Chapter 1) and Hughes Bennett's 'epileptic' (Chapter 4), the well-being of the woman at the centre of the medical gaze in the case reported by Fischer-Williams *et al.* is obscured by an assumption of essentialised epileptic abjectness. Hughes Bennett, while acknowledging the toxic side-effects of long-term or excessive bromide use on the healthy body, was able to dismiss these consequences for the epileptic body precisely because it was, after all, already diseased.[24] The Fischer-Williams team pathologise their patient's dis-ease as neurotic and attention seeking, merely part of her epileptic symptomatology. Integral to both assumptions is an implicit belief that somehow the essential state of being for those with a cerebral paroxysmal condition is such that any negative change wrought by intervention figured as therapeutic is surely 'better than to have epilepsy'.[25] The epileptic, if not already, will be eventually and hopelessly degraded by the disorder. Ironically, this negative view of convulsion is radically refigured by electroconvulsive therapy, in which medically controlled seizure episodes are used as therapy for persistent forms of depression resistant to other forms of therapeutic intervention. This recuperation of bodily abjection for therapeutic efficacy seems to beg the question about the relationships between seizure, control, loss of control and who 'can' control.

The woman's requests to the Fischer-Williams team for the process to be stopped, and her statements about feelings of physical and psychological discomfort resulting from the procedures, are ignored because her physicians adhere to the same paradigmatic frameworks as their nineteenth-century predecessors. In 1964 as in 1884, medicine's fight 'against epilepsy' is so rhetorically ennobled that any cost is sufficient to the victory. These twentieth-century physicians remain caught in a matrix of signification that prevents them from seeing beyond an adversarial response to the disorder. The seizure – the primary signifier of diagnosis – must be flushed into the open and eradicated from the affected body as proof positive of medical effectiveness. By the turn of the century and into the 2000s, technology placed many neurologists in a predicament not dissimilar to the one experienced by Fischer-Williams' patient: they appear incapable of altering the direction of their (medical) gaze. They see an 'epileptic' who is globally pathologised. From this perspective, all experience is somehow subjugated to and symptomatic of the greater disorder and therefore beyond the physician's responsibility; but not beyond diagnostic purview. Secondly, epilepsy has been historically figured as such a tenacious 'evil' that any and all measures to combat it are permissible. In this paradigm, the lived body of the individual with a cerebral paroxysmal disorder is reduced to the desensitised field of battle.

While not being able to prevent their patient from seizing, the medical technology deployed by the Fischer-Williams research team afforded other means of control. Adjustments to technological stimuli allowed them to dictate the woman's bodily movements, functions and perceptual world. At least within the context of the EEG series. The *Epilepsia* case history not only includes EEG records of the woman's activated seizures, but also notes her 'mumbling', 'jargon dysphasia', visual hallucinations, attempts to avoid photic stimulation (and, by inference, further seizures), expressions of distress, articulations of fear, groans and anger at the continued imposed loss of self-control.

Their focus on the performativity of disorder and the electronic text that inscribed it with meaning – at least from a medical perspective – rather than the consequences for the patient resonates with Charcot's visual fetishisation of the convulsive female body *in extremis*. Their recorded comments on her verbal behaviours are reminiscent of the French physician's observations about one of his female patient's verbal behaviours in a medically stimulated convulsive episode: 'You could say it is a lot of noise over nothing'.[26]

Many of Charcot's British and North American counterparts felt that the physician's methods were hysterogenic: that is, they caused the very disorder that Charcot purported to diagnose, record and theorise about. By the latter part of the twentieth century, with the advent of activation methods, British and North American researchers had themselves become epileptogenic: in Michel Foucault's words, they were not only producing through knowledge 'the disease "in its truth"' (see Chapter 2), but in ignorance were too often becoming the agents of propagation and dissemination.

After an initial diagnosis had already been secured by the first session of the EEG study, we might ask *why* the Fischer-Williams team continued to repeat the procedure five times. What exactly was the medical gaze striving to see and understand? Was there knowledge relevant to the woman's future wellness to be obtained by the repeated activation sessions? If so, this is not suggested by the team's conclusions, which affirm the diagnosis made on the basis of information recorded in the first session. That being the case, did the medical project cross a line into scopic fascination with its own creation? Read against the physicians' accompanying commentary, the woman's increased loss of bodily control in the face of activation testing equates with the increased control of the diagnosticians over her (epileptic) body. Her recorded 'eyelid flutters', incontinent verbal ejaculations, fearfulness and 'petulance' fetishise her body in a medically orchestrated symphony of unveiled disorder. What might *her* gaze have seen if she could have wrenched her eyes forward and turned them on her physicians?

In the thirteen years after the EEG series, the woman continued to have occasional seizure episodes. It is worth noting that only 'mild methods' of activation were used in this series. Fischer-Williams' patient was not subjected to chemical activation. In salient ways, my experience of provocative diagnosis in 1972 is not dissimilar to the one sketched above. However, I was subjected to a combination of 'mild methods' and chemical activation. A *grand mal* seizure episode – the first I had ever experienced – was successfully provoked on day two of the series. It took a while, but the medical compulsion to 'see' what previously had only been hypothesised was finally satisfied when, with the injection of an activating chemical followed by extensive photic stimulation, I finally seized at fourteen flashes per second. The process was repeated over the next three consecutive days, with similar success. Once 'outed' by that first medically induced *grand mal* seizure, and despite an increasingly complex medication regime, I continued to seize with regularity and gusto for the next twenty years. These two decades included prolonged episodes of *status epilepticus*. Since ceasing the medication regime in 1990, I have not experienced a *grand mal* seizure. Through the closing decades of the twentieth century, activation procedures remained part of standard diagnostic practice and usually comprised a combination of the gentle methods described above and chemical stimulation.

III

Pharmaceutical responses to the epilepsies by the mid twentieth century were also being reviewed and here, again, there is a sense of heroic response coupled with pioneering zeal. Donald Scott writes that 'When we attempt to clarify the nature of the discovery of anti-epileptic [medication], we enter an area more akin to the casino than the chemistry laboratory'.[27] According to Scott, the 'casino factor' in the development of epilepsy drug regimes entails elements of 'chance, luck and serendipity'.[28] With no sense of irony he notes that 'chance' is derived from the old French *cadare*, meaning 'to fall'. In following Scott's lead and consulting my own dictionary on the matter, I found that chance might also tell a sorrier tale for those on the receiving end of pharmaceutical research's 'luck'. 'Chance: the absence of design or assignable cause; the course of events regarded as power; a casual or fortuitous circumstance; an unfortunate event, mishap, mischance; = accident'.[29] Julia Kristeva notes that '*cadere*, to fall' also refers to 'cadaver': 'The corpse … that which has irremediably come a cropper, is cesspool, and death; it upsets even more violently the one who confronts it as fragile and fallacious chance'.[30] Luck, so Scott informs the reader, is from the German meaning prosperity, and is always positive, while 'serendipity' is a word coined by Sir Horace Walpole in 1754 to describe the fortunate Princes of Serendip, who were 'always making discoveries by accident and sagacity, of things they were not in quest of'.[31]

Chance, luck and serendipity. Scott's rather whimsical imagery of the casino evokes ideas of gambling, of risk taking; he in fact footnotes the phrase 'casino factor' to a book called *Easy Money: Inside the Gambler's*

Mind. It is a rather unfortunate connection, given the historical view in western medicine that to be beset by any form of cerebral paroxysmal condition is disastrous, and in the twentieth century warranted the most vigilant pharmaceutical response. Moreover, late twentieth-century medical orthodoxy held that for those with epilepsy not to take medication was to be negligent in the care of the self. This pressure to medicate (regardless of side-effects) is further complicated by the legal and social prohibitions still attached to an epileptic identity category in the twenty-first century. In this light, easy money might also refer to the development and marketing of anti-epileptic drugs for pharmaceutical companies. The gambling image is suggestive, of course, of winning and losing. Scott's analogy claims good fortune for medical technology's (and the pharmaceutical industry's) battle to control epileptic disorder, yet nevertheless remains silent about the costs of the gamble. Or, indeed, who bears the losses.

Lennox, in relating the costs of trying to achieve complete control of inter-seizure muscle spasms for a thirty-seven-year-old male patient (Merle McBride) who had already attained control of convulsions through the use of Dilantin, writes that after Phenurone was added to the medication regime the patient succumbed to liver toxicity and died. In the Kristeva sense, he was overtaken by chance – *cadere*. In words reminiscent of Henry Maudsley's more sentimental moments, Lennox concludes:

> Merle was cheerful and confident to the end. His parents expressed only gratitude for efforts spent in their son's behalf, their chief desire that his life, death, and the autopsy results should benefit others. His unswerving determination to fit himself for work against epilepsy was transferred to his devoted wife. Working at the time as our secretary, she put herself through college and a school of social work and now promises to accomplish more for the cause than Merle ever could have.
>
> Who will strike a balance between good and ill, between good health and illness? Was Merle's travail and death ordained for the glory of epilepsy? An experience such as this places on the physician the responsibility of keeping faith with persons who trust him even in the face of disaster and who work with him towards the end they all desire, the end of epilepsy.[32]

Across a time span of some nine decades, Lennox perpetuates Maudsley's narrative impulses and textually positions himself as being engaged in a morally elevated quest to rescue the epileptic from a metaphorical paroxysmal pit.

This rhetorical impulse allows Lennox to depict Merle McBride as a martyr to the cause. He continues his commemoration of the young man with the words of Robert Browning:

> One who never turned his back but marched breast forward,
> Never doubted clouds would break,
> Never dreamed, though right were worsted, wrong would triumph,
> Held we fall to rise, are baffled to fight better,
> Sleep to wake.[33]

Of course, Merle McBride may well have been so incapacitated by his muscle spasms that he thought the gamble, and the risk it entailed, was well worth his while. Unfortunately, his voice is absent from the recorded history of his illness. We have only his treating physician's perspective and, in the context of Lennox's militaristic imagery, Merle McBride has been reduced to the status of regrettable, but necessary, collateral damage in a war that medicine is yet to win.

By 1987 the British researcher Christopher Ounsted was claiming: 'In 1948, and for decades afterwards, the world of epileptology was wholly dominated by medical myths'.[34] Though seemingly grounded in medical science, many of these 'myths', according to Ounsted, could not be critically tested. Ounsted's observation regarding the 'tautological absurdities'[35] troubling medical models of epilepsy lends itself to further examination. It hinges on two crucial questions: what is epilepsy, and what is cerebral paroxysm? In other words, when does the defining marker of epilepsy – the seizure – point to an epilepsy condition and when is it the visible manifestation of some other underlying condition or pathology? Ounsted's remark concerns idiopathic epilepsy, which is not readily traceable to a known or specific pathogenic source. His claim for tautological absurdity seems attached to the view that to suggest that epilepsy *is* idiopathic – that is, not consequent on or symptomatic of another disease – is to ignore the fact that epilepsy can be its own distinct attribution. If we accept, though, that not all instances of cerebral paroxysm indicate an underlying pathology or disease process, and that not all seized states involve the debilitation and potentially dangerous consequences of a *grand mal* episode, it becomes possible to extend thinking beyond the current equation between some epilepsy syndromes, 'disease' and therapeutic intervention.

In a biographical study spanning the years 1948 to 1986, Ounsted and his team tested the 'tautological absurdities' that they identified as dominating modern epileptology. For all the children included in their study, EEG evidence of temporal lobe activity had to have been obtained. They insisted that 'This was the *sine qua non* of diagnosis'.

> In many children the first electroencephalographic examination showed *no abnormality*, but these children were repeatedly studied (many of them having more than 10 records) until *satisfactory* EEG support for

> the clinical diagnosis had been obtained. Activating methods were used when indicated, including sleep records, Megimide–Pentothal activation records and other activating techniques.[36]

If the brain is free of recurring excessive neuronal discharge until such time that recurring excessive neuronal discharge is medically activated, where is disorder located? Is neurological disorder in this instance endemic to the brain or the technological procedures and chemicals that seize the brain for EEG validation? The reasoning of Ounsted and his team – that to clinically diagnose epilepsy, one has to artificially produce the neuronal conditions denoting epilepsy – while keeping faith with stated research protocols, would appear to reproduce a tautological absurdity of the type that the team had been so anxious to dispel from epileptology.

As the twentieth century progressed, it became increasingly apparent that while some forms of epilepsy were well served by advances in medical technology, pharmaceutical developments and increased medical knowledge about brain function, other forms, particularly those paroxysmal conditions emanating from the limbic system and temporal lobes (those paroxysmal episodes now called partial seizures, complex partial seizures or temporal–limbic syndrome), had not been dealt with as efficaciously. This may be due, at least in part, to the fact that these forms of the condition often entail perceptual changes rather than generalised seizure episodes. These psychic epilepsies deflect comprehensive classification within either neurological or psychiatric diagnostic paradigms. A lack of clarity in categorisation, in turn, creates medical uncertainty as to the most effective forms of therapeutic response. As a consequence, there is a nascent if uncomfortable acknowledgement by some medical researchers that not only are those with temporal–limbic or temporal lobe syndromes not necessarily helped by orthodox medical therapies currently in use, but they may, in fact, be harmed by them.

In their study, Ounsted and his team point out that 'A single drug is both a convulsant and an anticonvulsant'. Further to this observation they reveal:

> In the present series, as in our wider experience, we *commonly* found that some children with habitual epilepsy were cured when we *withdrew* their drugs. Their *clean* brains then were free to inhibit seizures and their epilepsy troubled them no longer. For patients in our group A, *withdrawal of drugs may be life-saving*.[37]

Given these observations, the diagnostic practice of artificially provoking or chemically stimulating seizure activity where none had hitherto been discernible appears not to be in these children's best interests: as the researchers' findings suggest, once activated, treatment to control this activity is imprecise and sometimes epileptogenic. Taking direction from Ounsted's claim and leaving aside, for the moment, the very real medical emergency presented by *status epilepticus,* I again pose the question: are all cerebral paroxysmal conditions necessarily deleterious to health and long-term well-being, as current medical models of epilepsy would suggest?

In the late 1980s, medical writings on the subject of seizure and 'the epileptic' were again hedging towards clinically reductive representations reminiscent of the late nineteenth century. The impulse was to recuperate a silenced, deviant subject position for the epileptic. M.-Marsel Mesulam cites data from experiments on rhesus monkeys to reinforce his arguments for an epileptic social and intellectual pathology. The monkeys evidently had their responses to certain stimuli measured and interpreted after bilateral alterations to the amygdala and surrounding temporopolar cortex. Three 'dramatic' behavioural changes were noted: the animals exhibited 'incessant and inappropriate mouthing of inedible objects, attempts to copulate with animals of the same sex and even inanimate objects, and an uncharacteristic friendliness to human beings'.[38] I am tempted to ask of this last deviation, will they (the monkeys) never learn? As Mesulam notes, while these behaviours represent part of a 'normal' repertoire for the animals, 'they are no longer directed to the proper extrapersonal target'.[39]

From this model of an artificially provoked deviance in monkeys, Mesulam extends discussion to a human subject with epilepsy who manifests a variety of physical and psychical phenomena such as staring, lip smacking, hallucinations and sudden and unprovoked aggression, which can sometimes 'have major criminal consequences'.[40] In citing other 'anecdotal observations and quantitative studies', he informs the reader of another human subject who is prone to acting as though 'the entire world were saturated with intense emotional significance'.[41] Threading the final strand in the barbed-wired rhetoric of containment Mesulam goes on to write of his human patients:

> They may lack a sense of humor, become overly serious and brooding, develop excessive philosophical interests, an obsessive hyperreligiosity, and a curious tendency to write excessively. Many show difficulty in getting to the point during conversation, become lost in interminable detail, and display a characteristic circumstantiality of thought patterns.... The circumstantiality, obsessive rumination, humorlessness, and intense emotionality lead to a rather striking style of interpersonal interaction that has been described as interpersonal viscosity.[42]

The observations are 'uncannily' evocative of those recorded by his predecessors in late nineteenth-century editions of the *Lancet, British Medical Journal* and *Australasian Medical Gazette*.

Mesulam remains silent on whether or not these humourless, intensely emotional humans are currently adhering to a medication regime for the condition and, if so, what part the medications might play in this fragmentation and dulling of persona and impairment of intellectual function. Of the eighteen substances listed for the treatment of epilepsy syndromes in the 1988 abridged edition of *MIMS* (the year Mesulam publishes his observations), fourteen have listed among their adverse effects a range of functional and psychological disruptions, including drowsiness, ataxia, fatigue, emotional lability, disturbances to memory, depression, impaired mental acuity, behavioural disturbances, personality changes and psychiatric disturbances. One merely carries the advice 'complex' in the section on adverse reactions and, along with twelve of the listings which cite some of the adverse psychological and physiological side-effects of the substances, directs the reader to the *MIMS* annual for a more comprehensive account of these side-effects.[43]

In May 1980 Ian Curtis, poet and lead singer with the British band Joy Division, committed suicide at the age of twenty-three. Reportage on his death and Deborah Curtis's memoir describe the complex mix of professional and personal pressures bearing on his life leading up to the time of his demise. Sources also describe the significant side-effects he was experiencing from the medication regime prescribed to control his epilepsy seizures. These side-effects included a range of the functional and psychological disruptions sketched above. The medication regime, though, failed to control his seizures. Those close to the singer comment on his mood swings and his struggles to function beyond the constraints of his medication. It is impossible to say how much of Curtis's self-destructive despair was due to his personality and youth, how much due to the circumstances of his life. Certainly the combination of medications he was taking would have made coping with these circumstances extraordinarily difficult.

His suicide resonates with the death of Arthur Myers (Chapter 3) in that, a century apart, both men found themselves caught in a matrix of signification and pharmaceutical constraints that configured epilepsy in complex ways. We cannot but help return to the questions posed in relation to Myers' death: for Curtis, was the 'tragic' – and lethal – 'flaw' that caused his death the erratically discharging lesion in his brain or the problematic brew of medication that quelled his sense of self? It would seem that to answer via either of these options would be to reduce Curtis to the sum total of his symptomatology and medication regime, a point I return to below. For the moment, it is sufficient to point out that Ounsted claims that as late as 1987 there was no single drug used in the treatment of epilepsy 'whose mode of action is understood'.[44] To echo Scott, for Curtis and others experiencing epilepsy at the close of the twentieth century, it was still a case of chance, luck and serendipity.

Expressing reservations about the potential benefits of surgical intervention for some forms of epilepsy, Joel Reiter argued in 1995 that late twentieth-century neurology was still 'a long way from knowing what actually causes epilepsy' and any possible benefits offered by this sort of treatment needed to be weighed carefully against risks to faculties such as speech, memory and personality.[45] Reiter also pointed out that while there is no doubt that some anticonvulsant drug regimes are beneficial for some patients in controlling some seizure states, most of these drugs were discovered through trial-and-error pharmaceutical research, a fact that might go some way in explaining 'why they have so many serious side effects'.[46] Inadvertently, Reiter compounds the gambling motif appropriated by Scott with his advice to women planning a pregnancy that the risk of birth defects from anticonvulsants is probably less than six per cent and 'the risk of serious birth defects is less than 2 percent. Your odds of having a healthy child are very good.'[47]

Reiter confesses that 'In prescribing antiepileptic drugs I feel as if I am walking a tightrope between stopping seizures and producing side effects'.[48] When pressing the need for accurate and safe diagnostic testing he points out that 'less than ten percent of adults with epilepsy have tumors, blood vessel anomalies, or other abnormalities on their brain scans' and celebrates the fact that after an EEG recording, computerised tomography (CT) scan and magnetic resonance imaging (MRI) scan, he can usually reassure patients that in fact their brain structure falls well within normal ranges.[49]

The changes in medical approaches to epilepsy brought about by the technological developments and medical epilepsy narratives of the 1960s, '70s and '80s had consequences for the doctor–patient relationship beyond the environs of the diagnostic process. By the 1990s neuroscientists were becoming increasingly confident in their knowledge of what the electrical discharges denoting epilepsy activity looked like via EEG records and imaging technology. Moreover, treating physicians had recourse to a fairly extensive pharmacy of anticonvulsant drugs. If drug therapy failed, various surgical options were now also available to try to minimise the negative effects of epilepsy conditions for the patient and management problems for physicians. They had come to understand from the narrative history of their profession that the physician's duty was to somehow win out over this most stubborn and disturbing of disorders. These advances, however, did not always equate with increased control.

IV

In her 1997 book *The Spirit Catches You and You Fall Down: A Hmong Child, Her American Doctors, and the Clash of Two Cultures,* Anne Fadiman examines cross-cultural understandings of epilepsy and the consequences for all those involved in the case of Lia Lee, a Hmong child with epilepsy living in the United States.[50] I am not going to cover the same ground here: Fadiman presents a comprehensive account of the cross-cultural complexities that confronted both Lia Lee's physicians and her family. Rather, here I briefly examine the matrix of signification that these physicians were caught up in: the kinds of stories that shaped their medical identity; the kinds of stories they could tell, given the systems of representation they had available to them, about what they did and why they did it in relationship to epilepsy.

Lia Lee first came to the attention of the medical profession because of her seizures in 1982. She was three months old. Over the next four years of encounters between Lia and her medical carers at the Community Medical Center in Merced, California, a climate of distrust between the medical team and Lia's family develops apace with the child's management problems. Part of this mutual disaffection arises from different cultural understandings of what it means to have epilepsy. The Lee family, although unhappy that their child is suffering from the disorder and cognisant of the fact that she could die as a result of a seizure, do not adhere to a belief system that figures epilepsy as an enemy to be bested. They view it as a condition of life. To be sure, a condition that requires interventions that will hopefully alleviate (if not cure) the suffering of the affected individual, but not a condition that demands control at further cost to the quality of life for that individual.

This understanding and acceptance of their child's condition diametrically opposes the prevailing medical view. One of Lia's doctors observes that 'It was very foreign to me that [the Lees] had the ability to stand firm in the face of expert opinion' about their daughter's ongoing management.[51] His comment is sparked by the family querying the relationship between some of the treatments that Lia was receiving from the medical profession and the negative side-effects they were observing in her at home. He added:

> And the other thing that was different between them and me was that they seemed to accept things that to me were major catastrophes as part of the normal flow of life.... I felt a tremendous responsibility to stop the seizures and to make sure another one never happened again, and they felt more like these things happen, you know, not everything is in our control, and not every thing is in your control.[52]

The anxiety of Lia's treating health care professionals was exponential with the intractability of the child's seizure condition. It finally reaches a pitch of displaced and unremitting antipathy focused on the parent's racial and cultural differences.

Eventually, the battle fought over Lia's seizing body becomes as much about getting her parents to comply with a position demanded of them by the physicians at Merced as it does about controlling her seizures. The anxiety and antipathy felt by the paediatric physician in charge of her case was such that he had Lia removed, via the court system, from the care of her parents. At his behest, Lia was placed in an Anglo-American foster home. His reasons for doing this had nothing to do with the quality of parental care as such – there was no question that Lia's parents spent considerable time and energies on trying to maintain her general well-being. The issue at stake was their ongoing reservations about medical responses to Lia's seizure condition. Their reservations and misunderstandings are interpreted by the physician as wilful non-compliance and are extrapolated into a narrative of neglect. At the time of her removal from her familial home, the child was almost three years old and accustomed to functioning in an environment where Hmong was the primary language of communication.

Lia's foster mother noted the adverse side-effects that some of the treatments were having on the child and informed physicians that her current drug regimes 'were the worst combination for Lia. The *worst*.'[53] Ironically, it was Lia's mother's insistence that this combination was 'too strong' for her daughter and her refusal to administer the drugs that finally prompted the treating paediatrician's application to the court for Lia's removal from her home. It was noted by one of her case workers that Lia actually seized more frequently while in the care of her foster family than she did at home.

The whole sorry saga was resolved only after Lia succumbed to brain death as a consequence of septic shock. The infection was undiagnosed when she presented to Merced Medical Center because she was seizing. Staff in the emergency department assumed that this was the long-awaited and much dreaded 'big one':[54] the seizure episode that everyone had taken for granted *would* happen and that they had all been anticipating with great anxiety. Lia's epilepsy seized the medical gaze so effectively that, tragically, her physicians failed to see beyond her paroxysmal disorder. As one of Fadiman's interviewees commented when trying to understand the reasons for this crucial lapse in diagnostic awareness: '*No one* at [Merced Community Medical Center] would have noticed anything but her seizures. Lia *was* her seizures.'[55] On the occasion in question, however, rather than epilepsy causing the seizures, it turned out that they were symptomatic of *Pseudomonas aeruginosa* bacilli in her blood (possibly introduced via an earlier medical procedure). Moreover, her treating physician at the Valley Children's Hospital, to which she was transferred after being stabilised at Merced, told Fadiman that although Depakene (Lia's medication at the time of the medical catastrophe) was probably 'the drug of choice' for her epilepsy, it actually made her more susceptible to the ravages of *P. aeruginosa* because it 'can hamper the body's ability to fight infection'.[56]

In her conclusions Fadiman acknowledges the tragic consequences of the medical saga for Lia and her family. She argues that Lia's 'life was ruined not by septic shock or noncompliant parents but by cross-cultural misunderstanding'.[57] Indeed, the subtitle of her text informs the reader that it is an account of a 'clash of two cultures'. The phrase denotes the conflict between Hmong and North American Anglo culture as it also refers to the clash between medical and non-medical cultures. This conflict identified by Fadiman is complicated further, I argue, by the fact that the disorder at the centre of the collision is epilepsy.

It is worth recalling here the point made by Byron Good: medical language is not merely reflective of illness or disease processes, he argues, but is rather constituted by 'a rich *cultural language*, linked to a highly specialized version of reality and system of social relations, and when employed in medical care, it joins deep moral concerns with its more obvious technical functions'.[58] The medical language and culture of epilepsy as they have developed in a western context over the 150 years or so preceding the events recounted by Fadiman present physicians with an uncompromising model of the condition that demands nothing less than aggressive medical response. The physician is called upon to battle, control and conquer the seizure. Where the patient figures in this often violent process is not always clear. That physicians are trained to understand epilepsy seizures as a challenge and test of medical capability is evident in the comments recorded by Fadiman in her book. The physicians tell of their increased levels of anticipatory anxiety that Lia will be brought in while they are on duty, their acute stress when confronted by her seizing body, their euphoria when they control the seizures, and their belief that the ability to quell Lia's seizures is the mark of a skilled medical practitioner.

A medical practitioner, commenting on one of Lia's admissions to the hospital while he is on duty, acknowledges that, in their efforts to stop the seizures, physicians 'Sometimes ... have to give so much medicine' that the patient goes into a state of respiratory arrest.[59] When Lia finally has 'the big one' that her paediatrician has been dreading for months, he describes his entry into the emergency room where she is being treated as being 'like something out of *The Exorcist*'.[60] As I suggested in the Introduction, his description of the scene suggests the *unheimlich* effect of the seizing body on medical sensibilities.

Lia's condition appeared to be exacerbated by increased stress – her own, and that of those around her. It is suggestive that her seizure episodes increased when she was removed from her home and placed in foster care. It is worth noting that away from the ambient stress of the hospital environment Lia's seizure episodes were often (but not always) shorter and stabilised spontaneously. This phenomenon was also noticeable after the cerebral event that caused her brain death.

> On December 9, 1986, Lia had returned home from [Merced Community Medical Center] with a fever of 104 degrees, an irregular breathing pattern, an inability to cough up or swallow her own secretions, and a prognosis of imminent death. Within days, her temperature was normal, her breathing was regular, and her swallowing and gag reflexes were back. Scratching their heads, her doctors attributed these improvements to reduced swelling in the medulla and hypothalamus. Her parents attributed them to the herbal infusion with which they had bathed their daughter when she first came home, and for many days thereafter.[61]

Frequent tepid sponging for children with high temperatures has long been a faithful standby in paediatric nursing practice, particularly before the widespread availability of drugs that lower elevated body temperatures. That this type of attention helped Lia's condition is not surprising. It is also more than possible that the acute and life-threatening state of her brain, given time and opportunity, abated enough to facilitate return of her swallowing and gag reflexes.

Fadiman, the treating physicians at Valley Children's Hospital where Lia was transferred – myself – we all have the benefit of hindsight analyses conducted in quiet reflection. We can read about and comment on what happened in the emergency department at Merced when Lia was admitted in *status epilepticus*, unpressured by the medical emergency of recurring *grand mal* seizures that may end in death for the patient. We can, perhaps, imagine how the urgency and attendant stresses increase when the presenting patient is a child. And this is the complexity, I think, for these physicians: in that moment of emergency, there is no time for the luxury of reflection. There is only time to act on what is currently understood as recommended medical intervention.

In her conclusions Fadiman notes that western medicine's investment in a Cartesian model of knowledge production about the body may well produce 'excellent physicians', but it does not always produce 'good healers'. Citing Arthur Kleinman, she argues that biomedical culture, while 'eagerly embracing' changes produced from within its own boundaries (technologies, drugs, procedures), will still aggressively deflect cross-cultural innovations as 'an assault on rationality'.[62] I wonder, though, whether biomedical rationality has always been vulnerable to assault from its own repressed subconscious.

The perspectives explored in the preceding chapters of this book and sketched above suggest a complex and problematic dynamic operating in exchanges between physician and the patient with epilepsy. Vulnerability to an internally produced dis-ease is certainly noticeable when medical knowledge reaches its limits and is found wanting. Medical rationality is destabilised, for example, when biomedicine's highly specialised version of reality and system of social relations begin to break down in the face of disorders that will not be cured. An irrationally aggressive response is sometimes observable when a patient will not accept cure at any cost. When this dis-ease flares up in relation to intractable seizures, it infects an otherwise reasonable physician with unreasonable and paroxysmal behaviours mimetic of those ascribed to the epileptic patient. Perhaps this remains the dilemma for twentieth-first-century medical practitioners: how not to match neuronal chaos with epistemic violence; how not to respond with therapeutic regimes exponential to the explosive physiological violence of the seizure process.

An episode of the Australian television documentary series *RPA* broadcast in 1999 aptly demonstrates this dynamic.[63] A middle-aged male patient is brought by ambulance to the emergency department of Sydney's Royal Prince Alfred Hospital. He has been in *status epilepticus* for approximately ninety minutes. In the course of trying to bring his seizures under some sort of control, physicians administer various anticonvulsant preparations, all to no avail. The atmosphere around his unconscious, seized body is charged with the adrenaline of the medical emergency being played out in front of the cameras. Not to mention the bright lights needed to facilitate filming. Phones are ringing, pagers are beeping, various machines monitoring the man's vital signs are bipping: there is also the spectacle and theatre of the convulsing body being recorded by the cameras for the wider viewing audience. A young male medico in attendance intersperses his commentary for the camera by shouting repeatedly at the patient in a loud voice, 'What's your name, mate?' He also laments to the camera that the patient's workmates have taken a long time to send him to hospital. The man's seizures continue unabated. Eventually he is intubated, paralysed with a curare derivative and removed to a special care unit, where his seizures finally cease.

The episode is interesting for several reasons. If nothing else, it graphically illustrates the acute sense of impotence experienced by the observer of a *grand mal* seizure, even when that observer is medically trained. However, it also gestures towards a visual fascination with the seized body. Close-up shots of the man's convulsions play in concert with shots of the increasingly agitated body language of the attending physician. The interplay of intractable, somatic epileptic disorder and spasmodic therapeutic response provokes an endemic (and mutually produced) medical dis-ease. An obvious awareness of the critical nature of the man's condition fulminates in uncomfortable juxtaposition with the attending physician's complete 'bemazement' and mounting anxiety at the intractability of the man's seizures to therapeutic – pharmaceutical – control.

Filming in these circumstances also raises some pressing ethical questions. Although I assume the patient signed a release form before this episode could go to air, the act of filming his unconscious and seizing body prior to obtaining permission is problematic. That the filming process supplements those conditions which can exacerbate his seizure condition (bright lights needed for the camera work; increased ambient sound; increased performance pressure for the young physician, whose lamentations about workplace response to the patient's seizure episode were addressed to the camera rather than colleagues) would appear to bring the episode very close indeed to the ethical limits of 'duty of care' protocols.

Because the triggers for cerebral paroxysm are so varied, the public and private spaces of everyday life can present something of an obstacle course for those with an epilepsy condition. A vulnerability to photic stimuli – sunlight flickering through leaves, faulty fluorescent lights, neon displays, spontaneous red-light sales at any large department store – can provoke seizure with little warning. Auditory stimuli such as some forms of music, sudden or repetitive piercing sounds and sudden, loud noises can also have deleterious consequences.

Ironically, one of the most dangerous spaces for those with particular forms of neuronal sensitivity is the emergency department of any modern western hospital, with its flashing lights, beeping pagers, constantly ringing telephones and cacophony of busy, over-stressed voices.

This is particularly so if the subject is immediately post-ictal: a term that refers to the interval near or at the end of a seizure process, when sensitivity to seizure triggers can be unusually heightened. In general terms, when the neurones have discharged excess energy, the sensitive brain is protected from further immediate paroxysm. However, there are some forms of epilepsy (some types of complex partial epilepsy, for example) where this is not necessarily the case and this period of acute sensitivity post-seizure can render the brain more vulnerable to those triggers described above. Subsequent paroxysmal discharge can then result in ongoing seizures for the patient: *status epilepticus*.

This seems to be a foundational knowledge about seizure states associated with epilepsy: medical literature abounds with examples of the part that auditory and photic stimuli play in exacerbating neuronal paroxysm in the sensitised brain. As I have indicated above, in some epilepsy research and in some epilepsy diagnostic procedures these stimuli are used in conjunction with various chemicals to increase neuronal sensitivity in order to provoke medically controlled and monitored seizure states. Nevertheless, it is an awareness that seems to be overridden in medical practice in most, if not all, modern emergency departments, by the compelling urgency to quell the seizure, to win 'the war against man's ancient enemy' at all costs. It is not an uncommon occurrence for medicos to labour mightily to suppress repeated seizures with ever-increasing pharmaceutical and technological vigour on a patient located in the middle of the very conditions that trigger and prolong seizure states: as a therapeutic intervention, it might be likened to filling the *Titanic* with ice cubes after it has hit the iceberg.

Despite the proliferation of knowledge since the late 1800s about brain function in general, and paroxysmal cerebral discharge in particular, in the 1990s, when a neurologist told a meeting of the Epilepsy Association of Massachusetts that – in relation to epilepsy – 'We don't know anything', his statement was greeted with laughter and applause. His audience of physicians, health care workers and people with various epilepsy conditions seemed to ruefully acknowledge a basic if elusive truth in his claim. This anecdote is related by Adrienne Richard to illuminate the specific and limited model of the epilepsies circulating though late twentieth-century biomedical knowledge systems. She goes on to cite Oliver Sacks' view that medical knowledge is profoundly incomplete in 'the neurology of living experience'.[64]

Sacks argues that, in a sense, all neurological and psychological testing currently in use functions not merely to expose or uncover neurological deficits or anomalies but, in fact, reduces or decomposes the patient to the sum total of those deficits: an observation that resonates with Reen Carter's disavowal of her spiritual life in favour of the medical story offered by neurology (see Introduction). These deficits then become the field marked out by medical technology for therapeutic intervention, redress or supplement. As Sacks suggests, by reducing interpretation of bodily ability to an account of neurological deficit or otherness, medicine fails to comprehend a larger story of the ways in which individuals experience or live neurophysiological difference.[65] While acknowledging the undoubted benefits of some forms of testing and interpretation of results, Reiter expresses concern that, because biomedicine is still largely ignorant of the underlying neurological reasons for most forms of epilepsy, some current interpretative models actually limit understanding of compensatory or coping mechanisms in the human brain.[66] It is worth recalling that John Hughlings Jackson expressed similar concerns in the late nineteenth century when he noted that medical students were being routinely taught 'to study cases as the symptoms show *approaches* to certain clinical standards, and not as they show departures from healthy states'.[67] Sacks returns to this point throughout his writings; however, he perhaps encapsulates this idea most powerfully in *An Anthropologist on Mars*, especially in his discussion of the young English artist Stephen Wiltshire, who is affected by autism.

Medicine's impulse to visually record instances of unconventional physiology and culture's fascination with these images persist. In her analysis of the visual culture of medicine, Cartwright argues that by the early decades of the twentieth century 'cinematic inscriptions of physiology' had become part of public culture.[68]

V

In literature and film, the epileptic figure was not faring much better. Louis Nowra is an Australian playwright and novelist who focuses on the schismatic effects of social transition. His work draws on multiple literary forms and genres to examine and interrogate dominant systems of power and privilege. His plays and novels are peopled with the outcasts who become the human detritus of imperial excess; these characters are themselves often creatures of excess.[69] Passionate, irrational, violent, vulnerable, they embody all that has been excreted from the dominant order. Some of them also 'seize'.

One of Nowra's most striking representations of the hybrid figure in conflict with dominant ideologies is the character of Betsheb in the play *The Golden Age*. The 'lost tribe' found living in the wilds of

Tasmania have somehow slipped through the cracks of a developing colonial society. In their isolation they have remained true to a range of cultural and linguistic practices that mark them as the degenerate other. In *The Golden Age* Nowra explores the complexities of speaking out from a marginalised subject position. He inscribes the characterisations of Mac, Stef, Angel and Betsheb through a frame of late nineteenth-century discourses of degeneration to focus the tension between mainstream society and the tribe. The 'tribe' are the descendants of English society's outcasts: 'Criminals, retards, the lost, the desperate'.[70] Invoking the nineteenth-century eugenicist argument that the degenerate classes will breed themselves out over three generations, the tribe has finally come to the brink of extinction. Mac has a genital malformation that precludes him fathering offspring; Stef has intellectual disabilities and seizures. Although their language is a rich patois of Cockney and Irish English, they are speaking less.

Theirs is an oral culture and Betsheb is compelled by Queenie Ayre to learn and remember the stories of the tribe. Left to her own devices, though, the young woman prefers non-verbal communication. This non-verbal communication includes kinetic abilities and the mute gesture of the seizure. Mac and Angel have chosen not to speak at all. In *The Golden Age*, as in other Nowra texts that explore issues of meaning and identity, the mute gesture, that gesture for which there is no language, is ultimately signified by the convulsive moment. This moment of abjection is described by Kristeva thus:

> Mute protest of the symptom, shattering violence of a convulsion that, to be sure, is inscribed in a symbolic system, but in which, without either wanting or being able to become integrated in order to answer to it, it reacts, it abreacts.[71]

Nowra has said in interview: 'Language gives identity'.[72] Language and identity are a central theme of the play, which explores issues of how we speak ourselves and how we are constructed through the language of the dominant order. William Archer, a physician and father of one of the characters who 'discover' the lost tribe, is determined to understand the group, to unlock their secrets and make them intelligible to his society. He must decipher their language and translate their morphology into terms that render them accessible. His chosen interpretative mode is medical discourse. At one point he tells Mac, 'I'm going to conquer you. Understand you.... We'll get it right this time.'[73]

Housed in a psychiatric facility to keep them from becoming fodder for twentieth-century eugenic arguments, the tribe are finally 'understood' and re-sutured to a system of signification that renders them disordered. One by one they succumb to the culture of twentieth-century medicine and genetic ideals until only Betsheb remains alive. It is a dramatically grim outcome. However, it is a conclusion that refocuses those intersecting connections between language, knowledge and power explored throughout the present book in relationship to a developing discourse of epilepsy. Myshkin, Monks, Smerdyakov, Guster, Lucette Le Sueur, Yelena and Betsheb connote the violent struggles of cultures in transition, and the power of language to control and marginalise the disenfranchised. These representations also gesture to the power of language to inscribe meaning to the convulsive body in medical culture. The hybridity of these fictional characters resonates with the real, destabilising the dominant order and interrogating the conditions of their own production as 'other' within dominant social, ideological and political systems.

Despite a long cultural history of representation in theatre, from Shakespeare to Nowra, Martin Norden mentions only one film in his detailed (1994) examination of disability in Hollywood cinema in which a central character is depicted as living (and more or less coping) with a paroxysmal condition. To be sure, the title of Norden's text signals its focus on physical disability in film and his cursory discussion of epilepsy may well be due its liminal place in discourses of disability: it is both physical and psychical, both visible and hidden. Norden cites the 1970 film *Tell Me That You Love Me, Junie Moon* as 'dealing with the topics of deinstitutionalization and independent living, [which also offers] an exceptionally rare portrait of a person with epilepsy'.[74]

It was not that epilepsy had been completely absent from Hollywood film or wider visual culture prior to this overt (and institutionally related) treatment in 1970. Rather, the subject matter evoked a crisis of language that challenged representation. Nonetheless, in her comprehensive 2003 review of epilepsy in film, Sallie Baxendale from the Institute of Neurology in London identifies '62 movies produced over three-quarters of a century, across four continents, covering nine cinematic genres' that deal with epilepsy and various seizure disorders.[75] She finds evidence of all the historical stereotypes in her survey and concludes that, despite some advancement in understanding of the condition making it to the movies, there is still a pronounced tendency to portray seizure-prone females as vulnerably transgressive and their male counterparts as 'mad, bad, and … dangerous'.[76] Jennie Kerson *et al.* come to much the same conclusion and observe that, despite the enormous reach of cinema, mainstream film representations of epilepsy are more often than not the same old 'same old'. She and her colleagues find that epilepsy 'in film continues to be distorted, sensationalized, and presented in the most frightening and/or depressing ways'.[77]

In the 1995 television series *American Gothic*, Sheriff Lucas Buck, who is supposedly the devil incarnate, casually inflicts a seizure on a man about to cause him trouble.[78] The scene is brief and an almost casual invocation of seizure as a sign of demonic possession. The faked seizure makes an appearance in the 1989 film *Drugstore Cowboy* when one of the female characters, Dianne, feigns *grand mal* seizure in a store while her accomplice shop lifts. In an update of the sly Sleary's recourse to 'Pears's shaving sticks' to simulate the frothing at the mouth often associated with *grand mal* episodes (see Chapter 2), Dianne resorts to Alka Seltzer as her prop of preference.[79] In the 1993 film *The Fugitive*, the seizure is used as a device of transition. A prisoner on the bus taking Richard Kimble to prison after he is wrongly convicted of murdering his wife fakes a seizure to stage an escape. Before the prisoner can make good on this initiative, he is shot and dies. However, the bus subsequently crashes and, although some are killed, the event facilitates Kimble's escape, reinforces his essential goodness and launches his quest to prove his innocence.[80] Both representations reproduce links between the outward signifier of epilepsy – the seizure – and criminality.

The fit as a comic device appears in the television sitcom *Seinfeld*. A character on the show, Cosmo Kramer, experiences two seizures on hearing television presenter Mary Hart's voice on *Entertainment Tonight*.[81] The episode gestures beyond the parameters of the show to a 1991 report of an American woman who actually suffered seizures on hearing Hart's electronically transmitted voice. The presenter's voice was evidently an epileptogenic for the woman and triggered excessive cerebral electrical activity. The sitcom representation and the reportage of the woman's seizure episodes make much of Hart's *Entertainment Tonight* celebrity status, a rhetorical linkage that also foregrounds the vicarious entertainment value located with the spectacle of the convulsing body. In the *Seinfeld* episode, Kramer's seized episodes are represented as relatively benign extensions of the character's trademark explosive entrances into scenes throughout the overall series and his normal, if generally exaggerated, twitchy body language.

Undoubtedly, the body in seizure is rich with signifying possibilities and symbolic resonance. But what can a film character with epilepsy *do* when not fitting? The following discussion engages with a limited selection of films to explore this question.

VI

In 2007 two films dealing with the life, times and art of Ian Curtis were released. The documentary *Joy Division*, made nearly thirty years after Curtis's death, mimes the singer's dance and symptomatology with spasmodic lighting, in-frame multiple imaging and between-scene cutting. It foregrounds Curtis's epilepsy in a way that is absent from Anton Corbijn's film *Control*, released that same year, perhaps because they – the epilepsy and Curtis's death – remain such a central and still painful feature of the collective memory of the surviving band members and those interviewed for the documentary project. In a *fin-de-siècle* turn, the documentary also links Joy Division's music (and, by extension, Curtis's epilepsy) to the dying days of the Mancunian economy at the end of the 1970s. It is a classic triangulation of social, civil and embodied disorder that resonates with the metonymic and symbolic deployment of epilepsy at the end of the nineteenth century. In this context, epilepsy spins back into the circuit of culture with all the weighted symbolic celebrity accreted over the previous century of signification.

The power of this style of representation for the collective imagination also manifests in medical culture. In much the same way that Taylor and Marsh scrutinise the writings of Arthur Myers for definitive signs of pathology (Chapter 3), Zarko and Jasna Martinovic from the Department of Epilepsy, Institute for Mental Health, Beograd, Yugoslavia, examine Curtis's song lyrics for diagnostic evidence. In their abstract for the 1998 Third European Congress of Epileptology they argue:

> Presented with examples of painful expression of epilepsy in Curtis's poetic lyrics, combined with original innovative music, our analysis adds other evidence of the ways in which hyperemotionality in epilepsy leads to depression. Although a common but complex association of creativity with perceptual hypersensitivity and psychopathological susceptibility is apparent, their unique forms in each creative individual deserve separate analysis.[82]

Their observations invoke preoccupations expressed by Shahram Khoshbin in relation to Vincent van Gogh's creativity and the various debates about the possibility of connections between Dostoevsky's writing and his pathology (considered in the Introduction). 'Hyperemotionality [and the ways it] leads to depression' is figured here as signifier and evidence of epilepsy rather than considered as a by-product of treatment regimes or a factor related to age, gender, socialisation and the cultural context in which Curtis lives and understands his symptomatology.

I cannot help but wonder if this is still a productive direction in medical inquiry. Gastaut argued, after all, that Dostoevsky's creative capacities were 'in no way' derived from his epilepsy and should not be considered as merely a 'by-product' of disease. Moreover, the author was adept at exploiting his paroxysmal condition artistically. Jacques Catteau and James Rice agree. Indeed, Rice argues that Dostoevsky's acceptance and mastery of the cultural implications of his symptomatology allowed him to subvert and move beyond the normal/abnormal binary to a polymorphous and polyphonic expression of paroxysmal experience 'negotiated through art'.[83] As I have proposed earlier, it may well be the case that the cultural languages of creativity and spirituality offer a better rate of exchange than the medical languages of diagnosis and treatment in some instances.

Corbijn's film[84] presents Curtis's epilepsy as part of his life: not the central tenet, or a metaphor for wider instability. In this, it breaks new ground in epilepsy representation. When Sam Riley, as Curtis, is not seizing, he is participating – for better and worse – in all those social roles that comprise a life. Nevertheless, there are aspects of Curtis's epilepsy that are undeniably part of his public persona, most notably through his dancing. Susan Hawthorne's description of *grand mal* seizure reproduced at the outset of this chapter evokes both the event and the experience of observing outward signs of neuronal excitement which trigger the event. The analogy of the dance is seductive. Dance has long been associated with celebration, rituals of creation and metamorphosis. Friedrich Nietzsche associates dance with the desire for lightness and transcendence.[85] Anyone who has seen Curtis's live or filmed performances cannot but be transfixed by his dance.

Jon Savage has suggested that the singer's on-stage movements 'lacked fluidity': that somehow his 'dance' failed to transcend his essential embodiment.[86] Others have described his dance as 'other-wordly' and 'hypnotic'; one fan commented 'You would be drawn into it. It functioned like those shaman things do.'[87] I tend to agree with these latter views: it is difficult to watch Curtis's performances, even one step removed via the medium of film from the strobing lights that could only have exacerbated his symptomatology, without wanting to 'go all the way'. That is, without wanting to enter into the escalating journey to transcendence or, as Dostoevsky would have it, to those celebrated 'higher moments'. And for those with epilepsy vulnerabilities, this is precisely the temptation. And the danger. As, indeed, it was for Curtis: he suffered several on-stage seizures, at times losing control of his dance. Did he make the connection between the auto-stimulation of his performance and its potential to move him beyond, to that moment for which Dostoevsky 'would give ten years of his life, and perhaps all of it, for a few seconds of such bliss'?[88] Quite possibly.

To be clear, I am not suggesting that Curtis deliberately invoked seizures with his dance: I suspect that these events, when they occurred on stage or immediately following a performance, were triggered by a combination of lighting and the musical rhythms central to Joy Division's performances. I am suggesting that his capacity to get lost in the music was facilitated by his dance rhythms, and this in turn transported him closer to those pleasurable sensations 'of completeness, of proportion, or reconciliation', of ecstasy, identified by Dostoevsky through the pre-seizure states he associates with the character of Myshkin in *The Idiot* (see Chapter 3). The trick, as Dostoevsky notes through Myshkin, is to stay in the borderlands and not inadvertently fall into the darkness. The lyrics from the Joy Division song 'Atrocity exhibition' mark a critical and politicised awareness of the body as spectacle. They also express Curtis's quandary, simultaneously inviting the spectator to identify with both the ecstasy and the abjection of the paroxysmal moment, while insisting on its place in wider human experience: 'For entertainment they watch his body twist/Behind his eyes he says: "I still exist". This is the way, step inside.' There is potential in Curtis's performative to move like Dostoevsky beyond a normal/abnormal binary: had he, of course, been able to survive the combined circumstances of his life.

VII

Beyond these representations though, and as Baxendale notes, mainstream cinema tended to mobilise stereotypes already in circulation. The female figure coded 'epileptoid' often bears close resemblance to the medically reified image of a sexualised tendency to convulse. One of the early cinema versions of this type of visual representation appears in Hawks' film *The Big Sleep*,[89] although it must be said that Carmen Sternwood does not actually convulse in this version of the film (as she does in Chandler's text). Nor is the source of her 'disorder' directly named. Rather, it remains an inexpressible and uncanny presence lurking beneath much of the dialogue. Her innate 'wrongness' is conveyed through characterisation and half-formed phrases that, as Philip Marlowe concludes in Hawks' film, indicate she is 'that way'.

Carmen gambles, sucks her thumb, tries to sit on Marlowe's lap while he is 'still standing up' and generally runs around being, in turn, sexually provocative, linguistically repetitive ('you're cute!' is the stock utterance whenever she encounters Marlowe), childish and disorderly. She also has memory lapses that are extensive enough to make her and her sister vulnerable to blackmail attempts from casino boss Eddie Mars. He claims that she has killed Sean Regan, an ex-employee of her father, and simply 'remembers nothing about it'. In trying to convince Marlowe of Carmen's guilt despite her lack of memory of the event, he explains that she was 'pretty high', and 'you know. That way'. General Sternwood describes his daughters to Marlowe at the beginning of the film as being alike 'only in that they have the same corrupt blood'. Vivien is 'Spoilt; exacting; smart; ruthless', while Carmen, the younger of the two, is described as being still a child 'who likes to pull the wings off flies'. Although General Sternwood is being blackmailed to pay off some old gambling debts incurred by his younger daughter, he tells Marlowe that it is pointless asking her about them because 'she'll just suck her thumb and look coy'.

In a film notable for its sharp and explicit dialogue, much is said about Carmen's wayward tendencies. Whenever her behaviour is the subject of conversation, there are knowing nods between conversants: all understand something quite specific about the young woman's behavioural excesses. When General Sternwood tells Marlowe that it is futile to raise the gambling debts with Carmen, he replies 'Yeah. I know what you mean'. Near the end of the film, when Eddie Mars is finally cornered into talking to Marlowe about Regan's disappearance and tells the detective that Carmen killed him but had no memory of it because she was 'that way', Marlowe replies 'Yeah. We've all seen her that way. We know what she looks like.' Well, yes: but why can't they be straightforward about Carmen? There are so many words to choose from, yet because these characters persist in using words that convey much without actually naming, Carmen remains somewhat of an enigma. Marlowe tells Vivien at the end of the film:

> What I tell the police will be pretty close to the truth. You'll have to send Carmen away. From a lot of things. They have places for that. Maybe they can even cure her. It's been done before.

In the 1978 film of the same book, directed by Michael Winner,[90] the setting for the action has been moved to England and the 'wild' sisters are renamed Charlotte and Camilla. Again, a lot of dialogue deals with the younger sister's tendency to social excess and disorder. This version has her more overtly represented as being prone to violence and sexually 'perverse'. She poses naked for erotic photographs (as she does in the book) and tends to take rejection of her physical charms very badly indeed. Transgressively erotic she may be, but by no stretch of the imagination can she be seen as vulnerable. Unlike Carmen in Hawks' film, Camilla *is* guilty of murdering Regan (who in this version has been married to Charlotte) because he rejected her sexual advances. When Marlowe takes her to the old ruin near the Sternwood mansion to refine her shooting skills, he has already anticipated her lethal potential and loads the gun with blanks. She shoots at him and when the gun is empty devolves into a *grand mal* seizure. Suddenly all the talk from both film versions coalesces into definitive meaning. It took thirty-two years and an Atlantic crossing, but with that convulsive moment Carmen/Camilla's disorder, as it is in Chandler's text, is finally pathologised as epileptiform of uncertain aetiology: drugs, alcohol, 'corrupt blood'?

Unlike Humphrey Bogart's Marlowe in the 1946 film, whose efforts to deal with Carmen's problems are, in part, fuelled by his attraction to Vivien, Robert Mitchum's Marlowe is doing it for a standard fee and General Sternwood. His code of practice demands he save the dying old man (and fellow American expatriate) from the knowledge that 'his blood is poison' and that his daughters are 'perverts and killers'. This Marlowe gives Charlotte much the same advice that Humphrey Bogart's 'shamus' gave the elder Sternwood girl in 1946: Carmen/Camilla needs to be sent away; there 'are places for that.... Hell. She might even get herself cured, you know? It's been done.'

The Andromeda Strain[91] also features a female character with epilepsy and quite remarkably resists the lure of the female stereotypes already in circulation. Dr Ruth Leavitt is a microbiologist and one of a group of scientists attempting to contain the biological crisis sparked by a satellite falling onto a village in New Mexico. Located at the opposite end of the representational spectrum that produced Carmen/Camilla, Dr Leavitt is smart, career focused and opinionated. She is also still very much 'in the closet' about her epilepsy. She is seconded to an underground government facility (ironically dubbed 'Wildfire') as the only female member of a team trying to unlock the secret of the deadly organism that seems to have come to Earth with the satellite. Although at least two of her team personally know her quite well from past work alliances, neither is aware of her seizure condition. As the team moves through each level deeper into the high-security part of the facility to commence the task of saving human kind, they are identified by palm print, scanned internally and externally, and disinfected of as many potential contaminants as possible. Despite extensive and intrusive scrutiny of their bodies, Dr Leavitt's paroxysmal condition remains undetected. Her body becomes the literalisation of the facility's hidden potential to disorder.

A *petit mal* or absence seizure while she is reviewing data has her miss a vital piece of information about the organism. When the team is responding to an emergency caused by a breakdown in the integrity of the facility's sealing units, she again lapses into a *petit mal* episode, which this time develops into a *grand mal* seizure. The emergency is indicated by warning signals being activated and a nurse proclaiming 'Contamination!' As team member and physician Mark Hall runs along the corridor towards the site of the disaster (the autopsy suite), Ruth Leavitt joins him and asks for information on the situation. 'Infection spread', he replies. A moment later Leavitt lapses into a *petit mal* episode provoked by a red light flashing three times per second. When the *grand mal* seizure begins, a female co-worker exclaims 'She's got the germ!' Other co-workers start to flee. Hall, realising his colleague's problem, rushes to her aid, simultaneously reassuring the panicked co-workers 'There's no danger. She isn't contagious.' When a nurse finally arrives with a phenobarbitone injection to treat the seizing microbiologist, Hall reassures her that it is not contamination from the alien organism: 'Come on. She won't hurt you. It's epilepsy.' Up to this point in the film Leavitt's epilepsy can be read as dangerous and a potential contaminant for the purity of the scientific project. Her first (unobserved) seizure while reviewing the data places in jeopardy the project to understand and contain the organism.

In the middle sections of the film Leavitt's paroxysmal disorder (which is still hidden from her colleagues) is associated with a range of unpredictable technological factors that have, despite all efforts to the contrary, managed to degrade the integrity of what was thought to be a foolproof facility. The contamination scene towards the end of the film brings these associations into sharp focus, and projects the hitherto hidden and volatile properties located with Ruth Leavitt onto the mystery of the organism. A little time later, and still upset by the shocking revelation of Leavitt's epilepsy, Hall tells another team member that the microbiologist has just had a seizure and demands 'Why the hell didn't she tell us about it?' The pragmatic response is: 'Probably no top lab would have her if they knew. Insurance, prejudice, and all that crap'; to which Hall replies with some exasperation 'That's the middle ages'. The implication of the exchange is that once her paroxysmal condition has been recognised and medically understood for what it is, it no longer poses a threat. It is in this scene that the team finally begins to comprehend the mystery of the organism and its narrow range of viability. Once they are able to understand the limits and consequences of the Andromeda strain (and narrowly avert the auto-destruction of the facility) they are able to control its implications for human life. The film adopts a relatively enlightened approach to epilepsy. Dr Leavitt recovers from her seizure and continues in her role as team member to avert the disaster posed by the alien organism. At the film's conclusion she is very much part of the solution, although now her secret is out she may never work in a 'top lab' again.

VIII

The 1992 Australian film *Romper Stomper*[92] is one of the few mainstream films to deal with epilepsy at the level of characterisation and thematic structure. It is a boy-meets-girl, boy-loses-girl, boy-tries-to-kill-girl narrative set within the neo-Nazi counter-culture of multicultural Australia. In exploring the romantic triad of its main characters (Hando, Gabe and Davey), the film dwells on the social exigencies of power, disempowerment and alienation in the big city. It also reprises the figure of the eroticised female epileptic. Fraught with its multiple and often conflicting significations, the epileptic body with its *grand mal* 'dance' becomes a structuring motif of the film. Although a degenerative metamorphosis or perverse kind of transcendency may be seen as part of the synaptic event of seizure, the *grand mal* 'dance' is also disruptively primitive, signifying both physical and metaphysical transgression. Elaine Showalter argues that in folklore and medicine dance has a long tradition of special signification. Both 'the violent *chorea* of the asylum or the tarantella of legend' carried suggestions of Charcot's *grande hystérie* and so becomes associated with convulsive femininity.[93]

In many ways *Romper Stomper* can be read as a prolonged (hystero-) epileptoid event inflected through the pathology represented by the character of Gabe. On the run from the incestuous attentions of her father, Gabe drifts from one dysfunctional relationship to another until she finally captures the attention of Hando, leader of a skinhead gang. The character of Gabe is not only epileptic, she is infantilised through the semiotic coding of dress, recurring child-like body language and an ongoing dependency on her father. At the beginning of the film we see her call on him to rescue his 'little girl' from the violence of a disintegrating relationship. Gabe is constructed along the lines of Charcot's hystero-epileptic women. She is a child/woman, an 'innocent temptress'; both her father and Hando cast her as seductress.

The film's treatment of her epileptic body is also imbued with shades of Dickensian assumptions about indexical morphology. Gabe's epilepsy functions as an outward signifier of psycho-sexual trauma, genetic guilt, transgressive sexuality, not to mention a lack of homosocially validated codes of behavioural integrity. By 'dobbing' to the police about the skinheads' hideout location, she is implicated in the death of Bubsy, the gang's child member. And she ultimately dislocates the symbiotic relationship between Hando and Davey, irrevocably contaminating their bonds of loyalty. Her epileptic body is deployed as both a trope and the somatic site of the film's exploration of dysfunction and disorder. This strategy provides a problematic out for the film's representations of discursive and material violence, a point that will be considered further below.

Gabe's pattern of epilepsy conforms to the following phases: the prodromal or pre-seizure stage is marked by changes in emotional reactivity, restlessness, anxiety, depression, loss of motivation and disorientation. Medical research suggests that most paroxysmal behaviours are preceded by a prodromal phase of sorts. The convulsive phase involves loss of consciousness, tonic/clonic spasms, automatic movements and generalised muscular disturbance. The post-ictal, or post-seizure, phase is marked by some slowness in re-orienting, initial low energy and some automatic behaviour. However, this final stage alleviates the previous symptoms, at least temporarily; once the neurones have discharged excess energy, they enter a phase of normal function. This final stage has been referred to by Ounsted as a period of 'after-glow',[94] a descriptor that posits links between the paroxysms of epilepsy and orgasm.

Development of the film's crisis/resolution scenarios suggests the prodromal, ictal and post-ictal phases of an epileptic cycle: periods of relative calm or normality that explode into erratically charged and violent activity, to be followed by an almost euphoric peacefulness. For example, near the beginning of the film the comparative tranquillity of the room where Hando and Gabe have spent their first night together, and where casual post-coital dickering goes on between gang members about the street value of a Hitler Youth knife, is quickly followed by the leaping, colliding, thrashing bodies and driving music of a party scene. The explosive, chaotic activity of this latter scene suggests the paroxysmal electrical discharges registered in EEG readings of a brain in seizure pattern. In this scene, bodies violently erupt, clash together, bounce off each other; electrical impulses randomly discharging, escalating energy. Not all epileptic episodes are unpleasurable. *They dance. They rampage.*

Inter-cut shots link the dance with eroticism and transgression, the tempo of the music choreographing the sexual encounter between Hando and Gabe. Hando's pounding of Gabe's body in this sexual interlude is underscored by Davey's rhythmic pounding of the suggestively phallic punching bag. The driving music and disjointed, garbled speech are mimetic of the auditory and visual distortions associated with some epileptic symptomatology marking the transitional phase between prodrome and convulsion. A post-ictal 'afterglow' is choreographed in the scene's wind-down, with shots of Bubsy attempting to copulate with one of the gang's older female acolytes, Davey being sprayed with fluid from a bottle and Magoo lying unconscious on the floor.

In *Romper Stomper* the dance exceeds appropriate social boundaries, disrupting both temporality and spatiality. In a later scene, Gabe's frenetic movements during seizure embody the hyperkinetic and purposeless activity of the skinheads' dance party; as Gabe jerks through her *grand mal* dance on the floor, Sonny Jim mimics the movement of her flailing limbs, thus becoming explicitly identified with her loss of agency and control, her loss of bodily autonomy, her excess and stigmatisation. Part of Hando's signification can also be located with Gabe. Her seizure pattern may be read in conjunction with his spirals into confusion, loss of direction and paroxysmal rage: behaviours associated with prodromal and ictal phases. The sequential placement of Gabe's seizures also signals moments of resolution in gang conflict.

Notions of space and dispossession become crucial concerns in the film and within this milieu Gabe functions as both a conduit for masculine desire and a commodity within a homosocial economy. Dispossessed, yet embodying the signifiers of possession, simultaneously displaced within the terrains of the film's socialscape, Gabe symbolises and embodies spatial dislocation as she moves through, temporarily inhabits, taints and symbolically reconfigures masculine psychic space. In the initial encounter with the skinheads, one of the group's female members refers to Gabe as a 'space monster': an appellation that suggests her configuration as a monstrous creature of multiple spaces, a signifier of monstrous, alien spatiality.

The philosophy of Hando's group is defined by the territorial battles that they wage with the Vietnamese. Space and subjectivity become linked through these scenes and through Hando's reinvention of space: the Nazi paraphernalia that adorns the group's headquarters is echoed in the tattooed stigmata of their body decorations, which, in turn, reflect ideological loyalties. In her reading of Roger Callois's work on mimicry as luxury or excess, Elizabeth Grosz considers the reaction to spatial dislocation in association with psychasthenia. This discussion of Callois's work has implications for the film's treatment of space and territory. In response to their perceived territorial displacement by society, Hando and his group 'invent … space of which [they] are in *convulsive* possession'.[95] This space is charged with meaning and symbolic power for the group; it functions as a microcosmic reconstruction of an idealised, white supremacist, phallocentric world in which they rule.

In his biomedical account of the temporolimbic epileptic body, Mesulam argues that epileptics may 'saturate' their world with 'intense emotional significance' and become convinced of their own uniqueness within that context.[96] The narrative economy of Mesulam's mapping of epileptic space and spatiality foregrounds both its instability and its importance to psychic health. Spatial location and perceived control of space, the place of the material body in relationship to space, become inextricably bound up with perceptions of self and self in relationship to other. It is therefore significant that when the group's headquarters are destroyed and the skinheads are forcibly displaced from their spatial idea/l, Hando is thrown into crisis. He is dislocated from spatial privilege and control and cannot reorient himself.

The group consequently experience a disruption between subjectivity and their relationships to spatiality. When a warehouse is later commandeered to temporarily accommodate them, Hando slides from being the focus for group activity and cohesion to becoming decentred – displaced by Gabe's offerings of hot food and stories of her past life. She now occupies an equivalent spatial position to him at the table where they eat. Hando's spatial dislocation becomes focused on her and is again suggestive of the prodromal phase of the seizure process, with its anxiety, disorientation and disassociation from spatial realities.

He tries to re-establish centrality by rejecting her captivation of his narrative and psychic space at the table where they are eating; however, in the kitchen area Gabe remains the focus of group activity while he remains temporarily marginalised. It is while Gabe and Davey play and work in the kitchen that she falls to the floor and begins to seize. Although we have already been alerted to Gabe's epilepsy through oblique references to her medication regime, this is the first overt representation of symptomatology. Once her *grand mal* seizure has run its course, Hando's signs of disorientation alleviate. He returns to a state of relative normalcy, regaining focus and motivation. In the post-ictal afterglow, he is even able to sympathise with her transitory loss of self-control. It is after Gabe has this first seizure that the group re-mobilise and Hando re-establishes his focal position in its hierarchy.

Gabe's second seizure follows soon after Hando murders a Vietnamese shopkeeper. He, Davey and Gabe are fleeing to Adelaide in a stolen car; their physical movement is reactive to external conditions and their responses resemble the automatisms associated with furore and fugue states. Resolution for this current crisis is unimagined beyond their arrival in the new city. After this second seizure, both Hando and Davey begin to articulate plans for an ongoing survival. Davey's plan entails remaining with Gabe; Hando's requires her elimination from the space he seeks to dominate between himself and Davey.

Early in the film we see Hando dancing behind Gabe as they provocatively flirt/play with Davey in a shopping arcade. Hando drags Gabe's body between the two men, using her as both taunt and decoy. This positioning is suggestive of the spatial configuration that these three characters occupy in relation to each other and the pattern becomes a thematic device in the film. In the party scene referred to above, inter-cut shots are used to synchronise and sexualise the symbiotic relationship between the three characters. Significantly, we do not get the same sense of Hando's presence in the sexual encounter between Gabe and Davey.

In a sense, Hando can be seen to function as Gabe's disjunctive double. Together they suggest the duality of mixed-form epilepsy: a combination of *grand mal* and temporolimbic pathology. They contest the same psychic space, particularly in relationship to Davey, and when Hando is vanquished from that triad at the end of the film he assumes the outward signifiers of Gabe's stigma. While Gabe's body remains asymptomatic, Hando becomes inarticulate. He falls. Stabbed in the back by Davey. Saliva and blood dribble from his mouth. In the throes of death, he *dances*.

Gabe's epilepsy not only serves as an indexical signifier of the film's transgressive movements but ultimately functions as a containment of the film's violence, thus deferring the possibility for an ongoing reflexivity. Within the film's ideological economy, the epileptic body is constructed as other and becomes the repository for a host of displaced cultural anxieties. Gabe's disorder, as it is represented through the pathology of epilepsy, is symptomatically relocated with Hando. His death seizure, then, signals a symbolic end to the disorder and violence represented by his character. It is a problematic strategy. The phallocentric, white supremacist space of the film is semiotically coded epileptic. By associating representations of gang rage and racial violence with the organic disorder of Gabe's epilepsy, the film implicitly obviates the potential for further debate about agency and the politics of representation.

IX

The 1990s American television series *The X Files* draws on the trope of epilepsy to create two characters of note, Max Fenig and Robert Modell ('Pusher'). The characters are drawn from opposite – and extreme – ends of the signifying spectrum. In the episode 'Fallen angel', Max Fenig's seizures resonate with ancient beliefs that epilepsy results from some sort of assault from external forces. The title of the episode, although referring to unidentified flying objects (UFOs) that crash into the Earth, also invokes the semiotic legacy of epilepsy as a metaphysical event. Max is a member of the National Investigative Committee of Aerial Phenomenon and, like FBI agents Fox Mulder and Dana Scully, investigates extra-terrestrial phenomena.[97] As Scully notes when she and Mulder visit Max in his trailer home, he also takes the drugs Dilantin and Mellaril. The first substance is usually prescribed for epilepsy, the second – or so Scully tells Mulder – is only used to treat schizophrenia. She argues that because Max takes anticonvulsant and psychotropic medications, his perceptions and interpretation of events are quite probably unreliable.

When coming upon Max during one of his seizures, Mulder notices a small triangular scar behind his right ear and later tells Scully that this type of scar is common in UFO abductees. The episode resonates with contemporary alien abduction narratives circulating through the wider North American cultural circuit. In doing so, it gestures to government conspiracy theories and draws on wider cultural disaffection with 'official' responses to the possibilities of extra-terrestrial contact with the Earth. Whatever the aetiology, Max's 'otherness' is left in no doubt for the viewer when, towards the end of the episode, Mulder sees him suspended in the air surrounded by an eerie blue light. Seconds later Max mysteriously disappears in a flash of white light.

In contrast, Modell conforms to Baxendale's 'mad, bad and … dangerous' male stereotype: a sort of updated Monks or Edward Hyde for the twentieth century's *fin-de-siècle*. The character's temporal lobe epilepsy endows him with psychic abilities, which he uses to build up his kill rate by willing people to commit suicide.[98] The problem is that it just is not fun if there is nobody to appreciate his capabilities. Mulder and Scully become his adversaries of choice. When profiling Modell, Mulder discovers that he is an 'average man' who has a history of aiming above his abilities when it comes to career choices; at one point, he even applied to join the FBI but failed because testing concluded that he is egocentric and an inveterate liar. Scully comments that Modell is essentially a 'little man', whose epileptically enhanced psychic abilities allow him to be 'big'. The episode ascribes the character's late-onset temporal lobe epilepsy to a brain tumour, of which he is aware but has never had treated. In an inversion of Myshkin's celebration of the ecstatic aspects of his epilepsy, Modell values the murderous transcendence his disorder allows.

Modell has a contemporary in Princeton graduate James Walter Wayland, the protagonist of the 1997 film *Deceiver*. As with Modell, Wayland's purported murderous impulses are directly connected to his temporal lobe epilepsy. Wayland is a suspect in the murder of Elizabeth Loftus, a 'call girl'. Like *Romper Stomper, Deceiver* thematises epilepsy through characterisation and narrative structure. The narrative is largely developed within the confines of police procedure and organised around the interrogation of Wayland by Detectives Braxton and Kennesaw. The film uses elements of the discontinuous narrative form, a strategy that mimes spasmodic shifts between the ordered conventions of the police investigation, both Wayland's and Kennesaw's fragmented rememberings of past events, and the disorienting slippages between recall and murderous fantasy.

Much of the textual play in *Deceiver* focuses on ideas of truth. The opening scenes establish links between truth, lying and Wayland's as yet unidentified epilepsy with a series of close-up shots of the polygraph readout: a strategy that gestures – at least implicitly – to EEG technology. During these early scenes, Braxton asks Wayland if he has ever told lies: 'Now, I'm not talking about the kind of lie like when you tell your wife she's a good cook. I'm talking about malicious lies – devious lies – lies that deliberately conceal the truth. Do you understand the difference?'[99] As a polygraph expert, Kennesaw is an 'expert in truth' and tells Wayland that the technology is 'foolproof'; if he is only honest in his responses to police questioning, all will be fine. Wayland counters that the machine can measure and record only vital signs and levels of perspiration; he asks what they 'have to do with the truth'. It is a weighted moment that, at least notionally, indicates the limits of imaging technologies in general. Wayland and Kennesaw are linked in various ways, sharing similar gestures and via a range of in-frame juxtapositions. Both have degrees in psychology; both have above-average IQs – Wayland's is 151, Kennesaw's 122; and despite both having connections to the murdered woman, both exhibit signs of the hyposexuality supposedly characteristic of male temporal lobe symptomatology. Throughout the film these two characters occupy unstable positions of power in relationship to each other: Kennesaw, expert in polygraph testing and the identification of truth, eventually becomes, himself, subject to the process, with Wayland as his interrogator. The polygraph exposes the detective as a liar.

Wayland's epilepsy is revealed by increments and his medication implicated in a capacity to be less than honest without triggering polygraphic evidence of lying. He eventually admits to faulty memory about his actions on the night of Loftus's murder, to drinking absinthe, to taking anticonvulsant medication mid-way through an interrogation session. Finally, he tells the detectives: 'Epilepsy. I suffer from temporal lobe epilepsy. I'm not a well man.' The film maps his temporal lobe condition onto the more lurid (and fictionally licensed) aspects of van Gogh's symptomatology. Consulted by the detectives to help them better understand Wayland's psychology, psychiatrist Dr Simmons Banyard tells them: 'You see, van Gogh was an epileptic and like our friend Wayland, he had a fondness for absinthe: not such a good combination. For you see absinthe is an epileptogenic.'

Although there is a disjunctive doubling between Wayland and Kennesaw, the film ultimately recuperates a reductive and sensationalised representation of temporal lobe epilepsy. Banyard also informs Braxton and Kennesaw:

> Just don't forget the feeling this guy gives you. People with temporal lobe epilepsy make your skin crawl for a reason. If you think he's being seized – even if you suspect it – you treat him like you would a strange dog in an alley. Don't initiate any casual conversation; don't stare him in the eye; don't touch him. Whatever you do, don't turn your back on him.

After Kennesaw is attacked when trying to restrain Wayland while he is seizing, Banyard comments to Braxton: 'Ooops! Shouldn't have touched him. I warned you about that.... It's all chemicals Phil. It's all chemicals.'

By the last years of the twentieth century, nothing much had changed in medical–cultural stories of the epileptic since the late nineteenth century. Cultural representational systems still located epileptics in the borderlands at the limits of social experience and beyond. Medical representational systems, despite considerable advances in scientific understanding of neurophysiology, still subscribed to an epileptic figure narratively voided of all but disorder. Clearly, the keynote stories explored above present less than viable options for those living with an epilepsy condition. Interventions into stereotypical representations of folk with epilepsy are difficult to find and when they occur at all seem to beckon from unexpected directions, Corbijn's film a rare example.

X

In 1985 North American fantasy and science fiction author Whitley Strieber experienced what he was to describe in his book *Communion: Encounters with the Unknown. A True Story* as 'a shattering assault from the unknown'.[100] While staying in their log cabin in remote up-state New York with his wife and young son, on the night of 26 December,

Strieber's sleep was disturbed by a range of profound sensory disruptions that resulted in a prolonged altered state of consciousness. He was abruptly awoken by a 'peculiar whooshing, swirling noise'[101] that seemed to emanate from the downstairs section of the cabin. Although shocked and 'very curious' about the noise, rather than investigating its cause he settled back to resume sleep. He then experienced what appeared to him a visitation of 'small compact figures' rushing into his bedroom. Of the time immediately following this visual phenomenon Strieber only recalls 'blackness'.[102]

His next 'conscious recollection' is of an extended period of non-volitional movement: 'Something was hideously wrong, so wrong that my mind went blank. I couldn't think.'[103] He writes of coming into awareness from beneath a 'thick, suffocating curtain' of 'raw fear' to find himself in a facility surrounded by figures of the type that had heralded the onset of his episode.[104] This re-orientation to his surroundings was accompanied by olfactory sensations and bright flashing lights. The episode culminated in an invasive procedure which left him with the impression of being anally raped by some 'mechanical device' introduced into his body.[105] He awoke the next morning in his bed with a 'distinct sense of unease' but no immediate memory of the event, which he recalled later only under hypnosis. His wife, who had been occupying the same bed, slept through the disturbance.

Over the next few weeks Strieber's personality evidently underwent a significant deterioration. He writes: 'I became hypersensitive, easily confused, and, worst of all, short with my son. We have always been a happy family, and there was no change in our life condition or relationship to account for this personality shift.'[106] Difficulties in relating to his wife and son continued. In fact his behaviour became so intolerable that it threatened his marriage. Strieber finally sought outside advice in trying to understand what he was going through. He first contacted Bud Hopkins, a prominent researcher in the field of alien abduction and an abstract artist of some note. This meeting provided focus for his experience. Although he professed himself 'unwilling' to ascribe his sensory disturbances to UFO phenomena, he sought a therapist who was open-minded about the possibility.

In 1986 he met with Dr Donald Klein, a psychiatrist at Columbia University and the Director of Research at the New York State Psychiatric Institute. After listening to Strieber's accounts of his experiences over several months, some conducted while the author was under hypnosis, Klein suggested that these states of altered consciousness might be consistent with an 'abnormality' in the temporal lobe. Strieber subsequently underwent an EEG recording via a 'nasal probe' and returned a normal result. It should be noted that an EEG recording can register electrical disturbance only as it happens. During the recording Strieber manifested no symptoms of his previously reported altered states, so a normal EEG reading is not surprising. As the Ounsted research team reported in their study of children with temporal lobe epilepsy, a significant number of subjects recorded multiple normal EEGs before any abnormality was detected. And, in some cases, an EEG that 'satisfactorily' supported clinical diagnosis was obtained only after extensive sleep studies or after the administration of 'activating' agents such as Megimide–pentothal.

Initially, Strieber seized on the medical model as an explanation for his experiences; however, further research diminished his assurance:

> But the more I studied temporal-lobe disorder, the less it seemed an answer. It did not explain the overwhelming sense of the real connected with my experiences. It did not explain the physical consequences.... Temporal-lobe epilepsy was nothing more than another speculation, essentially no different and no more supportable than the visitor hypothesis or any other hypotheses that I had put forward. I had to fall back on the truth: I did not know what was happening, but it certainly appeared to be happening in the real world.[107]

Some years later, an MRI brain scan showed 'Occasional punctate foci of high signal intensity ... located in the cerebral white matter of the frontal lobes bilaterally, as well as the left temporo-parietal region'.[108] He was to later refer to the cerebral foci as the 'bright objects' in his brain and includes an image from his MRI scan in a series of 'Implant Photos' published in his 1998 novel *Confirmation: The Hard Evidence of Aliens Among Us*, as part of the 'hard evidence' for alien intervention into human life.[109] The foci, as Eve LaPlante argues, are also suggestive of scarring that could generate paroxysmal activity typically associated with temporal lobe phenomena.[110] At this point in time, Strieber declined further testing.

Strieber's rejection of a medical explanation for his phenomenological states gestures to the inadequacy of the model to account for his subjective experience. Like Arthur Myers a century before him, he appears to be searching for another way of living with temporal lobe phenomena, a way that will take him beyond a normal/pathological (good/evil) opposition – beyond the identity category 'epileptic'. His attempt is astutely attuned to wider cultural experiences of estrangement. He claims to receive 'fifty letters some days' from readers all describing experiences similar to his.[111] In a reversal of Dostoevsky's strategy of displacing epilepsy symptoms onto non-epileptic characters in his fiction, response to Strieber's narrative suggests that the signifiers of spasmodically disturbed identity are already there, disseminated throughout the North American population.

A Roper poll conducted in North America from July through to September 1991 concluded that nearly four million citizens had experienced 'indications' of alien abduction. The authors of the poll, which was published in 1992, are named as Bud Hopkins (painter and sculptor), David Jacobs (historian) and Ron Westrum (sociologist). John Mack, Pulitzer Prize winner and a professor of psychiatry at Harvard Medical School, wrote the introduction for the publication, in which he argued that hundreds of thousands of American men, women and children had been affected by UFO abduction and that clinical practitioners should educate themselves to 'the most common symptoms and indications in the patient or client's history' that point to mental health problems resulting from abduction.[112] A similar study in England found that subjects polled acquired knowledge of alien life forms from reading and watching television. Susan Blackmore points out that her own research would seem to nullify the Roper report findings. Although a stringent critical comparison of the two studies cannot definitively 'prove that no real abductions are occurring on this planet', she concludes that the North American evidence on abduction 'is false'.[113]

In her study of what she calls 'hysterical epidemics' in modern culture, Showalter argues that the alien abduction genre is one of the more recent 'hystories' in a tradition of personal narratives about social dislocation.

> Hysteria not only survives in the 1990s, it is more contagious than in the past. Infectious diseases spread by ecological change, modern technology, urbanization, jet travel, and human interaction. Infectious epidemics of hysteria spread by stories circulated through self-help books, articles in newspapers and magazines, TV talk shows and series, films, the Internet, and even literary criticism. The cultural narratives of hysteria, which I call *hystories*, multiply rapidly and uncontrollably in the era of mass media, telecommunications, and e-mail.[114]

She argues that the alien abduction narrative is highly conventionalised, having been shaped and validated since the 1970s by journalists and professionally invested academics like Professor John Mack and Professor David Jacobs, a historian at Temple University in Philadelphia. Although Strieber's accounts of altered states tangentially connect with many of the stories gathered by researchers such as Hopkins, Mack and Jacobs, Showalter argues that he is deemed an unreliable witness of his experiences. So much so that even Hopkins at one point evinced some doubt as to the veracity of Strieber's claims.[115]

While repeatedly proclaiming a qualified receptiveness to medical investigation and diagnostic procedures, Strieber simultaneously expresses his fear of brain anomaly, repeatedly stating 'I am not a temporal-lobe epileptic'. It is unclear whether Strieber is refuting a medical definition of what that entails – that is, the medical stereotype of 'the epileptic' – or whether he is claiming that there is no neurophysiological explanation for the phenomena he experiences. In utterly refusing the subject position of 'epileptic', he argues that a medical explanation 'could not account for the elaborate experiences [he] had undergone. Only a full-scale epilepsy could account for them.'[116] What is 'full-scale epilepsy'? It is an oddly uninformed statement from one who claims to have done so much research into the subject. Evidently after the possibility of temporal lobe epilepsy had been broached, Strieber read the medical literature on the subject and extended his reading to Dostoevsky's autobiographical and fictional accounts of the phenomena associated with the epilepsies. These genres of writing all attest to the elaborate detail of some temporal lobe phenomena.

On one level, *Communion* can be read as an autobiographical account of Strieber's attempt to re-articulate an experience for which there is no language but medical language. On another level, it reads as an analogy for its time and culture. That he finds medical language an unsatisfactory medium is evidenced by his statement that a medical explanation could not possibly capture or account for the rich detail of his experience. *Communion* is also riddled with sly allusions to a wider cultural disaffection with late twentieth-century medicine. Strieber's sense of helplessness when he is being studied by the aliens suggests a disempowerment akin to that experienced by patients undergoing some of the neurological testing procedures discussed above. Of visiting a research facility in San Antonio in his earlier years he writes:

> I saw monkey cages with rows of doctored capuchins, shaved, their pink heads sewn or laid delicately open, and the trembling brain probes and the gabble of noise when the vocalization center of one of them was stimulated for the information of graduate students. What did the monkey with the needle in its brain think of its observers? Were they gods to whom it submitted itself with a noble passivity because it could do nothing else?[117]

Is this what Strieber is resisting after all? The possibility of being just another primate with a 'needle in its brain'? And if so, why is this image any less confronting than being transported to an alien ship and being just another primate having an involuntary colon biopsy?

Strieber's irritating tendency to inconsistency while claiming reasoned argument would have us believe that the latter is infinitely preferable. He writes of protesting the colon biopsy procedure by telling an alien proctologist 'You have no right'. 'We do have a right' is the response:

> 'We do have a right.' Five enormous words. Stunning words. *We do have a right*. Who gave it to them? By what progress of ethics had they arrived at that conclusion? I wondered if it required debate, or seemed so obvious to them that they never questioned it.[118]

Although acknowledging a vague similarity between the laboratory monkeys in San Antonio and his own experience as an involuntary test subject, he concludes: 'Try as I might, I simply did not have the feeling that the visitors were applying the same cold ethic to their relationship with us as we did to ours with the animals'.[119] It is difficult to understand how this conclusion is supported by his observation that the aliens refuse to acknowledge that their test subjects have any rights superseding their own. Like Mesulam's laboratory monkeys, Strieber is wont to show an 'uncharacteristic friendliness' towards the agents of his experimental status.

Commenting on the alien abduction narrative that he has deployed to articulate his experiences, Strieber claims: 'I see no evidence that the visitors are real physical beings. I haven't the faintest idea what they really are. What interests me is what I do with my perceptions, not their origin. I resist explaining what happened to me.'[120] The last aspect of this claim seems disingenuous. Of course he attempts to 'explain' what happened to him – not only in *Communion* but also in the sequels elaborating his experiences – *Transformation: The Breakthrough*; *Confirmation: The Hard Evidence of Aliens Among Us*; *The Secret School: Preparation for Contact*; *The Grays* – and his website, 'Whitley Strieber's Unknown Country: daily news of the edge'.

In his journal entry to the website for 7 January 2009, 'The blue light', Strieber writes of his vivid and 'very peculiar dreams' of the night before, where he seemed to be searching among friends and relatives for 'something ... that I could not quite find'. He moves from discussion about the pain in his ear caused by the implant put there in 1989 to a contemplation of the sacred: that deep desire to 'understand' the 'grandeur of God.... Find the creator of the blue light, for example, and ask what has been done and why.'[121] In his entry for 30 January 2009, he insists that, despite books like *Communion*, he has come to no conclusions about his own experiences: 'for the simple reason that there is no scientific basis, as yet, for such conclusions'.[122] His journal entries are layered with complex meaning and convey both a sense of yearning for the something that has been lost (perhaps the comforting predictability of his psychic life prior to 1985?) and a stringent awareness of the limits of scientific narratives to provide satisfactory explanations for the phenomena he experiences.

In refusing a pathologised subject position and the therapeutic response that a diagnosis of epilepsy often demands, it might be argued that Strieber is taking a lead from Dostoevsky. By exploiting his dis-ease artistically and choosing instead to mythologise his altered states, Strieber's chosen response to his experiences attempts to negotiate a re-evaluation of his symptomatology. Obviously his account of prolonged periods of disempowerment, abjection, psychological fragmentation and feelings of being invaded by an alien force articulate some truth about cerebral phenomena as inflected by late twentieth-century North American cultural experience. Of his own decision to live his phenomenological experiences as he does, Strieber has said:

> It's a terribly important and fundamentally human experience – perceptions that come from the level of mind that isn't interrupted by the rational structures that animate most of our thought. It's a kind of memory, a form of perception, or a mechanism of consciousness, something inexplicable that the mind attaches an explanation to, probably the same thing that caused people to believe in the old gods and myths, in angels, resurrection, and even UFOs today.... It probably starts in the human mind.[123]

Voskuil noted that Dostoevsky's personality, intellectual life and cultural influences all significantly mediated how he experienced and interpreted the phenomenological aspects of his paroxysmal condition.[124]

XI

Despite appearing across a diversity of genres and time frames, representations of the epileptic figure discussed throughout this and other chapters perpetuate a tradition. But what is myth? And what is matter? Is all human experience, including illness and differentiated physical and psychological function, already so intextuated by master narrative systems that to extract authentic experience from the static of validated signifiers risks incoherence? It seems to me that this issue forms around the historically entrenched impulse within western medicine to conflate the neurological with the phenomenological. It is an impulse that seems to be at the heart of Khoshbin's medicalised account of Reen Carter's experiences and the brain mapping project being advanced by Michael Persinger (see Introduction).

Whether Strieber's altered states are due to neurological or extra-terrestrial disturbances remains open to debate. Despite experiencing similar phenomena on occasion, I remain unconvinced by his arguments for the latter possibility. However, his obvious dissatisfaction with medical explanations for the richness and 'reality' of his subjective experience has precedence in the experiences of Arthur Myers and Dostoevsky. Frederic Myers' efforts to find an explanation for the phenomenological experiences that, for his brother, Arthur, were named 'epileptic' generated controversy. Medical opinion on Frederic's research group, the Society for Psychical Research, was, as I have argued in Chapter 3, unreservedly vitriolic. Dostoevsky, while acknowledging the abject limits of some forms of epilepsy experience, tried to find ways to map the transcendent pleasures of other forms onto everyday lived experience. While he acknowledged the 'downside' of his seizure condition, he chose to walk a fine line between managing these more negative aspects and experiencing the more pleasurable without medication. His representations of ecstatic aura were persuasive enough to influence medical thinking. While we might question the applicability of the strategies adopted by Frederic Myers and Strieber, it is impossible to remain unsympathetic to the motivations fuelling their respective endeavours.

Susan Sontag insists that illness is not a metaphor, and yet medical writers persist in drawing on metaphor to enrich representation. Lauren Slater not only leaps unashamedly into the debate about the play of figurative language in medical discourse and illness narratives in her book *Spasm: A Memoir with Lies*, she ups the ante with a proliferation of metaphorical epilepsies. Slater says of her own illness experience that it was 'more than a physical thing; it was also a metaphor', and it is the metaphor that helps her 'make some sense' of it all.[125]

> I have epilepsy. Or I feel I have epilepsy. Or I wish I had epilepsy, so I could find a way of explaining the dirty, spastic glittering place I had in my mother's heart. Epilepsy is a fascinating disease because some epileptics are liars, exaggerators, makers of myths and high-flying stories. Doctors don't know why this is, something to do, maybe, with the way a scar on the brain dents memory or mutates reality. My epilepsy started with the smell of jasmine, and that smell moved into my mouth. And when I opened my mouth after that, all my words seemed colored, and I don't know where this is my mother or where this is my illness, or whether, like her, I am just confusing fact with fiction, and there is no epilepsy, just a clenched metaphor, a way of telling you what I have to tell you: my tale.[126]

For Slater, epilepsy functions in this text as a figurative representation of psychic fragmentation; a metaphor for maternal ambivalence;

a pathologised mimesis of coitus. She jerks: in literary, if not literal, spasm. She jerks us – the reader – around, playing promiscuously with our understanding of her meaning. In travelling the borderlands demarcated by the signifiers of epilepsy, she repeatedly transgresses the boundaries. Her epilepsy is simultaneously over-determined and leached of defining stability. It cannot be 'fixed'.

What *is* epilepsy? Having asked this question several times and in various ways in the preceding chapters, have the texts discussed so far yielded a definitive answer? Is it merely the sum total of a sequence of neurophysiological events that momentarily seize an individual in an attitude of bemazement? A catastrophic firing off of neurones that can propel people to lofty serenity or plummet them to the lowest mode of existence? An out-take of psycho-sexual trauma? The consequence of corrupted blood? Stress? To what degree is it defined by the social relations and competing power structures specific to a particular time and culture? Can it be all of these, overlaid with a thick veneer of symbolic and cultural meaning? Is it even possible to begin to understand epilepsy beyond its metaphors and myths and subjective particularities? In some sense, I think it is. At least some of the time.

Arthur Myers died in the borderlands, unable to find a metaphor that could carry him beyond a normal/abnormal opposition – beyond good and evil. Dostoevsky found a way to work with the medical language that figured him as pathologised, while simultaneously subverting the medico-social connotations of symptomatic signifiers. In the second half of the twentieth century, medicine, in the quest for a more clearly defined understanding of the matter, focused its efforts on definitively locating and fixing an epileptic threshold in the human brain. Curtis became fatally mired in a matrix of negative signification and draconian pharmaceutical regimes that precluded him from coming to grips with this aspect of his life. Strieber responded to the oppositional bind by categorically denying the possibility of epilepsy and shifting the debate off world. Slater presents a plethora of signifying possibilities that resist categorisation. The question remains: where will the circuit of culture locate epilepsy and those who experience any one of the multiple forms of cerebral paroxysm in twenty-first century narratives?

Notes

1 Raymond Chandler. *The Big Sleep*. 1939. New York: Random House, 1988.

2 Quoted in Lisa Cartwright. *Screening the Body: Tracing Medicine's Visual Culture*. 1995. Minneapolis, MN: University of Minnesota Press, 1997, p. 59.

3 Quoted in Cartwright, *Screening the Body*, p. 60.

4 Frederic A. Gibbs. 'William Gordon Lennox: 1884–1960'. *Epilepsia*, vol. 2, 1961, p. 1.

5 Quoted in Gibbs, 'William Gordon Lennox', p. 1.
6 William Gordon Lennox. *Epilepsy and Related Disorders.* 2 vols. London: Churchill, 1960, vol. 2, p. 779.
7 Lennox, *Epilepsy and Related Disorders*, vol. 2, pp. 779–84; J. Feuerstein, D. Kurtz and F. Rohmer. 'Activation by means of Megimide: indications, value, and limits in the electroencephalographic diagnosis of epilepsy'. *Epilepsia*, vol. 7, 1966, pp. 220–27.
8 See, for example: A. Schulze-Bonhage and C. E. Elger. 'Induction of partial epileptic seizures by flumazenil'. *Epilepsia*, vol. 41, no. 2, February 2000, pp. 186–92.
9 Lennox, *Epilepsy and Related Disorders*, vol. 2, p. 780.
10 F. Cirignotta, C. V. Todesco and E. Lugaresi. 'Temporal lobe epilepsy with ecstatic seizure (so-called Dostoevsky epilepsy)'. *Epilepsia*, vol. 21, 1980, pp. 705–10.
11 P. H. A. Voskuil. 'The epilepsy of Fyodor Mikhailovitch Dostoevsky (1821–1881)'. *Epilepsia*, vol. 24, 1983, pp. 658–67.
12 Henri Gastaut. 'New comments on the epilepsy of Fyodor Dostoevsky'. *Epilepsia*, vol. 25, 1984, pp. 408–11. His renunciation of his original theory appeared as 'Fyodor Mikhailovitch Dostoevsky's involuntary contribution to the symptomatology and prognosis of epilepsy'. *Epilepsia*, vol. 19, 1978, pp. 186–201. Gastaut's acceptance and then rejection of Dostoevsky's claims is discussed in Chapter 3.
13 David Armstrong. *Political Anatomy of the Body: Medical Knowledge in Britain in the Twentieth Century.* Cambridge: Cambridge University Press, 1983, p. 2.
14 M. Fischer-Williams, R. G. Bickford and J. P. Whisnant. 'Occipito-parieto-temporal seizure discharge with visual hallucinations and aphasia'. *Epilepsia*, vol. 5, 1964, p. 281.
15 Fischer-Williams, 'Occipito-parieto-temporal seizure discharge', p. 282.
16 Fischer-Williams, 'Occipito-parieto-temporal seizure discharge', p. 280.
17 Fischer-Williams, 'Occipito-parieto-temporal seizure discharge', p. 282.
18 Fischer-Williams, 'Occipito-parieto-temporal seizure discharge', p. 282.
19 Fischer-Williams, 'Occipito-parieto-temporal seizure discharge', p. 285.
20 Fischer-Williams, 'Occipito-parieto-temporal seizure discharge', p. 286.
21 Fischer-Williams, 'Occipito-parieto-temporal seizure discharge', p. 285.
22 Fischer-Williams, 'Occipito-parieto-temporal seizure discharge', p. 285.
23 Fischer-Williams, 'Occipito-parieto-temporal seizure discharge', p. 281.
24 A. Hughes Bennett. 'An inquiry into the effects of the prolonged administration of the bromides in epilepsy'. *Lancet*, 17 May 1884, p. 884.
25 Quote from an unnamed physician commenting on the adverse side-effects of prolonged high-dosage bromide administration, cited in Owsei Temkin. *The Falling Sickness: A History of Epilepsy from the Greeks to the Beginnings of Modern Neurology*. 2nd edition, revised. Baltimore, MD: John Hopkins University Press, 1971, p. 299.
26 Jean-Martin Charcot. 'Hysteroepilepsy: a young woman with a convulsive attack in the auditorium. February 7, 1888'. In *Charcot the Clinician: The Tuesday Lessons.* Trans. and commentary Christopher G. Goetz. New York: Raven, 1987, p. 106.
27 D. F. Scott. *The History of Epileptic Therapy: An Account of How Medication Was Developed.* Nashville, TN: Parthenon, 1993, p. 7.
28 Scott, *The History of Epileptic Therapy*, pp. 8–9.
29 *Oxford Dictionary of English Etymology.* 1966. Ed. C. T. Onions, *et al.* Oxford: Clarendon, 1967.
30 Julia Kristeva. *Powers of Horror: An Essay on Abjection.* Trans. Leon S. Roudiez. New York: Columbia University Press, 1982, p. 3.

31 Scott, *The History of Epileptic Therapy*, pp. 9–10.
32 Lennox, *Epilepsy and Related Disorders*, vol. 2, p. 791.
33 Lennox, *Epilepsy and Related Disorders*, vol. 2, p. 791.
34 Christopher Ounsted, Janet Lindsay and Peronelle Richards. *Temporal Lobe Epilepsy 1948–1986: A Biographical Study*. London: MacKeith Press, 1987, p. 118.
35 Ounsted *et al.*, *Temporal Lobe Epilepsy*, p. 118.
36 Ounsted *et al.*, *Temporal Lobe Epilepsy*, p. 10 (italics added).
37 Ounsted *et al.*, *Temporal Lobe Epilepsy*, p. 120 (italics added).
38 M.-Marsel Mesulam. 'Neural substrates of behaviour: the effects of brain lesions upon mental state', in Armand Nicholi and J. R. Nicholi, eds. *The New Harvard Guide to Psychiatry*. Cambridge, MA: Belknap-Harvard University Press, 1988, p. 100.
39 Mesulam, 'Neural substrates of behaviour', p. 100.
40 Mesulam, 'Neural substrates of behaviour', p. 101.
41 Mesulam, 'Neural substrates of behaviour', p. 101.
42 Mesulam, 'Neural substrates of behaviour', p. 101.
43 *MIMS Australia*, vol. 35, no. 5, October/November 1988, pp. 107–11.
44 Ounsted *et al.*, *Temporal Lobe Epilepsy*, p. 120.
45 Adrienne Richard and Joel Reiter. *Epilepsy: A New Approach*. 2nd edition. New York: Walker, 1995, pp. 53–54.
46 Richard and Reiter, *Epilepsy*, p. 58.
47 Richard and Reiter, *Epilepsy*, p. 68.
48 Richard and Reiter, *Epilepsy*, p. 57.
49 Richard and Reiter, *Epilepsy*, pp. 53–54.
50 Anne Fadiman. *The Spirit Catches You and You Fall Down: A Hmong Child, Her American Doctors, and the Clash of Two Cultures*. 1997. New York: Noonday Press, 1999.
51 Fadiman, *The Spirit Catches You*, p. 53.
52 Fadiman, *The Spirit Catches You*, p. 53.
53 Fadiman, *The Spirit Catches You*, p. 88.
54 Fadiman, *The Spirit Catches You*, p. 143.
55 Fadiman, *The Spirit Catches You*, p. 256 (original italics).
56 Fadiman, *The Spirit Catches You*, p. 255.
57 Fadiman, *The Spirit Catches You*, p. 262.
58 Byron J. Good. *Medicine, Rationality, and Experience: An Anthropological Perspective*. Cambridge: Cambridge University Press, 1994, p. 5.
59 Fadiman, *The Spirit Catches You*, p. 54.
60 Fadiman, *The Spirit Catches You*, p. 143.
61 Fadiman, *The Spirit Catches You*, pp. 211–12.
62 Fadiman, *The Spirit Catches You*, p. 273.
63 *RPA*. Medical documentary series. Nine Network, Australia, 1999.
64 Richard and Reiter, *Epilepsy*, p. 15.
65 Oliver Sacks, *The Man Who Mistook His Wife For a Hat*, 1985. London: Picador, 1986, pp. 171–73. See also: *An Anthropologist on Mars*, Sydney: Picador, 1999, especially pp. 179–232.
66 Richard and Reiter, *Epilepsy*, pp. 52–54, 79–80.
67 John Hughlings Jackson. 'Observations on the localisation of movements in the cerebral hemisphere, as revealed in cases of convulsion, chorea, and "aphasia"', 1873, in James Taylor, ed. *Selected Writings of John Hughlings Jackson*. 2 vols. London: Hodder and Stoughton, 1932, vol. 1, p. 79.
68 Cartwright, *Screening the Body*, p. 17.

69 Gerry Turcotte. '"Speaking the formula of abjection": hybrids and Gothic discourses in Louis Nowra's novels.' *Westerly*, vol. 3, September 1991, pp. 61–72.
70 Louis Nowra. *The Golden Age*. 1985. Introduction Gerry Turcotte. Sydney: Currency Press, 1992, p. 36.
71 Kristeva, *Powers of Horror*, p. 3.
72 Quoted in Gerry Turcotte. '"Perfecting the monologue of silence": an interview with Louis Nowra'. *Kunapipi*, vol. 9, no. 3, 1987, p. 54.
73 Nowra, *The Golden Age*, p. 46.
74 Martin F. Norden. *Cinema of Isolation: A History of Physical Disability in the Movies*. New Brunswick, NJ: Rutgers University Press, 1994, pp. 236–37.
75 Sallie Baxendale. 'Epilepsy at the movies: possession to presidential assassination'. *Lancet Neurology*, vol. 2, December 2003, p. 764.
76 Baxendale, 'Epilepsy at the movies', p. 770.
77 Jennie F. Kerson, Toba Schwaber Kerson and Lawrence A. Kerson. 'The depiction of seizures in film'. *Epilepsia*, vol. 40, no. 8, 1999, p. 1167.
78 *American Gothic*. Prod. Shaun Cassidy, *et al*. Perf. Gary Cole, Lucas Black, Paige Turco, Brenda Bakke, Sarah Paulson. CBS, 1995.
79 *Drugstore Cowboy*. Dir. Gus Van Sant. Perf. Matt Dillon, Kelly Lynch, James LeGros, Heather Graham. Avenue Pictures Production, 1989.
80 *The Fugitive*. Dir. Andrew Davis. Perf. Harrison Ford, Tommy Lee Jones, Sela Ward, Julianne Moore. Screenplay Jeb Stuart and David Twohy. Warner Bros. Pictures, 1993.
81 *Seinfeld*. 'The Good Samaritan'. Writer Peter Mehlman. Episode 37, Season 3, 1992.
82 Zarko Martinovic and Jasna Martinovic. 'Ian Curtis: epilepsy and creativity of a rock musician'. Abstract. Third European Congress of Epileptology. Warsaw, Poland, 24–28 May 1998. *Epilepsia*, vol. 39, suppl. 2, 1998, p. 113.
83 James L. Rice. *Dostoevsky and the Healing Art: An Essay in Literary and Medical History*. Ann Arbor, MI: Ardis, 1985, p. 234.
84 *Control*. Dir. Anton Corbijn. Perf. Sam Riley, Samantha Morton, Alexandra Maria Lara, Joe Anderson. Writers Deborah Curtis and Matt Greenhalgh. Based on the novel by Deborah Curtis, *Touching from a Distance*. Three Dogs and a Pony, 2007.
85 Friedrich Nietzsche. *The Portable Nietzsche*. Ed. and trans. Walter Kaufman. New York: Viking Penguin, 1982, pp. 242–45.
86 Jon Savage. 'Dark star: the final days of Ian Curtis by his Joy Division bandmates'. *Independent*, 7 October 2007.
87 *Joy Division*. Dir. Grant Gee. Writer Jon Savage. Prod. Tom Astor, Tom Altencio, Jacqui Edenbrow. Madman Films, Brown Owl Films, 2007.
88 Dostoevsky quoted in Gastaut, 'Fyodor Mikhailovitch Dostoevsky's involuntary contribution', p. 188.
89 *The Big Sleep*. Dir. and prod. Howard Hawks. Perf. Humphrey Bogart, Lauren Bacall, Martha Vickers. Screenplay William Faulker, Leigh Brackett, Jules Furthman. Based on the novel by Raymond Chandler. Warner Bros., 1946.
90 *The Big Sleep*. Dir. Michael Winner. Prod. Elliott Kastner and Michael Winner. Perf. Robert Mitchum, Sarah Miles, Candy Clark. Screenplay Michael Winner. United Artists, 1978.
91 *The Andromeda Strain*. Dir. and prod. Robert Wise. Perf. David Wayne, James Olson, Kate Reid. From the novel by Michael Crichton. Universal Pictures, 1971.
92 *Romper Stomper*. Dir. Geoffrey Wright. Prod. Daniel Scharf and Ian Pringle.

Perf. Russell Crowe, Daniel Pollock, Jacqueline McKenzie. Australian Film Commission and Film Victoria, 1992.

93 Elaine Showalter. *Hystories: Hysterical Epidemics and Modern Culture.* 1997. London: Picador, 1998, p. 101.

94 Ounsted *et al.*, *Temporal Lobe Epilepsy*, p. 4.

95 Callois quoted in Elizabeth Grosz. *Volatile Bodies: Toward a Corporeal Feminism.* Sydney: Allen and Unwin, 1994, p. 47 (italics added).

96 Mesulam, 'Neural substrates of behaviour', pp. 101, 104.

97 *The X Files*. 'Fallen angel'. Episode 9, Season 1, 1993–94.

98 *The X Files*. 'Pusher'. Episode 17, Season 3, 1995–96.

99 *Deceiver.* Written and dir. Jonas and Joshua Pate. Perf. Tim Roth, Chris Penn, Michael Rooker, Renee Zellweger. MDP Worldwide, 1997.

100 Whitley Strieber. *Communion: Encounters with the Unknown. A True Story*. London: Arrow Books, 1987, p. 13.

101 Strieber, *Communion*, p. 20.

102 Strieber, *Communion*, p. 24.

103 Strieber, *Communion*, p. 24.

104 Strieber, *Communion*, p. 26.

105 Strieber, *Communion*, p. 30.

106 Strieber, *Communion*, p. 33.

107 Strieber, *Communion*, pp. 128–29.

108 Whitley Strieber. *Confirmation: The Hard Evidence of Aliens Among Us*. London: Simon and Schuster, 1998, p. 160.

109 Strieber, *Confirmation*, p. 221.

110 Eve LaPlante. *Seized.* New York: HarperCollins, 1993, p. 107.

111 Quoted in LaPlante, *Seized*, p. 108.

112 B. Hopkins, D. M. Jacobs and R. Westrum. *Unusual Personal Experiences: An Analysis of Data from Three National Surveys Conducted by the Roper Organization.* Las Vegas, NV: Bigelow Holding Corporation, 1992, p. 8.

113 Susan Blackmore. 'Abduction by aliens or sleep paralysis?' *Skeptical Enquirer*, vol. 22, no. 3, May–June 1998. Accessed via Expanded Academic Index online, 15 January 2000, p. 5.

114 Showalter, *Hystories*, p. 5.

115 Showalter, *Hystories*, p. 198.

116 Strieber, *Communion*, p. 130.

117 Strieber, *Communion*, p. 108.

118 Strieber, *Communion*, p. 107.

119 Strieber, *Communion*, p. 108.

120 Quoted in LaPlante, *Seized*, p. 108.

121 'The blue light'. Whitley Strieber's Unknown Country: daily news of the edge, 7 January 2009. http://www.unknowncountry.com/journal. Accessed 10 February 2009.

122 '"Virtual" UFO disclosure already here'. Whitley Strieber's Unknown Country: daily news of the edge, 30 January 2009. http://www.unknowncountry.com/journal. Accessed 14 February 2009.

123 Quoted in LaPlante, *Seized*, pp. 108–9.

124 Voskuil, 'The epilepsy of Fyodor Mikhailovitch Dostoevsky', p. 664.

125 Lauren Slater. *Spasm: A Memoir with Lies*. London: Methuen, 2000, p. 156.

126 Slater, *Spasm*, pp. 5–6.

Where to next? The ongoing story of epilepsy

The epilepsies, like all other changes to physical and psychological health, are always experienced within a specific historical and cultural context. The specificities of these contexts will not only colour how an epilepsy is experienced and lived but also influence medical interpretations and responses to the syndrome: what the epilepsies meant to the physicians of ancient Greece is clearly not the same as their signification for the apostles of Jesus when he heals the afflicted son of a follower in the mountains of Bethsaida almost 500 years later. Within the spatiality of a late nineteenth-century mill, the seized body invokes a range of social responses, prohibitions and cultural meanings absent from these earlier interpretations. Similarly, understanding of epilepsy syndromes varies considerably between the neurologists of the late nineteenth century and their twenty-first-century counterparts.

The past twenty years or so have seen a large field of scholarship develop around social and culturally differentiated interpretations of illness, disease and what has become known in medical sociology as 'illness behaviour'. It is argued in this field of scholarship that the signification and experiences of illness and illness roles are understood and internalised (naturalised) through complex cultural and social processes. The research of Christopher Ounsted and his team affords insight here: 'Biographies and diseases can be understood only in the context of the historical period in which they occur'.[1] Theorists such as Oliver Sacks, Lisa Cartwright, Tom Shakespeare, Lennard Davis, Rosemarie Garland Thomson, Arthur Kleinman and Byron Good, to name just a few, have set about examining the relationships between medicine, disease and disability by analysing western medicine and its wider cultural framework, and examine the cultural contexts in which disease and disability are lived, comprehended and treated. Questions about the compliance of folk with chronic health problems such as diabetes, schizophrenia and epilepsy – those conditions with recommended therapeutic regimes – form a distinct and important area of concern for health care professionals. For example, what constitutes medical responsibility for a patient who, for various reasons, refuses to take long-term medication for a diagnosed disorder? What are the physician's duties of administration, if any, in the ongoing care of that patient? What are the medico-legal ramifications for the physician when a patient presents in medical crisis because of non-compliance with therapeutic regimes? What constitutes medical authority and when does it cross the boundaries into authoritarianism?

The ethical dilemmas posed by these questions represent a fraught site for physicians, not least in relation to increased medical litigation in many western countries. When the physician's dilemmas about the parameters of ethical care and responsibility come into conflict with a dissenting patient's autonomy or sovereignty, the convergence is usually volatile for all concerned and, quite often, traumatic. The dogmatic moral function of neurology in relation to the epilepsies had become a well established feature of western medicine by the early twentieth century. In part, this was due to the fashion of moral management so characteristic of British, American and Australian physicians of the day. However, it is also fair to claim that the medical language of epilepsy constructs a subject radically incapable of sustained self-awareness and self-management. This prevalent version of the social realities of epilepsy, twinned with the belief that the syndrome was one of the more intractable and fragmenting misfortunes to befall a person, not only invited but in fact demanded vigorous medical intervention and surveillance. A palpable impulse if not to morally manage the patient with epilepsy then at least to police medically mediated self-control persists into the twentieth-first century.

The neurophysiologically affected body can be disruptive and chaotic. It is also, and always, culturally and historically situated. Both over-determined and, in crucial ways, under-theorised, it is gendered, ethnicised, inscribed through the discourses of class and sexual orientation. Furthermore, up until that moment of diagnosis or embodied gesture of pathology, the body prone to the effects of sudden neuronal discharge is often perceived as abled or normal within dominant defining regimes. This ability to pass within the dominant regimes of signification and social orthodoxy generates a climate of suspicion and distrust for the subject marked by signs of cerebral paroxysm. More often than not, the legacy generated by the presence of those with epilepsy in a community includes a significant level of medical and social discomfort. Of course, once identification or diagnosis occurs, then the subject with epilepsy becomes fixed within the discursive mappings of the re-inscripted body. Once interpellated as 'epileptic', this body will then be subject to a range of social, medical and juridical prohibitions, regardless of the intensity or specificity of symptomatology. In Foucauldian terms, categorisation as epileptic incurs a range of regulatory practices with the facility to produce and govern. Like all marginalising categories in this type of system of production, demarcation and circulation, the category 'epileptic' is both reductive and exclusionary.

As the projects using chemical activation techniques begun in the 1950s gained momentum, Robert Efron was articulating the need for twentieth-century medicine to retain an awareness of patient safety in treatment regimes. His ideas do not seem to have found a particularly receptive audience within his profession until rediscovered some years after initial publication by Adrienne Richard in a search for alternative approaches to dealing with her own epilepsy. In her co-authored book with Joel Reiter, *Epilepsy: A New Approach,* she revisits Efron's work at length and ponders its disappearance from the main body of medical literature about the subject. As the twentieth century came to a close, Reiter was one of the few medical practitioners working in clinical neurophysiology who was prepared to explore a variety of methods *with* his patients to afford them the most valuable regime for living well with their tendency to neuronal paroxysm.

Reiter factors patients' subjective and physiological responses to treatment regimes into refining and personalising each phase of the therapeutic process. The methods he draws on include bio-feedback and various behavioural approaches. While he is interested in establishing control over neuronal paroxysm in the accepted biomedical sense, he is not convinced that medicine has or can provide all the answers for those who experience paroxysmal conditions. He also dares to question the cost–benefit equation of current orthodox treatment regimes. 'In recommending [a behavioural] approach', he rather wryly notes, 'I differ from the majority of my neurological colleagues'.[2] Unsurprising. Reiter's methods are predicated on an ultimately self-knowing, self-monitored, self-managed subject.

Richard's late twentieth-century intervention into medical talk about epilepsy as an affected advocate represents what has been, until fairly recently, an under-valued source of productive dialogue between the medical profession and those it treats. Richard has worked closely with receptive neurologists to negotiate a treatment regime that allows her to live well with a cerebral paroxysmal condition. She argues that it is through a rigorously developed understanding of their own condition, and the interactions (both positive and negative) of their bodies with medical and non-medical regimes, that those with a paroxysmal condition can increase their self-control. 'Epilepsy has not yielded to ... newer medical practices', she observes; 'Why it hasn't ... is a function partly of its history'.[3] This history has too often failed to engage the affected subject in a *mutually productive* dialogue. Dialogue of the type suggested by Richard's work has the potential to produce new knowledges about what it means to live with an epilepsy *and* the consequences of current therapeutic regimes drawn upon to treat the conditions. It also widens the scope of the medical gaze beyond paroxysmal symptomatology, to take in the view from the borderlands.

Brain mapping projects begun in the late nineteenth century continue into the twenty-first century, the work of Khoshbin and Persinger being key examples. Sophisticated imaging technology now augments the medical gaze. Much of the research conducted with this technology still attempts to formalise connections between mental activity, subjective experience and brain structure. These mapping projects draw critical engagement from within the boundaries of neuroscience as well as from other disciplinary perspectives. Elizabeth Wilson, for example, argues that the latter-day mapping projects reproduce the Cartesian dualism integral to the earlier projects:

> Rather than being simply inscriptive over an otherwise innocent organ, these mappings are constitutive of the brain itself. It is the hierarchical effects issuing forth from a generalized mind–body dualism that have materialized the neuropsychological brain as intelligible matter. The brain of contemporary neuropsychology is not a simple factual object. It has been constituted scientifically via the division of body from brain, and between upper cortex and lower brain stem; so too it is constituted via the dualistic relations of mind and body, intellect and emotion.[4]

Despite the instability of meaning and conceptual boundaries argued for above, most western medical practitioners in the early twentieth-first century would claim that they understand what is meant when they talk about epilepsy, and that they have access to a well developed prognostic picture of what epilepsy means for the persona of the affected individual. Most would claim to have a professionally reasonable idea of what the appropriate medical responses to the epileptic patient should be. Yet certain standard medical responses to the epilepsies (and the 'epileptic') have long been subjected to critical scrutiny from within medicine itself. The concerns expressed by late nineteenth-century physicians such as Joseph Williams, J. Thompson Dickson, Hughlings Jackson and William Broadbent failed to change the direction of medical engagement with 'the epileptic' because, as a representational device, this figure neatly conflated troublesome differences and erased irresolvable tensions between a textual rendering that promised containment, if not clarity, and an intractable corporeal resistance to precise definition.

Throughout this book I have raised questions about the relations between western medicine and those with paroxysmal conditions known as epilepsy. I make the claim that there is a belief encoded in the medical practices reviewed through the preceding chapters that the presence of any of the epilepsies is so catastrophic to human function that any response, diagnostic or therapeutic, is justifiable. This philosophical condition of medicine, when overlaid with the frustration of a physician unable to curtail a patient's seizures, generates some profoundly problematic issues for western biomedicine and those of us who access its services, not least when it comes to the matter of thinking through what possible costs these diagnostic and treatment practices might entail for the one affected.

There is no doubt that some manifestations of epilepsy present physicians with a range of medical problems and medical emergencies that demand all the skill that western medical training has to offer. There is no doubt that some forms of epilepsy have indeed benefited from the medical and pharmaceutical research of the past 150 years or more, and that individuals with these particular forms of the syndrome are able to lead more autonomous lives because of those developments. There is no doubt that some manifestations of cerebral paroxysm *do not* benefit from current orthodox therapeutic regimes. There is no doubt that some folk with particular forms of cerebral paroxysmal conditions are *damaged* by orthodox therapeutic regimes. The problem for the physician is one of differentiation and refinement. The latter epilepsies demand a radical altering in the refraction of the medical gaze: a change in refraction that permits a clear view of what symptomatology can be rationally attributed to a cerebral paroxysmal condition that will be benefited by medical intervention, and what symptomatology is the by-product of medical intervention. Rather than continuing to focus on the epilepsy formed through the representational history examined in this book, it is time to enrich the biomedical perspective with other narratives and other possible outcomes to the diagnosis 'epileptic'.

Finally, and to return for a moment to the preoccupations identified at the beginning of this book, after exploring its genesis, how do we exorcise 'the epileptic' still haunting medical–cultural systems of representation? How do we show this figure the exit from the cultural circuit once and for all and begin developing narratives that engage differently with how we conceptualise, think about, understand, respond to, experience the epilepsies? It seems to me that at least some forward momentum can be achieved by ongoing robust and engaged conversations across disciplinary borders: by thoughtfully transgressing long-accepted boundaries, in the spirit of widening the terms of engagement and opening up new terrains of theory and practice. Hopefully, for the benefit of all.

Notes

1 Christopher Ounsted, Janet Lindsay and Peronelle Richards. *Temporal Lobe Epilepsy 1948–1986: A Biographical Study*. London: Mac Keith Press, 1987, p. 118.
2 Adrienne Richard, and Joel Reiter. *Epilepsy: A New Approach*. 2nd edition. New York: Walker, 1995, p. 51.
3 Richard and Reiter, *Epilepsy*, p. 16.
4 Elizabeth A. Wilson. *Neural Geographies: Feminism and the Microstructure of Cognition*. New York: Routledge, 1998, pp. 131–32.

Bibliography

Adams, James. 'Should epileptics marry?' *Lancet*, 20 March 1897, p. 841.

Anderson, Mabel. 'Should epileptics marry?' *Lancet*, 10 April 1897, p. 1053.

Armstrong, David. 'Foucault and the sociology of health and illness: a prismatic reading', in A. Petersen and R. Bunton, eds. *Foucault, Health and Medicine*. London: Routledge, 1997, pp. 15–30.

——. *Political Anatomy of the Body: Medical Knowledge in Britain in the Twentieth Century*. Cambridge: Cambridge University Press, 1983.

Aston, W. B. 'Abilene State School 1901–1976'. Unpublished document. Abilene, TX: Special Library, Abilene State School, 1976.

Atrens, Dale, and Ian Curthoys. *The Neurosciences and Behaviour: An Introduction*. Sydney: Academic Press, 1982.

Bakhtin, M. M. *The Dialogic Imagination: Four Essays by M. M. Bakhtin*. 1981. Trans. Caryl Emerson and Michael Holquist. Ed. Michael Holquist. Austin, TX: University of Texas Press, 1994.

Banta, Martha. *Taylored Lives: Narrative Productions in the Age of Taylor, Veblen, and Ford*. Chicago, IL: University of Chicago Press, 1993.

Barraclough, B. 'Suicide and epilepsy', in E. H. Reynolds and M. R. Trimble, eds. *Epilepsy and Psychiatry*. Edinburgh: Churchill Livingstone, 1981, pp. 72–76.

Bass, T. B. 'Epilepsy'. *Texas State Journal of Medicine*, May 1930, pp. 1–4.

Batchelor, Ivor R. C. *Henderson and Gillespie's Textbook of Psychiatry for Students and Practitioners*. 10th edition, revised. London: Oxford University Press, 1969.

Baudrillard, Jean. *Simulacra and Simulation*. Trans. Shiela Faria Glaser. Ann Arbor, MI: Michigan University Press, 2000.

Baxendale, Sallie. 'Epilepsy at the movies: possession to presidential assassination'. *Lancet Neurology*, vol. 2, December 2003, pp. 764–70.

Bear, David, and Paul Fedio. 'Quantitative analysis of interictal behaviour in temporal lobe epilepsy'. *Archives of Neurology*, vol. 34, 1977, pp. 454–67.

Bear, David M., Roy Freeman and Mark Greenberg. 'Behavioural alterations in patients with temporal lobe epilepsy', in D. Blumer, ed. *Psychiatric Aspects of Epilepsy*. Washington, DC: American Psychiatric Press, 1984, pp. 197–227.

Bear, David M., Roy Freeman, David Schiff and Mark Greenberg. 'Interictal behaviour changes in patients with temporal lobe epilepsy', in R. E. Hales and

A. J. Frances, eds. *American Psychiatric Association Annual Review 4*. Washington, DC: American Psychiatric Press, 1985.

Beaulieu, Anne. 'The brain at the end of the rainbow: the promises of brain scans in the research field and in the media', in Janine Marchessault and Kim Sawchuck, eds. *Wildscience: Reading Feminism, Medicine and the Media*. London: Routledge, 2000, pp. 39–52.

Beaumont, Pierre J. V., and R. B. Hampshire, eds. *Textbook of Psychiatry*. Melbourne: Blackwell Scientific, 1989.

Bell, Diane, and Renate Klein, eds. *Radically Speaking: Feminism Reclaimed*. North Melbourne: Spinifex Press, 1996.

Belton, John, ed. *Movies and Mass Culture*. New Brunswick, NJ: Rutgers University Press, 1996.

Bennett, A. Hughes. 'An inquiry into the effects of the prolonged administration of the bromides in epilepsy'. *Lancet*, 17 May 1884, pp. 883–84; 24 May 1884, pp. 928–30.

Bhabha, Homi, K. *The Location of Culture*. London: Routledge, 1994.

Blackmore, Susan. 'Abduction by aliens or sleep paralysis?' *Skeptical Enquirer*, vol. 22, no. 3, May–June 1998, p. 23 (7 pages). Accessed via Expanded Academic Index online, 15 January 2000.

Bleier, Ruth, ed. *Feminist Approaches to Science*. New York: Pergamon Press, 1990.

Blumer, Dietrich. 'The illness of Vincent van Gogh'. *American Journal Psychiatry*, vol. 159, no. 4, April 2002, pp. 519–526.

——, ed. *Psychiatric Aspects of Epilepsy*. Washington, DC: American Psychiatric Press, 1984.

——. 'The psychiatric dimensions of epilepsy', in Dietrich Blumer, ed. *Psychiatric Aspects of Epilepsy*. Washington, DC: American Psychiatric Press, 1984, pp. 1–65.

Bouchard, Donald F., ed. *Language, Counter-Memory, Practice: Selected Essays and Interviews*. 1977. Trans. Donald F. Bouchard and Sherry Simon. Ithaca, NY: Cornell University Press, 1980.

Bradwell, Stephen. 'Mary Glovers late woeful case, together with her joyfull deliverance', 1603. Reprinted in Michael MacDonald, *Witchcraft and Hysteria in Elizabethan London: Edward Jorden and the Mary Glover Case*. London: Tavistock/Routledge, 1991, n.p.

Braidotti, R. 'Body-images and the pornography of representation', in Kathleen Lennon and Margaret Whitford, eds. *Knowing the Difference: Feminist Perspectives in Epistemology*. New York: Routledge, 1994, pp. 17–30.

——. *Nomadic Subjects: Embodiment and Sexual Difference in Contemporary Feminist Theory*. New York: Columbia University Press, 1994.

Bramble, Forbes. *The Strange Case of Deacon Brodie*. London: Hamilton, 1975.

Bristowe, John Syer. 'Clinical remarks on pseudo-peritonitis and epilepsy in hysteria'. *British Medical Journal*, 22 February 1890, p. 401–3.

Broadbent, Sir William H. 'A lecture on epilepsy'. *British Medical Journal*, 4 January 1902, pp. 1–5.

Brown, John. 'Charles Booth and labour colonies', *Economic History Review*, 2nd series, vol. 21, 2 August 1968, pp. 349–60.

Brundage, Anthony. *The Making of the New Poor Law: The Politics of Inquiry, Enactment and Implementation, 1832–39*. London: Hutchinson, 1978.

Buchanan, Neil. *Understanding Epilepsy: What It Is and How It Can Affect Your Life*. Sydney: Simon and Schuster, 1994.

Burden, G. 'Social aspects of epilepsy'. *Epilepsia*, vol. 3, no. 2, 1962, pp. 201–4.

Butler, Judith. *Bodies That Matter: On the Discursive Limits of 'Sex'*. New York: Routledge, 1993.

——. *Gender Trouble*. New York: Routledge, 1990.

——. *The Psychic Life of Power: Theories in Subjection*. Stanford, CA: Stanford University Press, 1997.

Cartwright, Lisa. *Screening the Body: Tracing Medicine's Visual Culture*. 1995. Minneapolis, MN: University of Minnesota Press, 1997.

Catteau, Jacques. *Dostoevsky and the Process of Literary Creation*. Trans. Audrey Littlewood. Cambridge: Cambridge University Press, 1989.

Chandler, Raymond. *The Big Sleep*. 1939. New York: Random House, 1988.

Charcot, Jean-Martin. *Charcot the Clinician: The Tuesday Lessons*. Trans. and commentary Christopher G. Goetz. New York: Raven, 1987.

——. *Lectures on the Diseases of the Nervous System*. Trans. and ed. George Sigerson. New York: Hafner, 1962.

——, Paul Richer, Gilles de la Tourette and Albert Londe. *Nouvelle Iconographie de la Salpêtrière*. 4 vols. Paris: Lecrosnier et Babe, Libraires-Editeurs, 1889.

Chesler, Phyllis. *Women and Madness*. New York: Avon, 1972.

Cirignotta, F., C. V. Todesco and E. Lugaresi. 'Temporal lobe epilepsy with ecstatic seizure (so-called Dostoevsky epilepsy)'. *Epilepsia*, vol. 21, 1980, pp. 705–10.

Cixous, Hélène. 'Fiction and its phantoms: a reading of Freud's *Das Unheimliche* (the 'uncanny')'. *New Literary History*, vol. 7, no. 1, 1975, pp. 525–48.

Clark, George. *A History of the Royal College of Physicians of London*. Vol. 1. Oxford: Clarendon, 1964.

Clutterbuck, Dr. 'Lectures on the diseases of the nervous system: lecture XVI'. *Lancet*, 23 June 1826–27, pp. 353–59.

Cook, Harold John. *The Decline of the Old Medical Regime in London*. Ithaca, NY: Cornell University Press, 1986.

Cosnett, J. E. 'Charles Dickens and epilepsy'. *Epilepsia*, vol. 35, no. 4, 1994, pp. 903–5.

Crary, Jonathan, and Sanford Kwinter, eds. *Incorporations*. New York: Zone, 1995.

Creed, Barbara. *The Monstrous-Feminine: Film, Feminism, Psychoanalysis*. London: Routledge, 1993.

Critchley, Macdonald. *Sir William Gowers 1845–1915: A Biographical Appreciation*. London: Heinemann, 1949.

Critchley, Macdonald, and Eileen A. Critchley. *John Hughlings Jackson: Father of English Neurology*. Oxford: Oxford University Press, 1998.

Curtis, Deborah. *Touching from a Distance: Ian Curtis and Joy Division*. London: Faber and Faber, 1996.

Daiches, David. *Robert Louis Stevenson and His World*. London: Thames and Hudson, 1973.

Davidson, Donald. 'What metaphors mean', in Sheldon Sacks, ed. *On Metaphor*. Chicago, IL: University of Chicago Press, 1978, pp. 29–46.

Davis, Lennard J. *Bending Over Backwards: Disability, Dismodernism and Other Difficult Positions*. New York: New York University Press, 2002.

——. *Enforcing Normalcy: Disability, Deafness and the Body*. New York: Verso, 1995.

Dawkins, Richard. Transcript, 'God on the brain'. *Horizon*, BBC 2, 17 April 2003. http://www.bbc.co.uk/science/horizon/2003/godonbraintrans.shtml.

de Berdt Hovell, D. 'Hysteria simplified and explained'. *Lancet*, 20 December 1873, pp. 872–74.

de Man, Paul. 'The epistemology of metaphor', in Sheldon Sacks, ed. *On Metaphor.* Chicago, IL: University of Chicago Press, 1978, pp. 1–28.

Debus, Allen G. *The English Paracelsians.* New York: Franklin Watts, 1966.

Derrida, Jacques. *Dissemination.* 1972. Trans. and introduction Barbara Johnson. Chicago, IL: University of Chicago Press, 1981.

——. *The Gift of Death.* 1992. Trans. David Wills. Chicago, IL: University of Chicago Press, 1995.

——. *Resistances of Psychoanalysis.* 1996. Trans. Peggy Kamuf, Pascale-Anne Brault and Michael Naas. Stanford, CA: Stanford University Press, 1998.

Descartes, René. *Discourse on Method and the Meditations.* 1637. Trans. and Introduction F. E. Sutcliffe. London: Penguin, 1968.

Dever, Carolyn. *Death and the Mother from Dickens to Freud: Victorian Fiction and the Anxiety of Origins.* Cambridge: Cambridge University Press, 1998.

Dewhurst, Kenneth. *Hughlings Jackson on Psychiatry.* Oxford: Sandford, 1982.

Diagnostic and Statistical Manual of Mental Disorders, 4th edition (DSM–IV). Washington, DC: American Psychiatric Association, 2000.

Dickens, Charles. *Bleak House.* 1853. Ed. Norman Page. Introduction J. Hillis Miller. London: Penguin Classics, 1985.

——. *The Life and Adventures of Martin Chuzzlewit.* 1843–44. Ed. and Introduction Patricia Ingham. London: Penguin, 1999.

——. *The Old Curiosity Shop.* 1841. Ed. A. Easson. London: Penguin Classics, 1972.

——. *Oliver Twist.* 1837–39. London: Octopus Books, 1983, pp. 13–285.

——. *Our Mutual Friend.* 1865. Ed. and Introduction Adrian Poole. London: Penguin Classics, 1997.

——. *The Personal History of David Copperfield.* 1849–50. Ed. Jeremy Tambling. London: Penguin Classics, 1996.

——. *The Posthumous Papers of the Pickwick Club.* 1836–37. Ed. and Introduction Mark Wormald. London: Penguin Classics, 1999.

Dickson, J. Thompson. 'On the nature of the condition called epilepsy'. *Lancet,* 24 August 1872, pp. 251–52; 31 August 1872, pp. 290–91.

Diprose, Rosalyn. 'The body biomedical ethics forgets', in Paul A. Komesaroff, ed. *Troubled Bodies: Critical Perspectives on Postmodernism, Medical Ethics, and the Body.* Melbourne: Melbourne University Press, 1995, pp. 202–21.

Dostoyevsky, Fyodor. *The Brothers Karamazov.* 1880. Trans. and Introduction David McDuff. London: Penguin Classics, 1993.

——. *The Idiot.* 1868. Trans. Constance Garnett. Melbourne: William Heinemann, 1961.

——. *The Insulted and Humiliated.* 1861. Trans. Olga Shartse. Foreword E. Starikova. Moscow: Progress Publishers, 1976.

Douglas, Mary. *Purity and Danger: An Analysis of Concepts of Pollution and Taboo.* 1966. London: Routledge and Kegan Paul, 1979.

Dreyfus, Hubert L., and Paul Rabinow. *Michel Foucault: Beyond Structuralism and Hermeneutics.* New York: Harvester Wheatsheaf, 1982.

Du Bois, W. E. Burghardt. *The Souls of Black Folk: Essays and Sketches.* 1903. New York: Johnson Reprint Company, 1968.

Dunlop, J. D. 'Two cases of hystero-epilepsy'. *Australasian Medical Gazette,* February 1883, pp. 101–2.

Dwyer, Ellen. *Homes for the Mad: Life Inside Two Nineteenth-Century Asylums.* New Brunswick, NJ: Rutgers University Press, 1987.

Efron, Robert. 'The conditioned inhibition of uncinate fits'. *Brain*, vol. 80, no. 2, 1957, pp. 251–61.

Eliot, George. *Silas Marner: The Weaver of Raveloe*. 1861. Ed. and Introduction Q. D. Leavis. Harmondsworth: Penguin, 1996.

Ender, Evelyne. *Sexing the Mind: Nineteenth-Century Fictions of Hysteria*. Ithaca, NY: Cornell University Press, 1995.

Epstein, Julia. *Altered Conditions: Disease, Medicine, and Storytelling*. New York: Routledge, 1995.

Estroff, Sue E. 'Identity, disability, and schizophrenia: the problem of chronicity', in Shirley Lindenbaum and Margaret Lock, eds. *Knowledge, Power, and Practice: The Anthropology of Medicine and Everyday Life*. Berkeley, CA: University of California Press, 1993, pp. 247–86.

Evans, Martha Noel. *Fits and Starts: A Genealogy of Hysteria in Modern France*. Ithaca, NY: Cornell University Press, 1991.

Fadiman, Anne. *The Spirit Catches You and You Fall Down: A Hmong Child, Her American Doctors, and the Clash of Two Cultures*. 1997. New York: Noonday Press, 1999.

Fee, Elizabeth. 'Nineteenth-century craniology: the study of the female skull'. *Bulletin of the History of Medicine*, vol. 53, 1979, pp. 415–33.

Feher, Michel, with Naddaff Ramona and Tazi Nadia, eds. *Fragments for a History of the Human Body, Part Two*. New York: Zone, 1989.

Felman, Shoshana. *Writing and Madness: Literature, Philosophy, Psychoanalysis*. 1985. Trans. Martha Noel Evans, Shoshana Felman and Brian Massumi. Ithaca, NY: Cornell University Press, 1989.

Feuerstein, J., D. Kurtz and F. Rohmer. 'Activation by means of Megimide: indications, value, and limits in the electroencephalographic diagnosis of epilepsy'. *Epilepsia*, vol. 7, 1966, pp. 220–27.

Fischer-Williams, M., R. G. Bickford and J. P. Whisnant. 'Occipito-parieto-temporal seizure discharge with visual hallucinations and aphasia'. *Epilepsia*, vol. 5, 1964, pp. 279–92.

Fisher, Sue, and Alexandra Dundas Todd, eds. *Discourse and Institutional Authority: Medicine, Education, and Law*. Norwood, NJ: Ablex Publishing, 1986.

Flinn, Michael W. 'Medical services under the New Poor Law', in Derek Fraser, ed. *The New Poor Law in the Nineteenth Century*. London: Macmillan, 1976, pp. 45–66.

Forrest, Derek. *Hypnotism: A History*. London: Penguin, 2000.

Foucault, Michel. *The Archaeology of Knowledge and the Discourse on Language*. 1969. Trans. A. M. Sheridan Smith. New York: Pantheon, 1972.

——. *The Birth of the Clinic: An Archaeology of Medical Perception*. 1963. Trans. A. M. Sheridan. London: Routledge, 1991.

——. 'Body/power', 1975, in Colin Gordon, ed. *Power/Knowledge: Selected Interviews and Other Writings 1972–1977*. Trans. Colin Gordon, Leo Marshall, John Mepham and Kate Soper. New York: Harvester Wheatsheaf, 1980, pp. 55–62.

——. *Discipline and Punish: The Birth of the Prison*. 1975. Trans. Alan Sheridan. London: Penguin, 1977.

——. *Ethics, Subjectivity and Truth*. Trans. Robert Hurley and others. Ed. Paul Rabinow. New York: New Press, 1997.

——. *The History of Sexuality, Volume 1: An Introduction*. 1976. Trans. Robert Hurley. London: Penguin Books, 1990.

——. *The History of Sexuality, Volume 2: The Use of Pleasure*. 1984. Trans. Robert Hurley. New York: Pantheon, 1985.

——. *The History of Sexuality, Volume 3: The Care of Self.* 1984. Trans. Robert Hurley. New York: Pantheon, 1986.
——. *Madness and Civilization: A History of Insanity in the Age of Reason.* 1961. Trans. Richard Howard. London: Routledge, 1993.
——. *Mental Illness and Psychology.* Trans. Alan Sheridan. New York: Harper and Row, 1976.
——. 'Nietzsche, genealogy, history', 1971, in Donald F. Bouchard, ed. *Language, Counter-Memory, Practice: Selected Essays and Interviews.* 1977. Trans. Donald F. Bouchard and Sherry Simon. Ithaca, NY: Cornell University Press, 1980, pp. 139–64.
——. *The Order of Things: An Archaeology of the Human Sciences.* 1970. London: Tavistock, 1974.
——. 'The subject and power' (Afterword), in Hubert L. Dreyfus and Paul Rabinow. *Michel Foucault: Beyond Structuralism and Hermeneutics.* New York: Harvester Wheatsheaf, 1982, pp. 208–26.
——. 'Truth and power', in Colin Gordon, ed. *Power/Knowledge: Selected Interviews and Other Writings 1972–1977.* Trans. Colin Gordon, Leo Marshall, John Mepham and Kate Soper. New York: Harvester Wheatsheaf, 1980, pp. 109–33.
——. 'Two lectures', 1976, in Colin Gordon, ed. *Power/Knowledge: Selected Interviews and Other Writings 1972–1977.* Trans. Colin Gordon, Leo Marshall, John Mepham and Kate Soper. New York: Harvester Wheatsheaf, 1980, pp. 78–108.
Fox, Nick J. 'Is there life after Foucault? Texts, frames and *diferends*', in A. Petersen and R. Bunton, eds. *Foucault, Health and Medicine.* London: Routledge, 1997, pp. 31–50.
Frame, Janet. *To the Is-Land.* 1983. London: Paladin, 1987.
Fraser, Derek, ed. *The New Poor Law in the Nineteenth Century.* London: Macmillan, 1976.
Fraser, Mariam. 'Creative affects'. *New Formations*, vol. 39, winter 1999–2000, pp. 55–69.
Freud, Sigmund. 'Dostoevsky and parricide'. *Standard Edition of the Complete Psychological Works of Sigmund Freud.* Ed. and trans. James Strachey. Vol. 21 (1927–31). London: Hogarth Press, 1961, pp. 175–96.
——. 'The interpretation of dreams'. *Standard Edition of the Complete Psychological Works of Sigmund Freud.* Ed. and trans. James Strachey. Vol. 4 (1900). London: Hogarth Press, 1953, pp. 1–627.
——. 'The "uncanny"'. *Standard Edition of the Complete Psychological Works of Sigmund Freud.* Ed. and trans. James Strachey. Vol. 17 (1917–19). London: Hogarth Press, 1955, pp. 219–52.
Friedlander, Walter J. *The History of Modern Epilepsy: The Beginning, 1865–1914.* London: Greenwood Press, 2001.
——. 'Shakespeare on epilepsy'. *Boston Medical Quarterly*, vol. 14, 1963, pp. 113–20.
Furnas, J. C. *Voyage to Windward.* London: Faber, 1952.
Gaiman, Neil. Neil Gaiman's Journal, 15 June 2004. http://journal.neilgaiman.com/2004/06/day-i-was-interviewed-by-maddy.asp. Accessed 7 October 2008.
Gallop, Jane. *Feminism and Psychoanalysis: The Daughter's Seduction.* London: Macmillan, 1982.
Galton, Francis. *Hereditary Genius: An Inquiry into Its Laws and Consequences.* London: Macmillan, 1869.
Gastaut, Henri. 'Fyodor Mikhailovitch Dostoevsky's involuntary contribution to the symptomatology and prognosis of epilepsy'. *Epilepsia*, vol. 19, 1978, pp. 186–201.

——. 'New comments on the epilepsy of Fyodor Dostoevsky'. *Epilepsia*, vol. 25, 1984, pp. 408–11.

——. 'Vincent van Gogh's disease seen in the light of new concepts of psychomotor epilepsy', *Annals of Medical Psychology (Paris)*, vol. 114, 1956, pp. 196–238.

——, and Yvette Gastaut. 'La maladie de Gustave Flaubert'. *Revue Neurologique*, vol. 138, no. 6/7, 1982, pp. 467–92.

Gatens, Moira. *Imaginary Bodies: Ethics, Power, and Corporeality*. London: Routledge, 1996.

Gennaro, Alfonso R., *et al.*, eds. *Blakiston's New Gould Medical Dictionary: Illustrated*. 4th edition. New York: McGraw-Hill, 1983.

Geschwind, Norman. 'Behavioural changes in temporal lobe epilepsy'. *Psychocological Medicine*, vol. 9, 1979, p. 217.

——. 'Dostoievsky's epilepsy', in D. Blumer, ed. *Psychiatric Aspects of Epilepsy*. Washington, DC: American Psychiatric Press, 1984, pp. 325–34.

——. 'Interictal behavioural changes in epilepsy'. *Epilepsia*, vol. 24, 1983, pp. 523–30.

Gibbs, Frederic A. 'William Gordon Lennox: 1884–1960'. *Epilepsia*, vol. 2, 1961, pp. 1–8.

Gibson, John S. *Deacon Brodie Father to Jekyll and Hyde*. Edinburgh: Paul Harris, 1977.

Gilbert, Sandra M., and Susan Gubar. *The Madwoman in the Attic: The Woman Writer and the Nineteenth-Century*. New Haven, CT: Yale University Press, 1979.

Gilman, Sander L. *Difference and Pathology: Stereotypes of Sexuality, Race, and Madness*. Ithaca, NY: Cornell University Press, 1985.

——, ed. *The Faces of Madness: Hugh W. Diamond and the Origin of Psychiatric Photography*. New York: Brunner/Mazel, 1976.

——. *Health and Illness: Images of Difference*. London: Reaktion Books, 1995.

——. *Seeing the Insane*. New York: John Wiley in association with Brunner/Mazel, 1982.

Goetz, Christopher, Michel G. Bonduelle and Toby Gelfand. *Charcot: Constructing Neurology*. New York: Oxford University Press, 1995.

Goffman, Erving. *Stigma: Notes on the Management of Spoiled Identity*. Harmondsworth: Penguin, 1963.

Goh, Robbie B. H. 'Textual Hyde and seek: "Gentility", narrative play and proscription in Stevenson's *Dr Jekyll and Mr Hyde*'. *Journal of Narrative Theory*, vol. 29, no. 2, spring 1999, pp. 158–83.

Good, Byron J. *Medicine, Rationality, and Experience: An Anthropological Perspective*. Cambridge: Cambridge University Press, 1994.

Gooding, Caroline. *Disabling Laws, Enabling Acts: Disability Rights in Britain and America*. London: Pluto Press, 1994.

Gordon, Amy Deborah. 'Postoperative outcome of temporal lobectomy: a multivariable model of cognitive, emotional and psychoanalytic functioning in epilepsy'. Dissertation, Drexel University, 1998.

Gordon, Colin, ed. *Power/Knowledge: Selected Interviews and Other Writings 1972–1977*. Trans. Colin Gordon, Leo Marshall, John Mepham and Kate Soper. New York: Harvester Wheatsheaf, 1980.

Gordon, Jan B. 'Narrative enclosure as textual ruin: an archaeology of Gothic consciousness', in Michael Timko, Fred Kaplan and Edward Guiliano, eds. *Dickens Studies Annual: Essays on Victorian Fiction*, vol. 11. New York: AMS Press, 1983, pp. 209–38.

Gowers, W. R. *The Border-Land of Epilepsy*. London: Churchill, 1907.

——. 'The Gulstonian lectures on epilepsy: lecture I – part I'. *Lancet*, 28 February 1880, pp. 315–18.

——. 'The Gulstonian lectures on epilepsy: lecture I – part II'. *Lancet*, 6 March 1880, pp. 353–55.

——. 'The Gulstonian lectures on epilepsy: lecture II – part I'. *Lancet*, 13 March 1880, pp. 391–93.

——. 'The Gulstonian lectures on epilepsy: lecture II – part II'. *Lancet*, 20 March 1880, pp. 433–36.

——. 'The Gulstonian lectures on epilepsy: lecture III – part I'. *Lancet*, 27 March 1880, pp. 473–75.

——. 'The Gulstonian lectures on epilepsy: lecture III – part II'. *Lancet*, 3 April 1880, pp. 515–17.

——. 'The Gulstonian lectures on epilepsy: lecture III – part III'. *Lancet*, 10 April 1880, pp. 552–54.

——. *A Manual of Diseases of the Nervous System*. 2nd edition. 2 vols. London: Churchill, 1893.

Grosz, Elizabeth. *Sexual Subversions*. Sydney: Allen and Unwin, 1989.

——. *Space, Time and Perversion*. Sydney: Allen and Unwin, 1995.

——. *Volatile Bodies: Toward a Corporeal Feminism*. Sydney: Allen and Unwin, 1994.

Gutting, Gary, ed. *The Cambridge Companion to Foucault*. Cambridge: Cambridge University Press, 1994.

Hahn, Robert A. *Sickness and Healing: An Anthropological Perspective*. New Haven, CT: Yale University Press, 1995.

Hall, Marshall. 'Lectures on the theory and practice of medicine'. *Lancet*, vol. ii, 14 April 1838, pp. 65–74.

Hall, Stuart. 'Introduction', in Stuart Hall, ed. *Representation: Cultural Representations and Signifying Practices*. London: Sage, 1997, pp. 1–12.

——, and Paul du Gay, eds. *Questions of Cultural Identity*. London: Sage, 1996.

Haraway, Donna. 'A manifesto for cyborgs: science, technology, and socialist feminism in the 1980s'. *Australian Feminist Studies*, vol. 4, autumn 1987, pp. 1–42.

——. *Primate Visions: Gender, Race, and Nature in the World of Modern Science*. London: Verso, 1992.

Hardwick, Michael, and Mollie Hardwicke. *The Charles Dickens Encyclopedia*. New York: Citadel Press, 1993.

Hardy, Thomas. *The Life and Death of the Mayor of Casterbridge: A Story of a Man of Character*. 1886. London: Macmillan, 1974.

Hawthorne, Nathaniel. *The Scarlet Letter: A Romance*. 1850. Introduction Douglas Grant. Oxford: Oxford University Press, 1965.

Hawthorne, Susan. 'Bird 1'. Unpublished paper from the International Epilepsy Conference, Sydney, September 1995.

——. *The Falling Woman*. North Melbourne: Spinifex Press, 1992.

——. 'From theories of indifference to a wild politics', in Diane Bell and Renate Klein, eds. *Radically Speaking: Feminism Reclaimed*. North Melbourne: Spinifex Press, 1996, pp. 483–501.

Heidegger, Martin. *Poetry, Language, Thought*. Trans. and Introduction Albert Hofstadter. New York: Harper and Row, 1971.

Heidel, William Arthur. *Hippocratic Medicine: Its Spirit and Method*. New York: Columbia University Press, 1941.

Henriques, Julian, *et al.* *Changing the Subject: Psychology, Social Regulation and Subjectivity*. London: Methuen, 1984.

Hippocrates. *On the Sacred Disease* (*c.* 400 BCE). Trans. Francis Adams. http://classics.mit.edu/Hippocrates/sacred.html. Accessed 12 August 2007.

Holmes, Oliver Wendell. 'Currents and counter-currents in medical science', in *Medical Essays*. Boston: Houghton-Mifflin, 1911.

Hopkins, B., D. M. Jacobs and R. Westrum. *Unusual Personal Experiences: An Analysis of Data from Three National Surveys Conducted by the Roper Organization*. Las Vegas, NV: Bigelow Holding Corporation, 1992.

Hughes, John R. 'A reappraisal of the possible seizures of Vincent van Gogh'. *Epilepsy and Behaviour*, vol. 6, 2005, pp. 504–10.

Hunter, Kathryn Montgomery. *Doctors' Stories: The Narrative Structure of Medical Knowledge*. Princeton, MA: Princeton University Press, 1992.

Hunter, R., Valentine Logue and W. H. McMenemy. 'Temporal lobe epilepsy supervening on longstanding transvestism and fetishism'. *Epilepsia*, vol. 4, 1963, pp. 60–65.

Imlach, Francis. 'A case of hystero-epilepsy of twenty years' duration, treated by removal of the uterine appendages'. *British Medical Journal*, 7 April 1888, p. 740.

Jackson, John Hughlings. 'An address on the psychology of joking', 1887, in James Taylor, ed. *Selected Writings of John Hughlings Jackson*. 2 vols. London: Hodder and Stoughton, 1932, vol. 2, pp. 359–64.

——. 'A digression on epilepsy', 1866, in James Taylor, ed. *Selected Writings of John Hughlings Jackson*. 2 vols. London: Hodder and Stoughton, 1932, vol. 1, pp. 4–5.

——. 'Extract from an article, "Notes on the comparison and contrast of regional palsy and spasm', in James Taylor, ed. *Selected Writings of John Hughlings Jackson*. 2 vols. London: Hodder and Stoughton, 1932, vol. 1, pp. 5–6.

——. 'Neurological fragments'. *Lancet*, 4 August 1894, pp. 252–53.

——. 'Observations on the localisation of movements in the cerebral hemisphere, as revealed in cases of convulsion, chorea, and "aphasia"', 1873, in James Taylor, ed. *Selected Writings of John Hughlings Jackson*. 2 vols. London: Hodder and Stoughton, 1932, vol. 1, pp. 77–89.

——. 'On the comparative study of diseases of the nervous system (Leeds address)', 1889, in James Taylor, ed. *Selected Writings of John Hughlings Jackson*. 2 vols. London: Hodder and Stoughton, 1932, vol. 2, pp. 393–410.

——. 'On epilepsies and on the after-effects of epileptic discharges (Todd and Robertson's hypothesis)', in James Taylor, ed. *Selected Writings of John Hughlings Jackson*. 2 vols. London: Hodder and Stoughton, 1932, vol. 1, pp. 135–61.

——. 'On a particular variety of epilepsy ("intellectual aura"), one case with symptoms of organic brain disease', 1888, in James Taylor, ed. *Selected Writings of John Hughlings Jackson*. 2 vols. London: Hodder and Stoughton, 1932, vol. 1, pp. 385–405.

——. 'Relations of different divisions of the central nervous system to one another and to parts of the body (Hughlings Jackson lecture)', in James Taylor, ed. *Selected Writings of John Hughlings Jackson*. 2 vols. London: Hodder and Stoughton, 1932, vol. 2, pp. 422–43.

——. 'Remarks on the diagnosis and treatment of diseases of the brain', 1888, in James Taylor, ed. *Selected Writings of John Hughlings Jackson*. 2 vols. London: Hodder and Stoughton, 1932, vol. 2, pp. 365–92.

——. *Selected Writings of John Hughlings Jackson*. 2 vols. Ed. James Taylor. London: Hodder and Stoughton, 1932.

——, and Walter S. Colman. 'Case of epilepsy with tasting movements and "dreamy state" – very small patch of softening in the left uncinate gyrus', 1898, in James Taylor, ed. *Selected Writings of John Hughlings Jackson*. 2 vols. London: Hodder and Stoughton, 1932, vol. 1, pp. 458–63.

James, William. 'Frederic Myers's service to psychology'. 1901. *Antimatters*, vol. 1, no. 1, August 2007, pp. 193–200.

Jones, Gareth Stedman. *Outcast London: A Study in the Relationship Between Classes in Victorian Society*. Oxford: Clarendon, 1971.

Jones, Kathleen and Aileen Tillotson. *The Adult Population of Epileptic Colonies*. London: British Epilepsy Association and International Bureau for Epilepsy, 1963.

Jordanova, Ludmilla. *Sexual Visions*. Madison, WI: University of Wisconsin Press, 1989.

Jorden, Edward. 'A briefe discourse of a disease called the suffocation of the mother'. London, 1603. Reprinted in Michael MacDonald, *Witchcraft and Hysteria in Elizabethan London: Edward Jorden and the Mary Glover Case*. London: Tavistock/Routledge, 1991, n.p.

Keller, Evelyn Fox. *Secrets of Life, Secrets of Death: Essays on Language, Gender and Science*. London: Routledge, 1992.

Kerson, Jennie F., Toba Schwaber Kerson and Lawrence A. Kerson. 'The depiction of seizures in film'. *Epilepsia*, vol. 40, no. 8, 1999, pp. 1163–67.

Kevles, Daniel J. *In the Name of Eugenics: Genetics and the Uses of Human Hereditary*. New York: Alfred A. Knopf, 1985.

Kiloh, L. G. 'Psychiatric problems associated with epilepsy', in Pierre J. V. Beaumont and R. B. Hampshire, eds. *Textbook of Psychiatry*. Melbourne: Blackwell Scientific, 1989, pp. 68–73.

Kingdon, Wilfred R. 'The diagnosis of hystero-epilepsy from status epilepticus'. *Lancet*, 6 August 1898, pp. 320–21.

Kipling, Rudyard. 'The post that fitted'. 1886. *A Complete Collection of Poems by Rudyard Kipling*. http://www.poetryloverspage.com/poets/kipling/kipling_ind.html.

Kirby, Vicki. *Telling Flesh: The Substance of the Corporeal*. New York: Routledge, 1997.

Kleinman, Arthur. *The Illness Narratives: Suffering, Healing, and the Human Condition*. New York: Basic Books, 1988.

Kohler, Christian G., Melissa A. Carran, Warren Bilker, Michael J. O'Connor and Michael R. Sperling. 'Association of fear auras with mood and anxiety disorders after temporal lobectomy'. *Epilepsia*, vol. 42, no. 5, 2001, pp. 674–81.

Komesaroff, Paul A., ed. 'From bioethics to microethics: ethical debate and clinical medicine', in Paul A. Komesaroff, ed. *Troubled Bodies: Critical Perspectives on Postmodernism, Medical Ethics, and the Body*. Melbourne: Melbourne University Press, 1995, pp. 62–86.

——. 'Introduction: postmodern medical ethics?', in Paul A. Komesaroff, ed. *Troubled Bodies: Critical Perspectives on Postmodernism, Medical Ethics, and the Body*. Melbourne: Melbourne University Press, 1995, pp. 1–19.

——. *Troubled Bodies: Critical Perspectives on Postmodernism, Medical Ethics, and the Body*. Melbourne: Melbourne University Press, 1995.

Koutroumanidis, Michael, and Shelagh Smith. 'Use and abuse of EEG in the diagnosis of idiopathic generalized epilepsies'. *Epilepsia*, vol. 46, suppl. 9, 2005, pp. 96–107.

Kristeva, Julia. *Powers of Horror: An Essay on Abjection.* Trans. Leon S. Roudiez. New York: Columbia University Press, 1982.

Kuhn, T. *The Structuring of Scientific Revolutions.* 2nd edition. Chicago, IL: University of Chicago Press, 1970.

Laidlaw, John, and Alan Richens, eds. *A Textbook of Epilepsy.* Foreword Denis Williams. Edinburgh: Churchill, Livingstone, 1976.

Lankester, E. Ray. 'Reply to letter from William G. Thistle, "Should epileptics marry?"' *Lancet,* 6 March 1897, p. 696.

LaPlante, Eve. *Seized.* New York: HarperCollins, 1993.

Larner, Christina. *Witchcraft and Religion: The Politics of Popular Belief.* Ed. and Foreword Alan Mcfarlane. New York: Blackwell, 1984.

Lary, N. M. *Dostoevsky and Dickens: A Study of Literary Influence.* London: Routledge and Kegan Paul, 1973.

Latour, B. 'Visualization and cognition'. *Knowledge and Science,* vol. 6, 1986, pp. 1–40.

Lennon, Kathleen, and Margaret Whitford, eds. *Knowing the Difference: Feminist Perspectives in Epistemology.* New York: Routledge, 1994.

Lennox, William Gordon. *Epilepsy and Related Disorders.* 2 vols. London: Churchill, 1960.

L'Estrange, Guy. 'Eugenics in the light of higher civilisation'. *Australasian Medical Gazette,* 20 January 1910, pp. 1–6.

Lewis, I. M. *Religion in Context: Cults and Charisma.* Cambridge: Cambridge University Press, 1986.

Lhatoo, Samden D., and Josemir W. A. S. Sander. 'Cause-specific mortality in epilepsy'. *Epilepsia,* vol. 46, suppl. 11, 2005, pp. 36–39.

Lindenbaum, Shirley, and Margaret Lock, eds. *Knowledge, Power, and Practice: The Anthropology of Medicine and Everyday Life.* Berkeley, CA: University of California Press, 1993.

Lloyd, G. E. R., ed. *Hippocratic Writings.* 1978. Trans. J. Chadwick and D. Mann. Harmondsworth: Penguin,1983.

Locke, John. *An Essay Concerning Human Understanding.* 1690. Ed. A. D. Woozley. Glasgow: Collins Fount Paperbacks, 1984.

Lombroso, Cesare. *Crime: Its Causes and Remedies.* Trans. Henry P. Horton. London: Heinemann, 1911.

——. *The Man of Genius.* London: Walter Scott, 1891.

——, and William Ferrero. *The Female Offender.* London: Fisher Unwin, 1895.

MacDonald, Michael. *Witchcraft and Hysteria in Elizabethan London: Edward Jorden and the Mary Glover Case.* London: Tavistock/Routledge, 1991.

MacKenzie, Donald A. *Statistics in Britain 1865–1930: The Social Construction of Scientific Knowledge.* Edinburgh: Edinburgh University Press, 1981.

Magli, Patrizia. 'The face and the soul', in Michel Feher, with Naddaff Ramona and Tazi Nadia, eds. *Fragments for a History of the Human Body, Part Two.* New York: Zone, 1989, pp. 86–127.

Manning, F. Norton. 'The epileptic: his treatment and care'. *Australasian Medical Gazette,* 20 June 1900, pp. 217–23.

Marchessault, Janine, and Kim Sawchuck, eds. *Wildscience: Reading Feminism, Medicine and the Media.* London: Routledge, 2000.

Martinovic, Zarko, and Jasna Martinovic. 'Ian Curtis: epilepsy and creativity of a rock musician'. Abstract. Third European Congress of Epileptology. Warsaw, Poland, 24–28 May 1998. *Epilepsia,* vol. 39, suppl. 2, 1998, p. 113.

Maudsley, Henry. *Life in Mind and Conduct: Studies of Organic in Human Nature*. London: Macmillan, 1902.

——. *Responsibility in Mental Disease*. London: C. Kegan Paul, 1876.

McCallum, David. 'Mental health, criminality and the human sciences', in A. Petersen and R. Bunton, eds. *Foucault, Health and Medicine*. London: Routledge, 1997, pp. 53–73.

McColley, Kevin. *Switch: A Mystery*. New York: Aladdin Paperbacks, 1997.

McDonald, C. 'Feigned epilepsy: case of James Clegg, *alias* James Lee, the "Dummy Chucker"'. *American Journal of Insanity*, vol. 37, 1880, pp. 1–22.

McKnight, Natalie. *Idiots, Madmen, and Other Prisoners in Dickens*. New York: St Martin's Press, 1993.

McLean, Teresa. *Seized: My Life With Epilepsy*. London: Richard Cohen, 1996.

McNeill, Pearlie. *Counting the Rivers*. Kent Town: Wakefield Press, 1998.

McTurk, William. 'The apparent increase of epilepsy among the working classes of the town of Bradford'. *Lancet*, 10 April 1859, pp. 831–37.

McWhorter, Ladelle. *Bodies and Pleasures: Foucault and the Politics of Sexual Normalization*. Bloomington, IN: Indiana University Press, 1999.

Mélèse, Lucien, *La Psychanalyse au Risque de L'épilepsie*. Collection 'Actualité de la psychanalyse'. Saint-Agne: Erès, 2000.

Mersky, H., and Lawton W. Tonge. *Psychiatric Illness*. Foreword E. Stengel. London: Bailliere, Tindall and Cox, 1965.

Mesulam, M.-Marsel. 'Neural substrates of behaviour: the effects of brain lesions upon mental state', in Armand Nicholi and J. R. Nicholi, eds. *The New Harvard Guide to Psychiatry*. Cambridge, MA: Belknap-Harvard University Press, 1988, pp. 91–127.

MIMS Australia, vol. 35, no. 5, October/November 1988, pp. 107–11.

Miola, Robert S. 'Othello *furens*'. *Shakespeare Quarterly*, vol. 41, 1990, pp. 49–64.

Money, Angel. 'A few remarks on epilepsy'. *Australasian Medical Gazette*, 20 July 1900, pp. 287–88.

Morris, Meaghan, and Paul Patton, eds. *Foucault, Power, Truth and Strategy*. Sydney: Feral Publications, 1979.

Myers, Frederic W. H. *Collected Poems: With Autobiographical and Critical Fragments*. Ed. Eveleen Myers. London: Macmillan, 1921.

——. *Human Personality and Its Survival of Bodily Death*. Ed. Leopold Hamilton Myers. 1903. London: Longmans, Green, 1907.

——. *Poems*. London: Macmillan, 1870.

Nettleton, Sarah. 'Governing the risky self: how to become healthy, wealthy and wise', in A. Petersen and R. Bunton, eds. *Foucault, Health and Medicine*. London: Routledge, 1997, pp. 207–22.

New Shorter Oxford English Dictionary. Ed. Lesley Brown. 2 vols. Oxford: Clarendon, 1993.

Nicholi, Armand, and J. R. Nicholi, eds. *The New Harvard Guide to Psychiatry*. Cambridge, MA: Belknap–Harvard University Press, 1988.

Nickell, Joe. 'Alien implants: the new "hard evidence"'. *Skeptical Inquirer*, vol. 22, no. 5, September–October 1998, p. 18 (3 pages). Accessed via Expanded Academic Index online, 15 January 2000.

Nietzsche, Friedrich. *The Portable Nietzsche*. Ed. and trans. Walter Kaufman. New York: Viking Penguin, 1982.

Nilsson, Lena, Anders Ahlbom, Bahman Y. Farahmand, Marie Asberg and Torbjorn

Tomson. 'Risk factors for suicide in epilepsy: a case control study'. *Epilepsia*, vol. 43, no. 6, 2002, pp. 644–51.

Nisbet, J. F. *The Insanity of Genius and the General Inequality of Human Faculty Physiologically Considered*. 1891. London: Stanley Paul, 1912.

Nordau, Max. *Degeneration*. London: Heinemann, 1895.

Norden, Martin F. *Cinema of Isolation: A History of Physical Disability in the Movies*. New Brunswick, NJ: Rutgers University Press, 1994.

Nowra, Louis. *The Golden Age*. 1985. Introduction Gerry Turcotte. Sydney: Currency Press, 1992.

——. *The Misery of Beauty: The Loves of Frogman*. Sydney: Angus and Robertson, 1981.

——. *Palu*. Sydney: Picador, 1987.

——. *Visions*. Sydney: Currency Press, 1979.

Osborne, Thomas. 'Of health and statecraft', in A. Petersen and R. Bunton, eds. *Foucault, Health and Medicine*. London: Routledge, 1997, pp. 173–88.

Ounsted, Christopher, Janet Lindsay and Peronelle Richards. *Temporal Lobe Epilepsy 1948–1986: A Biographical Study*. London: Mac Keith Press, 1987.

Ovsiew, F. 'A case of epilepsy and psychosis in the seventeenth century'. *Behavioural Neurology*, vol. 5, 1992, pp. 215–17.

Oxford Dictionary of English Etymology. 1966. Ed. C. T. Onions, *et al*. Oxford: Clarendon, 1967.

Oxford Dictionary of National Biography. Oxford: Oxford University Press, 2004.

Oxford English Dictionary. 2nd edition. 12 vols. Ed. James A. H. Murray, *et al*. Oxford: Clarendon, 1989.

Paracelsus. *Four Treatises of Theophrastus von Hohenheim Called Paracelsus*. Ed. Henry E. Sigerist. Baltimore, MD: Johns Hopkins University Press, 1941.

Perkin, G. D. 'Neurology in literature: epilepsy'. *Journal of Neurology, Neurosurgery, and Psychiatry*, vol. 57, 1994, pp. 632–34.

Petersen, Alan, and Robin Bunton, eds. *Foucault, Health and Medicine*. London: Routledge, 1997.

Pick, Daniel. *Faces of Degeneration: A European Disorder, c. 1848–c. 1918*. Cambridge: Cambridge University Press, 1989.

Radley, Alan, ed. *Worlds of Illness: Biographical and Cultural Perspectives on Health and Disease*. New York: Routledge, 1993.

Raichle, M. 'Images of the mind'. *Scientific American*, April 1994, pp. 36–42.

Redding, Paul. 'Science, medicine, and illness: rediscovering the patient as a person', in Paul A. Komesaroff, ed. *Troubled Bodies: Critical Perspectives on Postmodernism, Medical Ethics, and the Body*. Melbourne: Melbourne University Press, 1995, pp. 87–102.

Renan, Joseph Ernest. *History of the Origins of Christianity. Book 1: The Life of Jesus* and *Book 4: Saint Paul, The Antichrist*. London: Watts, 1864. http://www.infidels.org/library/historical/ernest_renan/life_of_jesus.html. Accessed 6 November 2007.

Reynolds, E. H., and M. R. Trimble, eds. *Epilepsy and Psychiatry*. Edinburgh: Churchill Livingstone, 1981.

Rice, James L. *Dostoevsky and the Healing Art: An Essay in Literary and Medical History*. Ann Arbor, MI: Ardis, 1985.

Richard, Adrienne, and Joel Reiter. *Epilepsy: A New Approach*. 2nd edition. New York: Walker, 1995.

Russell, Denise. *Women, Madness and Medicine*. Cambridge: Polity Press, 1995.

Russell, J. S. Risien. 'The management and education of idiots and epileptics at the Bicêtre Hospital in Paris'. *British Medical Journal*, 6 June 1891, pp. 1247–48.
Sacks, Oliver. *An Anthropologist on Mars*. Sydney: Picador, 1999.
——. *Awakenings*. 1973. London: Picador, 1990.
——. *A Leg to Stand On*. 1984. London: Picador, 1991.
——. *The Man Who Mistook His Wife For a Hat*. 1985. London: Picador, 1986.
——. *Migraine*. 1970. London: Picador, 1995.
Sacks, Sheldon, ed. *On Metaphor*. Chicago, IL: University of Chicago Press, 1978.
Sadoff, Dianne F. *Sciences of the Flesh: Representing Body and Subject in Psychoanalysis*. Stanford, CA: Stanford University Press, 1998.
Sandison, Alan. *Robert Louis Stevenson and the Appearance of Modernism*. Basingstoke: Macmillan, 1996.
Sansom, Dr, and Mr G. T. Stonham. 'A mirror of hospital practice, British and foreign'. *Lancet*, 5 March 1881, pp. 369–70.
Savage, Jon. 'Dark star: the final days of Ian Curtis by his Joy Division bandmates'. *Independent*, 7 October 2007.
Sawicki, Jana. *Disciplining Foucault: Feminism, Power and the Body*. New York: Routledge, 1991.
Scambler, Graham. *Epilepsy*. London: Tavistock/Routledge, 1989.
Schachter, Steven. *Brainstorms: Epilepsy in Our Words*. Philadelphia, PA: Lippincott-Raven, 1993.
Schacter, D. *Searching for Memory: The Brain, the Mind and the Past*. Dunmore: Harper Collins, 1996.
Schmitz, B. and M. Trimble. 'Epileptic equivalents in psychiatry: some 19th century views'. *Acta Neurologica Scandinavica*, vol. 86, suppl. 140, 1992, pp. 122–26.
Schrader, Paul. 'Notes on film noir', in John Belton, ed. *Movies and Mass Culture*. New Brunswick, NJ: Rutgers University Press, 1996, pp. 153–70.
Schulze-Bonhage, A., and C. E. Elger. 'Induction of partial epileptic seizures by flumazenil'. *Epilepsia*, vol. 41, no. 2, February 2000, pp. 186–92.
Scott, D. F. *The History of Epileptic Therapy: An Account of How Medication Was Developed*. Nashville, TN: Parthenon, 1993.
Sedgwick, Eve Kosofsky. *Between Men: English Literature and Male Homosocial Desire*. 1985. New York: Columbia University Press, 1992.
——. 'Epidemics of the will', in Jonathan Crary and Sanford Kwinter, eds. *Incorporations*. New York: Zone, 1995, pp. 582–95.
——. *Epistemology of the Closet*. 1990. London: Penguin, 1994.
Shakespeare, Tom. *Disability Rights and Wrongs*. London: Routledge, 2006.
Shakespeare, William. *Hamlet*. Ed. Horace Howard Furness. New York: Dover Publications, 1963.
——. *Julius Caesar*. Ed. John Dover Wilson. Cambridge: Cambridge University Press, 1968.
——. *King Lear*. Ed. Ralph E. C. Houghton. Oxford: Clarendon Press, 1967.
——. *Othello*. Ed. Kenneth Muir. Harmondsworth: Penguin, 1968.
Showalter, Elaine. *The Female Malady: Women, Madness and English Culture 1830–1980*. 1987. London: Virago, 1996.
——. *Hystories: Hysterical Epidemics and Modern Culture*. 1997. London: Picador, 1998.
Shuttleworth, G. E. 'A discussion on the treatment of epileptics and imbeciles'. *British Medical Journal*, 16 September 1899, pp. 711–12.
Slater, Lauren. *Spasm: A Memoir with Lies*. London: Methuen, 2000.

Snyder, Sharon L., and David T. Mitchell. *Cultural Locations of Disability*. Chicago, IL: Chicago University Press, 2006.

——, Brenda Jo Brueggemann and Rosemary Garland Thomson, eds. *Disability Studies: Enabling the Humanities*. New York: Modern Language Association, 2002.

Soja, Edward W. *Thirdspace: Journeys to Los Angeles and Other Real-and-Imagined Places*. Cambridge: Blackwell Publishers, 1996.

Solly, Samuel. 'A clinical lecture on epilepsy following injury to the cranium'. *Lancet*, 5 January 1850, pp. 8–10.

Sontag, Susan. *'Illness as Metaphor' and 'AIDS and Its Metaphors'*. New York: Anchor, 1990.

Spratling, William P. *British Medical Journal*, 28 October 1899, p. 1228.

——. *The Craig Colony for Epileptics: Bulletin of General Information*. Buffalo, NY: Matthews-Northrup, 1 October 1902.

——. 'The treatment of epileptics and imbeciles'. *British Medical Journal*, 28 October 1899, p. 1228.

Stanly, Liz. 'The knowing because experiencing subject: narratives, lives and autobiography', in Kathleen Lennon and Margaret Whitford, eds. *Knowing the Difference: Feminist Perspectives in Epistemology*. New York: Routledge, 1994, pp. 132–48.

Star, Susan Leigh. *Regions of the Mind: Brain Research and the Quest for Scientific Certainty*. Stanford, CA: Stanford University Press, 1989.

Stastny, Peter. 'From exploitation to self-reflection: representing persons with psychiatric disabilities in documentary film'. *Literature and Medicine*, vol. 17, no. 1, 1998, pp. 68–90.

Stevenson, Robert Louis. *Strange Case of Dr Jekyll and Mr Hyde*. 1886. *Dr Jekyll and Mr Hyde & The Merry Men and Other Tales and Fables*. Hertfordshire: Wordsworth Classics, 1999, pp. 3–54.

Stirling, Jeannette. 'Dementia, discourse, difference and denial: "Who did I become?"' *Law/Text/Culture*, vol. 2, 1995, pp. 147–59.

Strieber, Whitley. *Communion: Encounters with the Unknown. A True Story*. London: Arrow Books, 1987.

——. *Confirmation: The Hard Evidence of Aliens Among Us*. London: Simon and Schuster, 1998.

——. *The Grays*. New York: Forge Books, 2006.

——. *The Secret School: Preparation for Contact*. London: Simon and Schuster, 1997.

——. *Transformation: The Breakthrough*. 1988. London: Arrow Books, 1989.

——. Whitley Strieber's Unknown Country: daily news of the edge. http://www.unknowncountry.com/journal/. Accessed 1 February 2009.

Sturken, Marita, and Lisa Cartwright. *Practices of Looking: An Introduction to Visual Culture*. London: Oxford University Press, 2001.

Summers, Montague. *The History of Witchcraft and Demonology*. New York: University Books, 1956.

Swan, John. 'A true and briefe report of Mary Glovers vexation, and of her deliverance by fastings and prayer', 1603. Reprinted in Michael MacDonald, *Witchcraft and Hysteria in Elizabethan London: Edward Jorden and the Mary Glover Case*. London: Tavistock/Routledge, 1991, n.p.

Szasz, Thomas S. *The Manufacture of Madness: A Comparative Study of the Inquisition and the Mental Health Movement*. 1973. London: Paladin Granada, 1977.

Szondi, L. *Lehrbuch der Experimentellen Trebdiagnostik*, 3rd edition. Bern: Huber, 1972.

——. *Schicksalsanalytische Therapie* Bern: Huber, 1963.

Taylor, David C., and Susan M. Marsh. 'Hughlings Jackson's Dr. Z: the paradigm of temporal lobe epilepsy revealed'. *Journal of Neurology, Neurosurgery and Psychiatry*, vol. 43, 1980, pp. 758–67.

Taylor, Frederick Winslow. *Scientific Management*. 1910. Westport, CT: Greenwood Press, 1972.

Taylor, James, ed. *Selected Writings of John Hughlings Jackson*. 2 vols. London: Hodder and Stoughton, 1932.

Temkin, Owsei. *The Falling Sickness: A History of Epilepsy from the Greeks to the Beginnings of Modern Neurology*, 2nd edition, revised. Baltimore, MD: Johns Hopkins University Press, 1971.

Thistle, William G. 'Should epileptics marry?' *Lancet*, 13 February 1897, pp. 480–81.

——. 'Reply to letter from W. R. Gowers'. *Lancet*, 27 February 1897, p. 621.

——. 'Reply to letter from E. Ray Lankester, "Should epileptics marry?"' *Lancet*, 20 March 1897, p. 841.

Thomson, Rosemarie Garland. *Extraordinary Bodies: Figuring Physical Disability in American Culture and Literature*. New York: Columbia University Press, 1997.

——. 'The politics of staring: visual rhetorics of disability in popular photography', in Sharon L. Snyder, Brenda Jo Brueggemann and Rosemary Garland Thomson, eds. *Disability Studies: Enabling the Humanities*. New York: Modern Language Association, 2002, pp. 56–75.

Thornton, E. M. *Hypnotism, Hysteria and Epilepsy: An Historical Synthesis*. London: Heinemann, 1976.

Thurschwell, Pamela. 'Ferenczi's dangerous proximities: telepathy, psychosis, and the real event'. *Differences: A Journal of Feminist Cultural Studies*, spring 1999, p. 150 (17 pages). Accessed via Expanded Academic Index online, 19 April 2001.

Todd, Dennis. *Imagining Monsters: Miscreations of Self in Eighteenth-Century England*. Chicago, IL: University of Chicago Press, 1995.

Todd, Dr. 'Epileptic mania'. *Lancet*, vol. ii, 1851, pp. 372–73.

Toga, A., and J. Mazziotta. *Brain Mapping: The Methods*. San Diego, CA: Academic Press, 1996.

Trenité, Dorothée G. Kasteleijn-Nolst, Renzo Guerrini, Colin D. Binnie and Pierre Genton. 'Visual sensitivity and epilepsy: a proposed terminology and classification for clinical and EEG phenomenology'. *Epilepsia*, vol. 42, no. 5, 2001, pp. 692–701.

Trimble, Michael R. 'Neuropsychiatry or behavioural neurology'. *Neuropsychiatry, Neuropsychology, and Behavioural Neurology: A Journal of Clinical Neuroscience*, vol. 6, no. 1, 1993, pp. 60–64.

Turcotte, Gerry. '"The circle is burst": eschatological discourse in Louis Nowra's *Sunrise* and *The Golden Age*'. *Span*, vol. 24, 1987, pp. 63–80.

——. '"Perfecting the monologue of silence": an interview with Louis Nowra'. *Kunapipi*, vol. 9, no. 3, 1987, pp. 51–66.

——. '"Speaking the formula of abjection": hybrids and Gothic discourses in Louis Nowra's novels'. *Westerly*, vol. 3, September 1991, pp. 61–72.

Turner, Aldren William. 'The care and management of epileptics in colonies'. *Lancet*, 26 June 1897, pp. 1733–35.

Turner, Bryan S. 'From governmentality to risk, some reflections on Foucault's contribution to medical sociology', in A. Petersen and R. Bunton, eds. *Foucault, Health and Medicine*. London: Routledge, 1997, pp. ix–xxi.

——. *Medical Power and Social Knowledge.* London: Sage Publications, 1987.

Vajda, Frank J., Terence J. O'Brien, Alison Hitchcock, Janet Graham, Mark J. Cook and Cecile Lander. 'The establishment of a prospective nationwide study of the consequences of the use of antiepileptic drugs in pregnancy'. *Headlines* (magazine of the Australian Epilepsy Association), no. 57, 2000, p. 11.

Veeder, William, and Gordon Hirsch, eds. *Dr Jekyll and Mr Hyde: After One Hundred Years.* Chicago, IL: Chicago University Press, 1988.

Voskuil, P. H. A. 'The epilepsy of Fyodor Mikhailovitch Dostoevsky (1821–1881)'. *Epilepsia*, vol. 24, 1983, pp. 658–67.

Ward, Colleen A., ed. *Altered States of Consciousness and Mental Health: A Cross-Cultural Perspective.* London: Sage Publications, 1989.

Watzman, H., and P. Aldhous. 'Have the mind mappers lost their way?' *New Scientist*, 4 May 1996, p. 12.

Wendell, Susan. *The Rejected Body: Feminist Philosophical Reflections on Disability.* New York: Routledge, 1996.

Weyer, Johann. *De praestigiis daemonum.* 1583. *Witches, Devils, and Doctors in the Renaissance.* Ed. George Mora. Trans. John Shea. Binghamton, NY: Medieval and Renaissance Texts and Studies, 1991.

Whetham, W. C. D., and Catherine D. Whetham. *The Family and Nation.* London: Longmans, Green, 1909.

—— and ——. *Hereditary and Society.* London: Longmans, Green, 1911.

Wilks, S. 'An address on some of the more unusual phenomena of epilepsy'. *British Medical Journal*, 2 January 1892, pp. 2–5.

Williams, Joseph. 'Practical observations on the cure of epilepsy'. *Lancet*, vol. i, 1854, pp. 128–30.

Wilson, Elizabeth A. *Neural Geographies: Feminism and the Microstructure of Cognition.* New York: Routledge, 1998.

Wolf, Peter. 'Epilepsy in literature'. *Epilepsia*, vol. 36, 1995, pp. 12–17.

——. 'Historical aspects of idiopathic generalized epilepsies'. *Epilepsia*, vol. 46, suppl. 9, 2005, pp. 7–9.

Wright, Daniel. '"The prisonhouse of my disposition": a study of the psychology of addiction in Dr. Jekyll and Mr. Hyde'. *Studies in the Novel*, vol. 26, no. 3, autumn 1994, pp. 254–67.

Wright, Hamilton. 'Abilene State Hospital in top rank of its type'. *Abilene Reporter News*, 14 May 1944.

Wynter, Andrew. *The Borderlands of Insanity.* 2nd edition. London: Robert Hardwicke, 1875.

Zielinski, Janusz, J. 'Epidemiologic overview of epilepsy: morbidity, mortality, and clinical implications', in D. Blumer, ed. *Psychiatric Aspects of Epilepsy.* Washington, DC: American Psychiatric Press, 1984, pp. 67–97.

Zilboorg, Gregory. *The Medical Man and the Witch During the Renaissance.* New York: Cooper Square Publishers, 1969.

Editorials

'Bite of an epileptic'. *Lancet*, 12 January 1884, p. 82.

'Care of epileptics'. *British Medical Journal*, 30 November 1895, p. 1386.

'Care of epileptics'. *Lancet*, 22 December 1881, p. 1104.

'Colony for epileptics'. *British Medical Journal*, 27 March 1897, p. 814.

'Correspondence: London'. *Australasian Medical Gazette*, 20 June 1911, pp. 348–50.

'Declining birth-rate'. *Australasian Medical Gazette*, 21 March 1904, p. 120.

'Discussion on the relation of epilepsy and insanity'. Introduced by W. R. Gowers. *British Medical Journal*, 28 September 1895, pp. 774–76.

'Employment of epileptics'. *British Medical Journal*, 22 May 1886, pp. 995–96.

'Epidemic of hystero-epilepsy'. *Lancet*, 16 October 1880, pp. 624–25.

'Epileptic colonies'. *Lancet*, 16 April 1892, pp. 881–82.

'Epileptic colony at Chalfont'. *Lancet*, 17 November 1894, pp. 1178–79.

'Eugenics'. *Australasian Medical Gazette*, 20 April 1912, pp. 414–15.

'Farm colonies for epileptics'. *British Medical Journal*, 3 November 1894, p. 1000.

'Farm colony for epileptics'. *British Medical Journal*, 18 August 1894, p. 380.

'Gleanings from the journals'. *Australasian Medical Gazette*, March 1882, p. 85.

'Home for epileptics'. *Lancet*, 6 August 1892, p. 319.

'Homicidal epilepsy'. *Lancet*, 14 September 1889, p. 554.

'Hospital-workshops for the epileptic'. *British Medical Journal*, 6 February 1886, p. 262.

'Hypochondria and hysteria in men and women'. *British Medical Journal*, 9 November 1889, p. 1054.

'Hysteria and tremulousness in males'. *British Medical Journal*, 18 July 1891, pp. 135–36.

'Hystero-epilepsy cured by a sham operation'. *Lancet*, 8 October 1887, p. 726.

'Importance of shampooing and gymnastic exercises in the treatment of epilepsy'. *British Medical Journal*, 2 May 1885, p. 890.

'Labour colony for epileptics'. *Lancet*, 12 November 1892, p. 1112.

'Marriage of female epileptics'. *Lancet*, 23 January 1897, pp. 260–61.

'Medical Association of Victoria'. *Australasian Medical Gazette*, 14 September 1912, p. 283.

'Medical miscellany'. *Australasian Medical Gazette*, 13 December 1913, p. 548.

'Minutes from a meeting of the Clinical Society of London. Friday, February 8, 1889'. *British Medical Journal*, 16 February 1889, pp. 358–59.

'National Society for the Employment of Epileptics'. *British Medical Journal*, 7 January 1893, pp. 31–32.

'National Society for the Employment of Epileptics'. *Lancet*, 1 October 1892, p. 787.

'No poison in the bite of an epileptic'. *Lancet*, 19 January 1884, p. 131.

'Physical conditions and conduct'. *Australasian Medical Gazette*, 19 October 1912, p. 407.

'Psychical research'. *Lancet*, 22 December 1881, p. 1104.

'Talbot colony for epileptics, Victoria'. *Australasian Medical Gazette*, 7 December 1912, p. 590.

'Treatment of pauper imbeciles and epileptics'. *British Medical Journal*, 1 October 1898, p. 996.

'Visit to the new colony for epileptics'. *British Medical Journal*, 29 December 1894, p. 1502.

Film and television

Alien. Dir. Ridley Scott. Prod. Gordon Caroll, *et al*. Perf. Sigourney Weaver, Tom Skerritt, John Hurt. Screenplay Dan O'Bannon. Twentieth Century Fox, 1979.

American Gothic. Prod. Shaun Cassidy, *et al*. Perf. Gary Cole, Lucas Black, Paige Turco, Brenda Bakke, Sarah Paulson. CBS, 1995.

The Andromeda Strain. Dir. and prod. Robert Wise. Perf. David Wayne, James Olson, Kate Reid. From the novel by Michael Crichton. Universal Pictures, 1971.

The Big Sleep. Dir. and prod. Howard Hawks. Perf. Humphrey Bogart, Lauren Bacall, Martha Vickers. Screenplay William Faulker, Leigh Brackett, Jules Furthman. Based on the novel by Raymond Chandler. Warner Bros., 1946.

The Big Sleep. Dir. Michael Winner. Prod. Elliott Kastner and Michael Winner. Perf. Robert Mitchum, Sarah Miles, Candy Clark. Screenplay Michael Winner. United Artists, 1978.

Brain Story. Series prod. Sam Roberts. Written and presented by Professor Susan Greenfield. BBC Worldwide, 2001.

Control. Dir. Anton Corbijn. Perf. Sam Riley, Samantha Morton, Alexandra Maria Lara, Joe Anderson. Writers Deborah Curtis and Matt Greenhalgh. Based on the novel by Deborah Curtis, *Touching from a Distance*. Three Dogs and a Pony, 2007.

Deceiver. Written and dir. Jonas and Joshua Pate. Perf. Tim Roth, Chris Penn, Michael Rooker, Renee Zellweger. MDP Worldwide, 1997.

Dr Jekyll and Mr Hyde. Dir. Victor Fleming. Perf. Spencer Tracy, Ingrid Bergman, Lana Turner. Screenplay John Lee Mahin. Metro-Goldwyn-Mayer, 1941.

Drugstore Cowboy. Dir. Gus Van Sant. Perf. Matt Dillon, Kelly Lynch, James LeGros, Heather Graham. Avenue Pictures Production, 1989.

The Fugitive. Dir. Andrew Davis. Perf. Harrison Ford, Tommy Lee Jones, Sela Ward, Julianne Moore. Screenplay Jeb Stuart and David Twohy. Warner Bros. Pictures, 1993.

Horizon, 'God on the brain'. BBC 2, 17 April 2003.

Joy Division. Dir. Grant Gee. Writer Jon Savage. Prod. Tom Astor, Tom Altencio, Jacqui Edenbrow. Madman Films, Brown Owl Films, 2007.

Romper Stomper. Dir. Geoffrey Wright. Prod. Daniel Scharf and Ian Pringle. Perf. Russell Crowe, Daniel Pollock, Jacqueline McKenzie. Australian Film Commission and Film Victoria, 1992.

RPA. Medical documentary series. Nine Network, Australia, 1999.

Seinfeld. 'The Good Samaritan'. Writer Peter Mehlman. Episode 37, Season 3, 1992.

The X Files. 'Fallen angel'. Episode 9, Season 1, 1993–94.

The X Files. 'Pusher'. Episode 17, Season 3, 1995–96.

Index

Page references for notes are followed by n and the note number, e.g. 78n63.